Executing Lean Improvements

Also available from ASQ Quality Press:

The Lean Handbook: A Guide to the Bronze Certification Body of Knowledge
Anthony Manos and Chad Vincent, editors

Lean Doctors: A Bold and Practical Guide to Using Lean Principles to Transform Healthcare Systems, One Doctor at a Time
Aneesh Suneja and Carolyn Suneja

The Lean Doctors Workbook: An Application Guide for Transforming Outpatient Clinic Systems with Lean
Aneesh Suneja and Carolyn Suneja

Lean Acres: A Tale of Strategic Innovation and Improvement in a Farm-iliar Setting
Jim Bowie

Advanced Quality Auditing: An Auditor's Review of Risk Management, Lean Improvement, and Data Analysis
Lance B. Coleman

The Certified Six Sigma Black Belt Handbook, Third Edition
T.M. Kubiak and Donald W. Benbow

The Quality Toolbox, Second Edition
Nancy R. Tague

Root Cause Analysis: Simplified Tools and Techniques, Second Edition
Bjørn Andersen and Tom Fagerhaug

The Certified Six Sigma Green Belt Handbook, Second Edition
Roderick A. Munro, Govindarajan Ramu, and Daniel J. Zrymiak

The Certified Manager of Quality/Organizational Excellence Handbook, Fourth Edition
Russell T. Westcott, editor

The ASQ Auditing Handbook, Fourth Edition
J.P. Russell, editor

The ASQ Quality Improvement Pocket Guide: Basic History, Concepts, Tools, and Relationships
Grace L. Duffy, editor

To request a complimentary catalog of ASQ Quality Press publications, call 800-248-1946, or visit our website at http://www.asq.org/quality-press.

Executing Lean Improvements

A Practical Guide with Real-World Healthcare Case Studies

Dennis R. Delisle

ASQ Quality Press
Milwaukee, Wisconsin

American Society for Quality, Quality Press, Milwaukee 53203
© 2015 by ASQ
All rights reserved.
Printed in the United States of America
20 19 18 17 16 15   5 4 3 2 1

Library of Congress Cataloging-in-Publication Data
Delisle, Dennis R., 1984– , author.
  Executing lean improvements : a practical guide with real-world healthcare case studies / Dennis R. Delisle.
    p. ; cm
  Includes bibliographical references and index.
  ISBN 978-0-87389-909-3 (alk. paper)
  I. American Society for Quality, issuing body. II. Title.
[DNLM: 1. Thomas Jefferson University. 2. Cost Control—methods—Pennsylvania.
3. Health Care Costs—Pennsylvania. 4. Organizational Case Studies—Pennsylvania.
5. Quality Improvement—economics—Pennsylvania. W 74 AP4]
  R728
  362.1068—dc23
                                                                        2015007112

No part of this book may be reproduced in any form or by any means, electronic, mechanical, photocopying, recording, or otherwise, without the prior written permission of the publisher.

Publisher: Lynelle Korte
Acquisitions Editor: Matt Meinholz
Managing Editor: Paul Daniel O'Mara
Production Administrator: Randall Benson

ASQ Mission: The American Society for Quality advances individual, organizational, and community excellence worldwide through learning, quality improvement, and knowledge exchange.

Attention Bookstores, Wholesalers, Schools, and Corporations: ASQ Quality Press books, video, audio, and software are available at quantity discounts with bulk purchases for business, educational, or instructional use. For information, please contact ASQ Quality Press at 800-248-1946, or write to ASQ Quality Press, P.O. Box 3005, Milwaukee, WI 53201-3005.

To place orders or to request a free copy of the ASQ Quality Press Publications Catalog, visit our website at http://www.asq.org/quality-press.

∞ Printed on acid-free paper

Quality Press
600 N. Plankinton Ave.
Milwaukee, WI 53203-2914
E-mail: authors@asq.org

The Global Voice of Quality™

This book is dedicated to my family, friends, students, colleagues, and mentors.

Table of Contents

List of Figures and Tables ix
List of Case Studies xv
Foreword by David B. Nash, MD, MBA xvii
Foreword by David P. McQuaid, RPh, MBA, FACHE xxi
Introduction xxv

Chapter 1 Lean Thinking **1**
   Performance Improvement Methodologies 1
   The Lean Thinking Philosophy 3
   Roadmap for Creating a Lean Process 7

Chapter 2 Principle #1: Define Value **9**
   Determine Scope 9
   Define Value through Customer's Eyes 12
   Identify Waste 17

Chapter 3 Principle #2: Map the Value Stream **31**
   Map the Current State 32
   Value Stream Maps 38
   Collect and Analyze Data for VSM 50
   Putting the Pieces Together 56

Chapter 4 Establish the Lean Fundamentals **61**
   5S 62
   Layout 67
   Visual Management 70

Chapter 5 Principle #3: Establish Flow **83**
   Determine Customer Demand 86
   Balance the Process 87
   Standardize the Work 96

Chapter 6 Principle #4: Implement Pull **101**
   Create a Pull System 102
   Reduce Batching 108
   Manage Inventory 110

Chapter 7 Principle #5: Strive for Perfection 117
Identify Root Causes 117
Error-Proof Processes 123
Sustain Improvements 127

Chapter 8 Executing a Project through Lean DMAIC 133
Kaizen 133
Lean DMAIC Model 136

Chapter 9 Facilitating Rapid Improvements 157
Facilitation Guidelines 158
The Kaizen Problem-Solving Process 159
Facilitator's Role in Group Dynamics 173

Chapter 10 Leading Change: Lessons from the Road 177
Lean Management 178
Leading Change 181
Lessons from Jefferson Lean Leaders 184

Appendixes 189

Appendix A Rapid Improvement Event Portfolio 191
High-Level Project Plan 191
Define 191
Measure 200
Analyze 204
Improve 207
Control 212

Appendix B Define Folder 215
DOWNTIME Matrix 215
Lean Engagement Communication Plan 215
Lean Opportunity Guide 220
VOC Waste Questionnaire 221

Appendix C Measure Folder 223
Process Value Analysis 223
Workflow Value Analysis 224

Appendix D Analyze Folder 225
5S Audit Tool 225
Swimlane Template 226

Appendix E Improve Folder 227
RIE Presentation 227
RIE Facilitator Evaluation Form 227

Appendix F Control Folder 229
Kaizen A3 Report 229
Control Phase Action Plan 229
Control Phase Action Plan—Gantt Template 232

References 235
Index 241
About the Author 247

List of Figures and Tables

Figure I.1	Roadmap for creating a lean process (based on the Lean Roadmap from BMGI)	xxvi
Table 1.1	Performance improvement methodologies	2
Figure 1.1	Purpose, process, people, and the leadership system	5
Figure 1.2	Lean thinking flowing horizontally	5
Figure 1.3	Strategy deployment (hoshin kanri)	6
Table 1.2	Lean project opportunity guide	7
Figure 2.1	Roadmap: Define value	10
Figure 2.2	Roadmap: Determine scope	10
Figure 2.3	Process map structure	10
Figure 2.4	Process scoping	11
Figure 2.5	SIPOC diagram	12
Figure 2.6	Lab receiving process SIPOC	12
Figure 2.7	Sterile processing SIPOC	12
Figure 2.8	Roadmap: Define value through customer's eyes	13
Table 2.1	Examples of VA, NVA, and NVA-R activities	14
Table 2.2	Physician's office visit example	15
Figure 2.9	VA versus NVA time for the physician's office visit	15
Figure 2.10	Before/after assessment of VA and NVA activities	16
Figure 2.11	Roadmap: Identify waste	17
Table 2.3	DOWNTIME waste matrix	18
Figure 2.12	Preliminary waste diagnostic tool	22
Figure 2.13	Lean thinking process	23
Figure 2.14	Operating room turnover (wheels out to wheels in) value analysis	24
Figure 2.15	Surgical equipment sterilization value analysis	24
Figure 2.16	Oncology infusion center patient flow value analysis	24
Figure 2.17	Clinical lab workflow process	25
Figure 2.18	Clinical lab receiving process for specimen throughput value analysis	26
Figure 2.19	Workflow value analysis for a lab technician	26
Figure 2.20	Rapid improvement event pictures of the clinical lab project	27
Figure 2.21	Results of the clinical lab project	28

List of Figures and Tables

Figure 3.1	Roadmap: Map the value stream	31
Figure 3.2	Roadmap: Map the current state	32
Figure 3.3	High- and midlevel process maps	33
Figure 3.4	Process map of physician's office visit	34
Figure 3.5	High-level process steps for physician's office visit	33
Figure 3.6	High- and midlevel process steps for physician's office visit	35
Figure 3.7	Cycle times for physician's office visit	36
Figure 3.8	First-pass yield	37
Figure 3.9	Value stream map for physician's office visit	40
Figure 3.10	First-pass yield for physician's office visit	41
Figure 3.11	VA and NVA categorization for physician's office visit	42
Figure 3.12	Identified opportunities for improvement for physician's office visit	43
Figure 3.13	Example of VSM with improvement (kaizen) prioritization	45
Figure 3.14	Example of VSM created by improvement team	46
Figure 3.15	Swimlane map template	46
Figure 3.16	Swimlane map example with position	47
Figure 3.17	Swimlane map example with patient flow process	47
Figure 3.18	Swimlane map example with process steps by position	48
Figure 3.19	Example of swimlane map created by improvement team	49
Figure 3.20	Roadmap: Collect and analyze data for VSM	50
Figure 3.21	Process value analysis screenshot	52
Figure 3.22	Process value analysis output example	53
Figure 3.23	Process value analysis output for PTC patient flow	54
Figure 3.24	Workflow value analysis screenshot	55
Figure 3.25	Workflow value analysis output example	56
Figure 3.26	Sterile processing SIPOC	57
Figure 3.27	Sterile processing VSM	58
Figure 3.28	Sterile processing process value analysis output	59
Figure 4.1	Roadmap: Establish lean fundamentals	61
Table 4.1	Lean fundamentals	62
Table 4.2	5S approach for organizing physical space and systems/processes	63
Figure 4.2	Example of process 5S	64
Figure 4.3	5S audit tool for physical space and layout assessment	65
Figure 4.4	5S audit tool output (radar chart)	66
Figure 4.5	Layout example	67
Figure 4.6	Example of current state layout	68
Figure 4.7	Example of current state layout with labeled processing areas	68
Figure 4.8	Example of spaghetti diagram of current state	68
Figure 4.9	Example of spaghetti diagram of improved state	68
Figure 4.10	Comparison of spaghetti diagrams before and after improvement	68
Figure 4.11	Layout improvement 1 of 3	69
Figure 4.12	Layout improvement 2 of 3	70

Figure 4.13	Layout improvement 3 of 3	71
Figure 4.14	Example of visual management in the Clinical Lab	72
Figure 4.15	PTC current state swimlane map	74
Figure 4.16	PTC current state process value analysis	75
Table 4.3	Pre-/post-intervention process	76
Figure 4.17	Redesigned process swimlane map	77
Figure 4.18	Length of stay results	78
Figure 4.19	Length of stay results by hour	79
Figure 4.20	PTC visual management example	79
Figure 4.21	Process from value analysis to solution development	80
Figure 5.1	Roadmap: Establish flow	83
Figure 5.2	Roadmap: Determine customer demand	86
Figure 5.3	Takt time equation	87
Figure 5.4	Roadmap: Balance the process	88
Figure 5.5	Process value analysis example	89
Figure 5.6	Workload balance example: Before intervention	90
Figure 5.7	Workload balance example: After intervention	90
Figure 5.8	Workload balance example: Before/after comparison	91
Figure 5.9	How to analyze a workload balance chart	92
Figure 5.10	Process value analysis of OR turnover	94
Figure 5.11	Improvement team creating a swimlane map of OR turnover	95
Figure 5.12	Next case checklist	95
Figure 5.13	Roadmap: Standardize the work	96
Table 5.1	Standard work template	98
Figure 5.14	Standard work and continuous improvement	99
Figure 6.1	Roadmap: Implement pull	101
Figure 6.2	Roadmap: Create a pull system	102
Figure 6.3	Push process	103
Figure 6.4	Push process example	103
Figure 6.5	Push process example: WIP	104
Figure 6.6	Push versus pull	104
Figure 6.7	Pull process	105
Figure 6.8	Pull process example	106
Table 6.1	Transportation pilot results	107
Figure 6.9	Roadmap: Reduce batching	108
Figure 6.10	Batching versus single-piece flow	109
Figure 6.11	Roadmap: Manage inventory	111
Figure 6.12	Kanban template	112
Figure 6.13	Kanban example	112
Figure 6.14	Pharmacy storeroom before improvements	113
Figure 6.15	Pharmacy storeroom after improvements	113
Figure 6.16	Pharmacy storeroom shelves after improvements	114

xii   List of Figures and Tables

Figure 6.17	Pharmacy decentralized storerooms before and after improvements	114
Figure 7.1	Roadmap: Strive for perfection	118
Figure 7.2	Roadmap: Identify root causes	119
Figure 7.3	Example of 5 Whys	120
Figure 7.4	Fishbone problem	121
Figure 7.5	Fishbone body structure	121
Figure 7.6	Fishbone categories	121
Figure 7.7	Fishbone with potential causes	122
Figure 7.8	Example of fishbone with potential causes	123
Figure 7.9	Roadmap: Error-proof process	124
Figure 7.10	Progression of error reduction	126
Figure 7.11	Roadmap: Sustain improvements	127
Table 7.1	Threats to sustainability	128
Table 7.2	Performance update table	129
Figure 7.12	Run chart examples	130
Figure 7.13	Bar chart example	130
Figure 7.14	Pie graph example	131
Table 7.3	Performance dashboard example	131
Figure 7.15	Performance dashboard example in the OR	132
Figure 8.1	PDCA cycle	134
Figure 8.2	Improvement kata model	135
Figure 8.3	Types of kaizen	136
Figure 8.4	Roadmap with DMAIC overlay	137
Figure 8.5	DMAIC checklist	138
Figure 8.6	Define phase checklist	139
Figure 8.7	Change readiness profile tool	141
Figure 8.8	Systems and process profile tool	142
Figure 8.9	Measure phase checklist	143
Figure 8.10	Analyze phase checklist	144
Figure 8.11	Improve phase checklist	146
Figure 8.12	Control phase checklist	148
Figure 8.13	Example of run chart, post-improvement	149
Figure 8.14	Example of a kaizen A3 report	151
Figure 8.15	Current state process map for OR patient flow	152
Figure 8.16	Value analysis breakdown for OR patient flow	153
Figure 8.17	Post-intervention process for OR patient flow	153
Figure 8.18	Improvement team piloting changes	154
Figure 8.19	Monthly average of SPU processing time	154
Figure 8.20	Process value analysis before and after intervention	155
Figure 9.1	Five-step kaizen problem-solving process	160
Figure 9.2	Step 1: Brainstorm issues and barriers	161
Figure 9.3	Examples of improvement teams brainstorming	162

Figure 9.4	Example of a fishbone diagram	163
Figure 9.5	Step 2: Filter and prioritize issues and barriers	163
Figure 9.6	In-control or out-of-control template	164
Figure 9.7	Example of categorizing issues and barriers	165
Figure 9.8	Examples of improvement teams voting	165
Figure 9.9	Step 3: Brainstorm solutions	166
Figure 9.10	Example of direct issue-to-solution brainstorming	167
Figure 9.11	Example of reverse engineering	168
Figure 9.12	Step 4: Filter and prioritize solutions	169
Figure 9.13	Payoff matrix	170
Figure 9.14	Example of Lamina tree of low-hanging fruit	170
Figure 9.15	Inventor of the Lamina tree	171
Figure 9.16	Step 5: Develop and implement an action plan	172
Table 9.1	Action plan template	172
Table 9.2	Recommendation template	172
Figure 9.17	Control phase action plan screenshot	173
Table 9.3	Stages of group dynamics	174
Figure 10.1	Change model	177
Table 10.1	States of change at the macro and micro levels	178
Figure 10.2	Segmenting roles and responsibilities	180
Figure 10.3	Change model with leadership responsibilities	181
Figure 10.4	Lean thinking summarized as 5-8-4	186
Figure A.1	Organization of CD documents	189
Table A.1	High-level project plan	192
Figure A.2	Project charter	194
Table A.2	Communication plan	195
Table A.3	Waste observations	196
Figure A.3	Waste diagnostic	197
Figure A.4	High-level process map	197
Table A.4	High-level SIPOC	198
Figure A.5	Change readiness profile	199
Figure A.6	System and process profile	200
Figure A.7	Process value analysis results example	201
Figure A.8	Workflow value analysis results example	201
Figure A.9	Current state VSM template	202
Table A.5	Voice of customer summary	203
Table A.6	Voice of customer more of/less of	204
Table A.7	Stakeholder analysis	205
Table A.8	RACI chart	206
Figure A.10	Fishbone diagram template	207
Table A.9	RIE agenda template	208
Figure A.11	Payoff matrix template	209

Table A.10	Action plan template	210
Table A.11	Recommendation template	211
Figure A.12	Future state VSM template	211
Figure A.13	Kaizen A3 report template	213
Table A.12	DOWNTIME matrix	216
Table A.13	Lean engagement communication plan	218
Table A.14	Lean opportunity guide	220
Figure A.14	VOC waste questionnaire	221
Figure A.15	Process value analysis Excel screenshot	223
Figure A.16	Workflow value analysis Excel screenshot	224
Figure A.17	Audit tool Excel screenshot	225
Figure A.18	Swimlane Excel screenshot	226
Figure A.19	RIE facilitator evaluation form	228
Figure A.20	Kaizen A3 report example: Phlebotomy 5S event	230
Figure A.21	Kaizen A3 report example: Rapid responses	231
Figure A.22	Control phase action plan screenshot	232
Figure A.23	Example of control phase action plan	232
Figure A.24	Gantt chart screenshot	233

List of Case Studies

Presurgery Patient Flow	16
Clinical Lab Workflow	25
Patient Flow in the Patient Testing Center	54
OR/SPCC Value Stream Mapping Event	57
Patient Flow in the Patient Testing Center	73
Evaluating Gastroenterology Physician's Office Visit	88
Rapid Changeover in the OR	94
Patient Transportation	107
Pharmacy Batching	110
Pharmacy Inventory	112
Inpatient Admission from the Emergency Department	122
Operating Room Performance Dashboards	131
Patient Flow through the Short-Procedure Unit (SPU)	152

Foreword
by David B. Nash, MD, MBA

I have the privilege of being the founding dean of the School of Population Health on the campus of Thomas Jefferson University in Philadelphia, the only school of its kind in the nation. In this capacity, I have come to know Dennis Delisle as one of our best teachers in several different capacities. First, I was one of a small group of mentors for Dennis as he began his management career following his health administration fellowship at our institution. It quickly became apparent to me that Dennis was not your average fellow! He had a burning passion for improving the outcomes of medical care, even as a non-clinician.

He rapidly became an expert in the concept of lean improvements, and I watched him quickly mature as a recognized campus-wide leader in the science of lean thinking. Our school was so impressed with his fund of knowledge and his enthusiasm that, together, we thought launching a graduate-level course as an elective in our School of Population Health (focused exclusively on lean improvement in healthcare) might be of interest to prospective students. Boy, was that a good decision!

Dennis's course quickly became one of the most highly sought after and most lauded electives in our school's portfolio. It therefore did not come as much of a surprise to me when Dennis, having just completed his doctorate, decided to write a textbook—hence, *Executing Lean Improvements: A Practical Guide with Real-World Healthcare Case Studies*. One might ask, "Another book on lean? Can we sort out all of the jargon from lean to Six Sigma to business process redesign?" The answer is a resounding yes, and this is the book that delivers the goods.

From my perch, "lean" means eliminate waste, and after 30 years in academic medicine, I'm convinced that a third of all the procedures my clinical colleagues order, and the money we collectively spend as a society, are wasteful. A good portion of what we do is not based on solid scientific evidence, but rather on a collection of the opinions of experts and the guild-like nature of our hierarchical training process. In a word, it still seems to me to be a world filled with "see one, do one, and teach one," with little regard for "Is that the right one in the first place?"

Executing Lean Improvements is not a clinical guide but rather a new mind-set, a paradigm shift, a sea change, a new lens with which to view waste.

Imagine the clinically integrated delivery system of the future. The chief medical officer makes regular gemba walks to see for herself where inefficiencies in the hospital's complex process might be lurking. Imagine, too, the daily huddle where clinicians, administrators, and others reflect on what occurred the day before and how they can make the process safer for all their patients. Admittedly, there are some organizations that embrace the gemba walk and the daily huddle for safety, but they are few and far between. This book will go a long way toward educating a large number of people who, in turn, can help their organizations catapult into such a future vision.

The book is well organized, and the figures and tables are clear and easy to grasp. The chapters walk us through the beginning of lean thinking and, in turn, define the key principles, such as value stream mapping, flow, and perfection. In fact, my favorite chapter is Chapter 10, and I agree with Dennis where he notes that the most salient take-away message of the book is "5-8-4." The "5" represents the five lean principles and the kaizen problem-solving process. The "8" represents the eight types of waste, and the "4" represents Spear's four rules. While some may balk at 5-8-4, I'm confident that we could reduce waste, improve outcomes, save money, and make patient care safer if every clinician and administrator embraced 5-8-4.

Lean thinking is not just a destination; it is a new way to view the world. As a dean, I have sent faculty for training in lean and have actively promoted enrollment in Dennis's graduate-level course. I'm supremely confident that lean thinking is one of the key tools that will help us implement healthcare reform. I'm equally confident that such implementation will put us on the road to redemption—a road paved with an increased attention to measurement, accountability, and closure of the feedback loop.

Who should read this book? I believe everyone in a leadership role in our increasingly complex delivery system would benefit from at least a rudimentary understanding of lean, and at best, a deep dive into each chapter in this helpful treatise. Kudos to Dennis Delisle for his many accomplishments, most especially this important new book. The only question I have is, Are we courageous enough, as practitioners, to embrace lean and to actually change our thinking in order to reduce the waste that surrounds so many of our processes?

As our school enters its next phase of growth and development, I'm confident that we will expand our course offerings in lean thinking and move to a world characterized by operational excellence. I'm sure that Dennis will help lead us in this important journey.

David B. Nash, MD, MBA
Dean, Jefferson School of Population Health

ABOUT DAVID B. NASH, MD, MBA

David B. Nash was named the founding dean of the Jefferson School of Population Health (JSPH) in 2008. This appointment caps a 25-year tenure on the faculty of Thomas Jefferson University. He is also the Dr. Raymond C. and Doris N. Grandon Professor of Health Policy. JSPH provides innovative educational programming designed to develop healthcare leaders for the future. Its offerings include master's programs in public health, healthcare quality and safety, health policy, and applied health economics. JSPH also offers a doctoral program in population health science.

Dr. Nash is a board certified internist who is internationally recognized for his work in public accountability for outcomes, physician leadership development, and quality-of-care improvement. He has been repeatedly named to *Modern Healthcare*'s list of Most Powerful Persons in Healthcare, and his pro bono national activities cover a wide scope. Currently he is on the VHA Center for Applied Healthcare Studies Advisory Board. He is a principal faculty member for quality-of-care programming for the American Association of Physician Leaders (AAPL) in Tampa, Florida, and leads the academic joint venture between AAPL and the JSPH. He is on the National Quality Forum task force on improving population health and is on the John M. Eisenberg Award Committee of the Joint Commission. He is also a founding member of the AAMC-IQ Steering Committee, the group charged with introducing the tenets of quality and safety into medical education. Dr. Nash has chaired the Technical Advisory Group (TAG) of the Pennsylvania Health Care Cost Containment Council (HC4) for more than 15 years, and he is widely recognized as a pioneer in the public reporting of outcomes.

Dr. Nash has governance responsibilities in both the not-for-profit and for-profit healthcare sectors. In the not-for-profit sector, Dr. Nash served on the board of trustees of Catholic Healthcare Partners in Cincinnati, Ohio, from 1998 to 2008, where he was the inaugural chair of the board committee on Quality and Safety. Currently, he is on the board of Main Line Health, a four-hospital system in suburban Philadelphia, Pennsylvania, where he also chairs the board committee on Quality and Safety. He is a member of the board of directors of the Population Health Alliance (PHA; formerly DMAA) in Washington, DC, and edits the official journal of the PHA.

In the for-profit sector, Dr. Nash was named to the board of directors for Humana, one of the nation's largest publicly traded healthcare companies, in 2009. He recently retired from the board of Endo Health Solutions, a publicly traded pharmaceutical company, now headquartered in Dublin, Ireland. In October 2013 he joined the board of Vestagen Technical Textiles, a privately held advanced medical textile company in Orlando, Florida. Recently, he joined the board of InfoMC in suburban Philadelphia, a leading information technology company.

Among his many awards are the following: In 1995 he received the top recognition award from the Academy of Managed Care Pharmacy. He received the Philadelphia Business Journal Healthcare Heroes Award in October 1997, and was named an honorary distinguished fellow of the American College of Physician Executives in 1998. In 2006 he received the Elliot Stone Award for leadership in public accountability for health data from NAHDO. In 2009 Dr. Nash received the Wharton Healthcare Alumni Achievement Award. In 2012, he received both the Joseph Wharton award in recognition of his social impact and the Philadelphia Business Journal innovation award.

Through publications, public appearances, his "Nash on the Road" blog, and an online column on MedPage Today, Dr. Nash routinely reaches more than 100,000 people every month. He has authored more than 100 articles in major peer-reviewed journals. He has edited 23 books, including *Connecting with the New Healthcare Consumer*, *The Quality Solution*, *Population Health: Creating a Culture of Wellness*, and most recently, *Demand Better*. From 1984 to 1989 he was the inaugural deputy editor of *Annals of Internal Medicine*. Currently, he is editor-in-chief of four major national journals: *American Journal of Medical Quality*, *Population Health Management*, *Pharmacy and Therapeutics* (*P&T*), and *American Health and Drug Benefits* (*AHDB*).

Dr. Nash received his BA in economics (Phi Beta Kappa) from Vassar College, his doctor of medicine from the University of Rochester School of Medicine and Dentistry, and his MBA in health administration (with honors) from the Wharton School at the University of Pennsylvania. While at Penn, he was a Robert Wood Johnson Foundation Clinical Scholar and medical director of a nine-physician faculty group practice in general internal medicine.

Dr. Nash lives in Lafayette Hill, Pennsylvania, with his wife of more than 34 years, Esther J. Nash, MD. They have 27-year-old fraternal twin daughters and a 23-year-old son. Dr. Nash enjoys jogging, biking, and playing tennis.

Visit the Jefferson School of Public Health at http://Jefferson.edu/population_health/ and his blog at http://blogs.jefferson.edu/nashhealthpolicy/.

Foreword
by David P. McQuaid, RPh, MBA, FACHE

This book represents the evolution of an organization's journey to excellence. In this practical guide, readers walk through a systematic approach to implement lean thinking in the healthcare environment, accompanied by real-world examples. Since my arrival at Thomas Jefferson University and Hospitals (Jefferson) in 2007, we have been committed to driving quality through proven methodologies and performance excellence frameworks. We have made incredible strides along the way and continue to strive to be the best in all that we do.

My initial role at Jefferson was in the capacity of chief operating officer. During my four-year tenure, I focused on building strong operational performance by enhancing a culture that expects superior results in patient and employee satisfaction, quality of care, and efficient patient access and throughput. Additionally, there was special emphasis on meaningful and productive partnerships between administrative and physician leadership in order to grow clinical service offerings and market share.

Central to this effort was the development of an organization-wide balanced scorecard (BSC) in 2007. The BSC provides leadership and staff a way to monitor and improve outcomes through targeted improvement activities. I brought the BSC approach to Jefferson to lay the foundation for the key organizational structures, processes, and systems needed to address complex operational challenges, improve accountability, and drive results.

Through various roles in my career, from pharmacy technician to pharmacist to chief executive officer, I have learned that it is impossible to effect change without structure and discipline. To this end, we began the development of the core competencies needed to leverage and optimize the BSC approach. In 2008, Jefferson introduced lean, Six Sigma, and change management to the organization. The chairman of the board at that time, Robert S. Adelson, challenged Jefferson leadership to accelerate the pace of change through proven performance excellence strategies. Those methodologies were chosen to help align hospital quality and business activities with the vision and strategy of the organization, improve internal communication, and monitor organizational performance. Select employees were trained and certified, leading the charge in a new way of doing business.

As time progressed, we realized there was a growing need to educate more staff and emphasize the use of lean thinking, which included accessible, logical tools for anyone to use. To accomplish this we needed to have a person with expertise in lean, Six Sigma, change acceleration, and project management. One of my mentees, Dr. Dennis Delisle, fit the description. Dennis worked under me while I served as Jefferson's COO. During that time, we began exploring the Malcolm

Baldrige National Quality Award program. As a national examiner, I knew the Baldrige Healthcare Criteria would help us create the structures and processes needed to drive meaningful results. Under my leadership, Dennis facilitated the writing and production of six applications over four years (four at the state level through the Keystone Alliance for Performance Excellence [KAPE] and two at the national level). In 2012, Jefferson received the Mastery Award recognition from KAPE. The Mastery Award honors organizations that demonstrate high-quality results that are directly attributable to the deployment of systematic approaches.

A critical element in our execution approach is the use of employees trained in Lean-Six Sigma. When Lean-Six Sigma was first introduced in 2008, Jefferson trained 42 change agents and 6 lean leaders ("lean leader" is a term Jefferson uses for an individual certified as a lean practitioner). These individuals serve full-time roles in other departments (e.g., nurses, pharmacists, physicians, administrators) and volunteer their time to work on team-based improvement projects. Over time there was a growing demand for these resources. I charged the department responsible for Lean-Six Sigma education and project execution to redefine the model and expand its ability to drive organizational results. This is where Dennis and his team stepped up to the challenge.

Since 2009, the program has grown almost exponentially. To date, Jefferson has certified over 200 staff as change agents and over 100 as lean leaders. Additionally, the education model has evolved into a robust program offering 15 courses in lean, change leadership, and project management, among others. Nearly 1000 employees have participated in at least one of these course offerings. The dramatic growth in certified facilitators and trained staff has positioned the organization to effect change rapidly, in a systematic fashion. Further advancements in the education program include the development of undergraduate and graduate courses in lean thinking and accelerating transformation as well as a graduate certificate in operational excellence through the Thomas Jefferson University School of Population Health. These courses and the graduate certificate provide opportunities for individuals within or outside Jefferson to learn the strategies and tactics that lead to successful integration of performance excellence methodologies in the healthcare environment.

In my new role as president and CEO of Thomas Jefferson University Hospitals, I have responsibilities for the organization's integrated clinical enterprise consisting of all its hospitals, its 640-member physician practice plan, multiple ambulatory and clinic sites, its clinically integrated network, and home healthcare services. As a member of Jefferson's executive team, I am also responsible for executing the strategic plans of the organization, providing management oversight for improving the patient experience and population health, and developing safe, high-quality, cost-effective patient care and integrated clinical programs. To this end, we rely on the lean thinking philosophy to guide our approach toward problem solving and execution.

I hope the insight offered in this book will help you leverage the power of lean thinking, whether it is on the front line or at the organizational level. Over the course of my career, from frontline pharmacy technician to executive, I have not found a more effective method to engage and empower staff to solve their own problems, enhance the patient experience, and achieve quality outcomes that exceed the competition. Best of luck on your journey to excellence!

David P. McQuaid, RPh, MBA, FACHE
President and CEO, Thomas Jefferson University Hospitals
Executive Vice President, Clinical Affairs, Jefferson Health System

ABOUT DAVID P. MCQUAID, RPh, MBA, FACHE

David P. McQuaid is an accomplished 35-year veteran of healthcare and healthcare administration. His value to healthcare systems is his exceptionally strong experience in operational and financial improvement. Over the years he has demonstrated success in building collaborative teams and sophisticated process and measurement systems in highly challenging environments. A mentor and developer of talent, he has been cited for his skill in developing and executing strategy, and partnering and engaging with physicians to develop high-quality market-leading services. His action orientation inspires and ignites competitive drive and focus for organizations, resulting in significantly improved outcomes and results.

He has been in executive leadership and operating positions with nationally prominent, complex community and academic healthcare systems and currently is president and CEO of Thomas Jefferson University Hospitals in Philadelphia, Pennsylvania. He received his BS degree in pharmacy from MCPHS University in Boston, Massachusetts, and his MBA degree from the University of New Hampshire in Durham.

Introduction

1 + 1 or ((97 − 88)*65/(1 + 4) − 17)^(1/2) − (64^(1/2) + 73 − 12*3 + 6*8 − 85)
You decide . . . both equal 2.

—Dennis R. Delisle

Without the vocabulary it is difficult to even start the conversation. In my experience, I have had an exponentially easier and more productive time discussing problems and developing and implementing solutions with fellow lean thinkers compared with individuals with no exposure to lean. This book focuses on the model, strategy, and lessons learned in implementing lean thinking in a healthcare organization. Using Jefferson's real-world case studies, the book provides approaches and tools to catalyze rapid improvements. The core goal is to create an accessible and usable guide for beginner through more advanced lean improvement practitioners.

Continuous improvement promotes the relentless refinement of systems and processes. Today's challenge in the healthcare environment lies in an organization's ability to rapidly improve at a greater rate than surrounding competitors. The goal is not simply to get better, but rather "become the best at getting better." This phrase serves as the vision for Jefferson's performance excellence journey. But to achieve this, the traditional problem-solving paradigm needs to shift.

I teach both undergraduate and graduate courses in lean thinking. At the beginning of each semester I tell the students, "If you like the way you think now and do not want to change, drop this class. Because once we get started, you will see the world through a different lens. You will fundamentally think and problem solve differently, and you will not be able to go back." Though slightly exaggerated, my goal as a teacher is to change the way my students see the world. I am not interested simply in the acquisition of knowledge, but rather the application and synthesis of that knowledge into their lives, both at work and at home. By changing the way people think, you can change the way they behave. As it relates to continuous improvement (the premise of the book), readers must shift their minds from simple observation to critical analysis and problem-solving strategies.

To me, the most important stage of learning is knowing why—understanding the significance and meaning of concepts at a fundamental level. I approach teaching from the ground up. Laying and solidifying a foundation is the critical first step. From there, layers of complexity are added and interrelationships established.

Readers can readily apply knowledge to the real-world setting with concepts and tools emphasizing meaning and use in a variety of situations.

There are so many books about lean on the market. Entire books are dedicated to specific tools (e.g., value stream mapping, A3 problem solving) as well as the philosophy and influences that led to the development of lean thinking. This book is different. From years of experience with over 100 projects and dozens of educational courses, I have refined the content in order to simplify concepts and tools, boiling it down to practical application. There are a lot of different ways to skin a cat. I prefer to highlight and use one or two concepts and/or tools that have proven effective, rather than present every possible or known way. This is not a book on theory. It is about action. The book provides readers the knowledge and ability to develop and implement meaningful change in the most simple and straightforward manner. It is a big challenge!

To meet this challenge, the book requires an organized and logical model for improvement. The roadmap for creating a lean process serves as the book's framework (Figure I.1). The model is an adaptation of the Lean Roadmap from Breakthrough Management Group International (BMGI). This framework provides the backdrop for systematic process evaluation and improvement within the five principles of lean: (1) define value, (2) map the value stream, (3) establish flow, (4) implement pull, and (5) strive for perfection. Chapters 2–7 construct the roadmap one block at a time. Readers will gain a comprehensive understanding of each element within the model.

The Five Principles of Lean

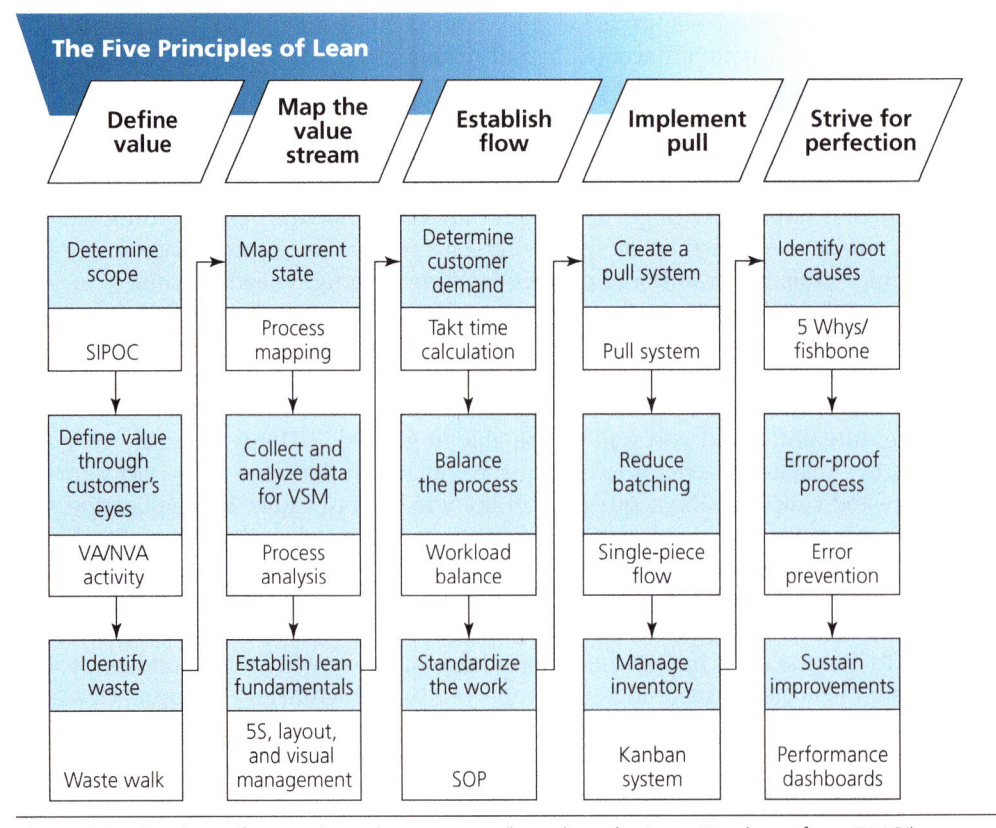

Define value	Map the value stream	Establish flow	Implement pull	Strive for perfection
Determine scope	Map current state	Determine customer demand	Create a pull system	Identify root causes
SIPOC	Process mapping	Takt time calculation	Pull system	5 Whys/ fishbone
Define value through customer's eyes	Collect and analyze data for VSM	Balance the process	Reduce batching	Error-proof process
VA/NVA activity	Process analysis	Workload balance	Single-piece flow	Error prevention
Identify waste	Establish lean fundamentals	Standardize the work	Manage inventory	Sustain improvements
Waste walk	5S, layout, and visual management	SOP	Kanban system	Performance dashboards

Figure I.1 Roadmap for creating a lean process (based on the Lean Roadmap from BMGI).

In this book you will find the following:

- A structured approach to executing lean improvements
- Relevant real-world case studies
- Examples of tools and templates along with downloadable files via CD
- Hints, tips, and lessons learned
- Chapter challenges aimed at giving the reader assignments to apply key concepts and tools in the work setting

WHO THIS BOOK IS FOR

The primary audience for this book is individuals responsible for improvement in healthcare settings, such as lean practitioners, Six Sigma belts, quality improvement specialists, and project managers. Additional health professionals will benefit from the practical application and guidance. Positions include frontline managers and supervisors, improvement teams, professors teaching quality improvement and/or operations management, healthcare professionals responsible for performance improvement, and students in all related health professions (clinical and administrative).

The book promotes practical application. Readers are equipped with the skills to implement lean concepts and tools within their work setting. Additionally, the book provides insight and strategies for avoiding failure and developing buy-in. Remember, every organization is unique. You know your organization's history and culture. Use that knowledge to adopt and adapt certain tools and techniques that fit the environment.

HOW THIS BOOK IS ORGANIZED

Chapter 1 provides an overview of lean thinking. The chapter introduces readers to the roadmap for creating a lean process. The roadmap provides the framework for systematically implementing lean improvements and serves as the foundation of the book. Chapters 2–7 dive into the five principles of lean thinking. Readers explore each specific principle along with the associated concepts and tools. Case studies support tools, highlighting their use, as well as hints and tips to consider when using the tools. This comprehensive section of the book serves as the core to practical implementation.

The final section of the book, Chapters 8–10, ties execution and lessons learned to the tools and approach provided within Chapters 2–7. Chapter 8 defines the lean DMAIC (Define, Measure, Analyze, Improve, Control) model. Readers learn the standardized approach for rapid improvements, which includes a checklist as a reference guide for project execution. Chapter 9 reviews the five-step kaizen problem-solving process. This structured model includes effective brainstorming and prioritization tools along with instructions for facilitating them. This chapter provides readers with practical tips and techniques to lead multidisciplinary teams through problem solving and action plan development. The final chapter discusses strategies and challenges in leading change as well as offers lessons learned from Jefferson's improvement journey. The chapter also integrates practical application with the leadership skills required to implement and sustain meaningful improvements. Readers will be able to identify, develop, implement, and sustain improvement efforts within their area of responsibility at the conclusion of this book.

As stated in the beginning of this section, once you learn how to see things through the lean thinking lens, you will not be able to turn it off. Waste is everywhere, and at times it will frustrate you. However, my goal is to show you not only to see it but to do something about it. The appendixes and accompanying CD of templates provide the necessary resources to get started. Keep this book close by your side as you start or continue executing lean improvements.

ACKNOWLEDGMENTS

Special thanks to Jean and Dennis Delisle, Rachel Eirich, Robert Bartosz, David McQuaid, and David Nash.

Chapter 1
Lean Thinking

Seek first to understand, then to be understood.

—Stephen Covey

Changes in the healthcare landscape have led to innovative and adaptive efforts of organizations to stay afloat (Martin, Neumann, Mountford, Bisognano, & Nolan, 2009). Current healthcare reform, with its focus on value-based reimbursement, serves as a catalyst for institutional and industry-wide change. Healthcare organizations are now starting to leverage improvement methodologies proven effective in other industries like manufacturing (de Souza, 2009; McConnell, Lindrooth, Wholey, Maddox, & Bloom, 2013). This effort is akin to evidence-based medicine, where organizations develop a systematic structure and process to produce high-quality results (Bradley et al., 2012; Bradley et al., 2006; Curry et al., 2011; Shojania & Grimshaw, 2005; Shortell, Rundall, & Hsu, 2007; Shortell & Singer, 2008).

Though improvements in quality have been slower than desired (Brennan, Gawande, Thomas, & Studdert, 2005; Classen et al., 2011; Dentzer, 2011; Leape & Berwick, 2005; Wachter, 2004), lean has shown to be effective in improving various healthcare processes, including operating rooms, emergency departments, and clinical labs (Aronson & Gelatt, 2006; Farrokhi, Gunther, Williams, & Blackmore, 2013; Martin et al., 2009; Vermeulen et al., 2014). Having a structured approach is essential since most problems relate to management and system/process design (Chalice, 2007). A silver bullet does not exist. The only way to be successful in this ever-changing environment is to be purposeful and agile in strategy and execution (Zidel, 2012). Limited resources require a thoughtful, methodical way to evaluate opportunity areas and develop high-impact solutions.

PERFORMANCE IMPROVEMENT METHODOLOGIES

There are many performance improvement methodologies. Each methodology provides some degree of structure and guidelines for using tools to improve processes. The focus of this book is lean thinking. However, various tools and concepts influenced by methods like Six Sigma, quality assurance, and total quality management also appear (Pande & Holpp, 2002). Table 1.1 depicts the more common approaches to performance improvement. The point is not to elaborate on

Table 1.1 Performance improvement methodologies.

Method	Problem	Goal	Implementing improvements	Approach	One-line description
Lean	Process inefficiencies, space/layout issues, poor quality	Reduce/eliminate waste	Frontline-based improvements or 2-hour to 3-day rapid improvement with solutions implemented during and within 30 days	Frontline improvement through PDCA, project execution through DMAIC model	Identify and eliminate non-value-adding activity (waste)
Six Sigma	Variation in outcomes, complex processes	Reduce variation	Complex problem resolution, may take 3–9 months	Project execution through DMAIC model	Comprehensive statistical process improvement approach to reduce variation
Business process redesign	Not achieving desired outcomes with current process, want dramatic results	Fundamental rethinking and radical process redesign	Teams redesign process, no defined timeline	Identify processes, review/update/analyze, design future state, test and implement	Complete process redesign
Quality assurance	Not meeting standards, errors	Fit for purpose and right the first time	Systematic measurement and monitoring	Feedback loop, no defined approach	Error prevention, ensuring quality requirements are met
Total quality management	Poor quality	Quality of products and processes	All employees participate daily in improving processes, services, etc.	Management approach—everyone's responsibility	Quality is everyone's responsibility

each; dozens of texts are available for that. There is not a singular best approach. Ideally, the most effective method is a combination of many (Smith, 2003).

A great analogy is the mixed martial arts. There are many techniques and styles of martial arts. Some emphasize using hands or legs, while others focus on grappling and ground control. The most effective martial artist is one who has competencies in all areas (i.e., skilled on his or her feet and adept on the ground). Depending on the situation, he or she will utilize certain tactics and techniques from the appropriate method/style to gain advantage over an opponent.

The perspective is similar for performance improvement methodologies. The approach varies depending on the organizational needs and current state of operations. This book takes concepts from other practices and incorporates them into the lean thinking framework. Fundamentally, though, there are elements that need to be present in order to ensure successful adoption and utilization. These elements include a clear purpose and direction, leadership support and staff empowerment, and a commitment to continuous improvement (Niemeijer, Trip, de Jong, Wendt, & Does, 2012).

Project and change management are two approaches that have the greatest impact on executing lean improvements. Project management provides the structure to implement improvement projects. Defined phases compose the project management approach to initiate, plan, execute, and then close. The DMAIC (Define, Measure, Analyze, Improve, Control) framework deconstructs these phases into specific deliverables and outputs. Chapter 8 describes executing lean improvements through DMAIC in detail.

Change management is the underlying model for driving transformation. Sustainable change does not happen through happenstance or luck. There are defined and proven strategies to facilitate the assessment and subsequent management of interventions. Chapter 10 reviews such strategies as well as lessons learned along the way.

THE LEAN THINKING PHILOSOPHY

This book will challenge you to see the world differently. It provides the tools and knowledge to effect positive change. Derived from Toyota, lean is an underlying management philosophy and way of thinking that permeates both professional and personal interactions (Womack & Jones, 1996). Defining value through the eyes of the customer (i.e., patient, specimen, or department) exemplifies lean thinking (Graban, 2012). The primary goal of lean is the identification and elimination of waste or those activities that do not add value to the process.

Empowering frontline employees to solve problems at the source and improve their workflow and quality is at the core of lean thinking (Graban & Swartz, 2012; Tapping, Kozlowski, Archbold, & Sperl, 2009). The focus of lean in the healthcare arena is not money and time. It is safety, quality, and service delivery (Graban, 2012). Focusing on quality as the highest priority leads to cost reductions (e.g., reduces rework and inefficiencies and improves productivity and throughput) (Imai, 1997; Langley et al., 2009; Liker, 2004). A continuous improvement framework and respect for people establish the foundation (Toussaint & Gerard, 2010). To this end, lean tools identify and eliminate the interruptions, errors, and other tasks that take away from the main goal at hand. These concepts and tools apply anywhere, from work to personal activities (Jones & Mitchell, 2006). We do not just want to do more with less; we want to do *better* with less.

Lean thinking requires a different approach toward management. The emphasis in a lean management environment is to ask the right questions rather than provide answers (Bicheno & Holweg, 2004; Womack, 2011). The systematic nature of implementing lean thinking leads to effective problem assessment and resolution through this method (Joint Commission on the Accreditation of Healthcare Organizations, 2006). Incremental improvements help make the current situation better while striving for perfection.

The ability to execute strategy and continuously improve enables an organization to achieve its vision (Hrebiniak, 2013). Essential to this is leveraging human resources and optimizing their potential through education and hands-on problem solving. Lean thinking promotes the method of establishing purpose, process, then people (Womack, 2011):

- *Purpose:* Where are we going? The purpose serves as the destination (future state). Customers are central to the purpose (in healthcare this is usually the patient).
- *Process:* How will we get there? A process is the stream of value from start to finish, envisioning how to move from the current state to the future state.
- *People:* Who do we need to get us there, and what skills should they have? Educate and empower employees to solve problems. Effective management systems position employees in systems and processes that enable quality, not produce errors and inefficiencies.

> *"Purpose comes first, then the processes to achieve the purpose, then engaged people to conduct the processes needed to achieve the purpose."*
>
> —James Womack

Organizations can develop a leadership system that leverages the purpose, process, people framework (Figure 1.1) (Meyer, 2010). The mission and vision define the purpose of an organization and articulate the customer-centric description of why the organization exists and what it aspires to become. Without purpose there is no direction. If employees do not understand how their contributions and roles fit into an overall strategy, their work feels directionless (Kotter, 1995). The lean philosophy is top-down driven, bottom-up executed. Leaders communicate where the organization is going and what needs to get done, but staff define how the organization will get there. To this end, without commitment from leadership, teams may not have the required resources, priorities, and focus needed to move an initiative forward. From a leadership perspective, the challenge is to clearly define and communicate the purpose (vision) and align and integrate the work systems and processes to achieve it.

The mission and vision are realized through the process of strategic planning and execution of key initiatives aligned with the organization's short- and longer-term objectives. Processes flow horizontally across functions, departments, and/or teams (Figure 1.2). Process design and execution contribute to the overall

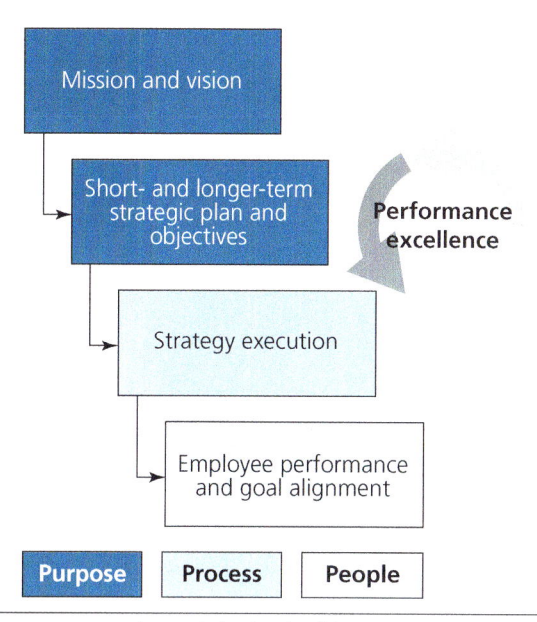

Figure 1.1 Purpose, process, people, and the leadership system.

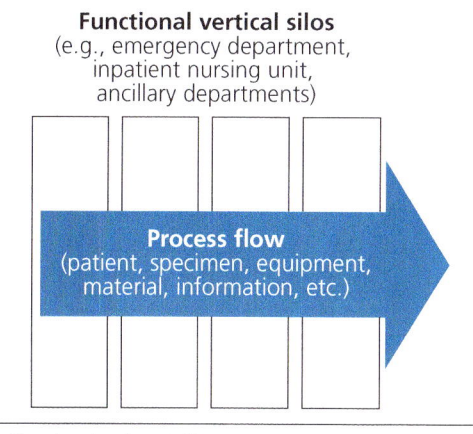

Figure 1.2 Lean thinking flowing horizontally.

impact and consistency of outcomes. Lean thinking targets the purpose and identifies the best, most efficient way to achieve it (process). When issues arise, lean thinkers systematically evaluate and identify ways to limit or reduce the likelihood of future occurrences (Wysocki, 2004).

The people component aligns and cascades organizational goals down to the individual employee. This enables strategic management of human resources to optimize quality, productivity, and efficiency (Swensen, Dilling, Harper, & Noseworthy, 2012). Employees can link their value to and impact on the organization through alignment of their tasks and responsibilities to overarching organizational goals.

The performance excellence framework activates the leadership system. The organization's improvement philosophy directs the systematic approach to align

6   Chapter One

and integrate purpose, process, and people. Hoshin kanri is a lean concept that drives the purpose, process, people approach. It represents the strategic deployment of projects to drive the organization's vision. Originally derived from Dr. Yoji Akao (Bicheno & Holweg, 2004), the approach aligns all three elements into tangible tactics. Strategic objectives articulate the vision. High-level performance metrics (also known as key performance indicators, or KPIs) translate strategic objectives into measurable variables. KPIs are typically lagging metrics in nature, meaning they are the outcomes or end results of processes. Examples include revenue, market share, and customer satisfaction (McChesney, Covey, & Huling, 2012). Operational and strategic projects focus on impacting the KPIs. Each project has its own defined metrics.

Unlike lagging metrics, project metrics are leading in nature. This means that leading metric performance should indicate the direction of the lagging outcome. For example, if your goal is to lose weight (lagging metric), you have to decrease your calorie consumption or increase calories burned (both leading metrics). Leading metrics tend to be within our operational control and, as a consequence, should be the focus of improvement efforts. They should be high-impact processes or behaviors that improvement teams can affect. The pivotal characteristics of good leading metrics are predictability of achieving the goal and being within the team's influence (McChesney et al., 2012). In other words, if you improve the leading metric, the lagging metric should likewise improve.

The hoshin kanri cascade from strategic objectives to project KPIs portrays the flow of the organizational vision down through improvement projects. Figure 1.3 is a simplified model that demonstrates the necessity to align and integrate activities to achieve results. Identifying the appropriate leading metric(s) is an essential skill that ultimately results in meeting, exceeding, or falling short of the strategic objectives or overall performance metrics (Hrebiniak, 2013).

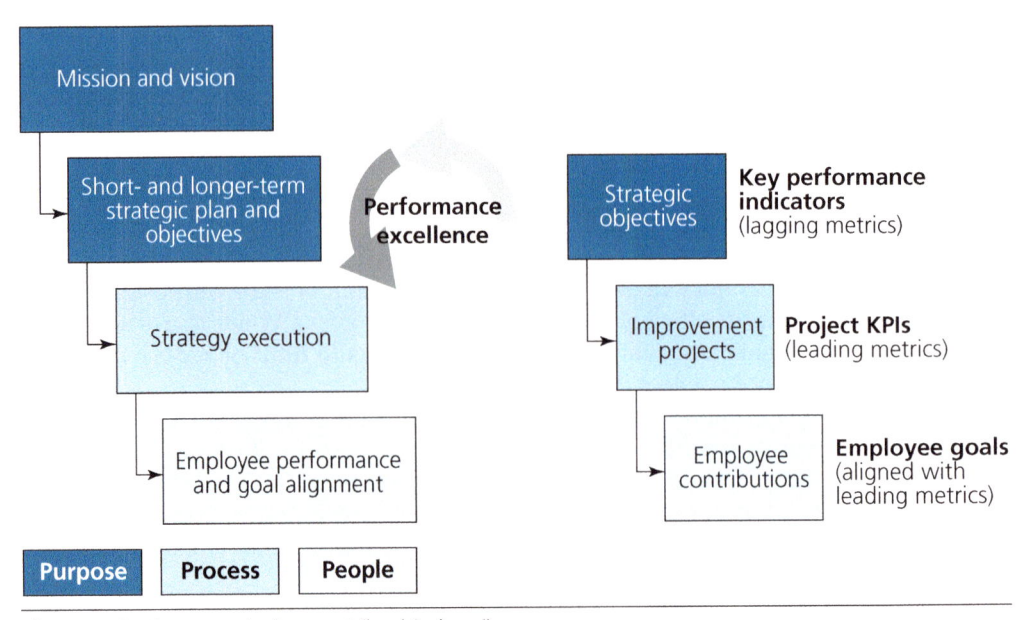

Figure 1.3   Strategy deployment (hoshin kanri).

ROADMAP FOR CREATING A LEAN PROCESS

The roadmap for creating a lean process functions as the model for the performance excellence framework (Figure I.1). The model, when implemented, can contribute to strong performance, wise resource utilization, and ultimately a competitive advantage. Atop the model are the five principles of lean: (1) define value, (2) map the value stream, (3) establish flow, (4) implement pull, and (5) strive for perfection (Womack & Jones, 1996). Each principle has three components. Each component represents a particular deliverable or concept with a corresponding tool (indicated in the white box below the component). The components are sequential, beginning with scope definition and ending with sustainability strategies. Chapters 2–7 construct the roadmap one block at a time. It is essential to have a comprehensive understanding of both the sequence and the significance of the model's elements.

The lean project opportunity guide (Table 1.2) provides a reference for healthcare processes that are appropriate for applying the roadmap. Remember, improvements are not only formal projects but any activity that reduces inefficiencies and waste, resulting in better processes and outcomes (Graban & Swartz, 2012). The scope of identified opportunities varies; however, the improvement approaches described throughout the book are consistent.

Table 1.2 Lean project opportunity guide.

General improvement opportunities		
Staffing	Workflow Workflow balancing	Time management Productivity
Physical organization/ inventory management	Ordering processes/par levels Space allocation	Visual management Physical layout/organization
Examples of lean project metrics		
Turnaround time Cycle/processing time	Throughput time (lead time) Customer, patient, employee satisfaction	Quality output Cost savings/avoidance

Examples of department/function-specific improvement opportunities		
Business services	Timeliness and accuracy of results/reports Transactional throughput	Request turnaround time
Emergency department	Length of stay Door to triage Door to physician	Door to disposition Door to discharge Admission order to transfer from ED
Diagnostic and ancillary departments	Patient transportation Patient registration Order to result	Request to completion Exam/procedure/testing scheduling Work assignments

(continued)

Table 1.2 Lean project opportunity guide. *(Continued)*

Examples of department/function-specific improvement opportunities		
Nursing and clinical units	Bed availability Bed empty to fill turnaround time	Patient flow Workload balance
Physician practice	Exam room utilization Access/scheduling	Patient flow Workload balance
Supply chain	Par levels Product standardization Space allocation/organization	Inventory locations Distribution process
Surgical services	Decontamination and sterilization processes Instrument availability Case assembly Operating room utilization	First case on-time start Scheduling process Operating room turnover Patient flow

CHAPTER CHALLENGE

Think of a work-related problem you would like to improve (refer to Table 1.2 for ideas). Identify an area within your scope of control that could benefit from lean thinking. Where is it? What improvement opportunities exist? What are the expected benefits?

QUESTIONS

1. What performance improvement methodologies would fit your organization/department/area of responsibility?
2. Have you seen projects or decisions that were based on people, process, then purpose (rather than the other way around)?
3. Why is establishing the purpose an integral first step?
4. What aspect of managing/implementing change is most critical in your workplace or chosen scenario?
5. What are your strategic objectives?
6. Are employee goals aligned with organizational objectives?
7. What leading metrics can you address in order to drive key lagging indicators?

Chapter 2
Principle #1: Define Value

It is not the employer who pays the wages. Employers only handle the money. It is the customer who pays the wages.

—Henry Ford, Sr.

Chapter 1 discussed the framework of lean thinking—the roadmap for creating a lean process. The five principles provide the structure for initiating, executing, and sustaining process improvements. This section is the beginning of lean thinking. Defining value is the most fundamental of the principles. Central to the lean philosophy are our customers and how they define value (Womack & Jones, 1996).

The focus of this chapter is on shifting your thinking from worker-centric to customer-centric process evaluation. Defining customer value is an essential step toward identifying and eliminating those activities that do not add value (synonymous with waste) (Graban, 2012; Womack & Jones, 1996). Three components are core to defining value (Figure 2.1):

1. Determine scope
2. Define value through the customer's eyes
3. Identify waste

These components, completed in sequence, provide an initial assessment of the current state (how the process is currently performing). In order to effect change, we must first understand the problems we are facing. To do this, we must go to the gemba (where the work takes place) to observe processes, ask questions, and engage staff in developing solutions (Womack, 2011).

DETERMINE SCOPE

Every project needs to have a scope (Figure 2.2). The scope is a well-defined description or depiction of the project boundaries (Project Management Institute, 2008). For process improvement projects, the best way to display the scope is through process maps. Process maps show what is happening through a visual breakdown of steps or activities (Figure 2.3). The map helps define the steps to evaluate and target for improvement.

10 Chapter Two

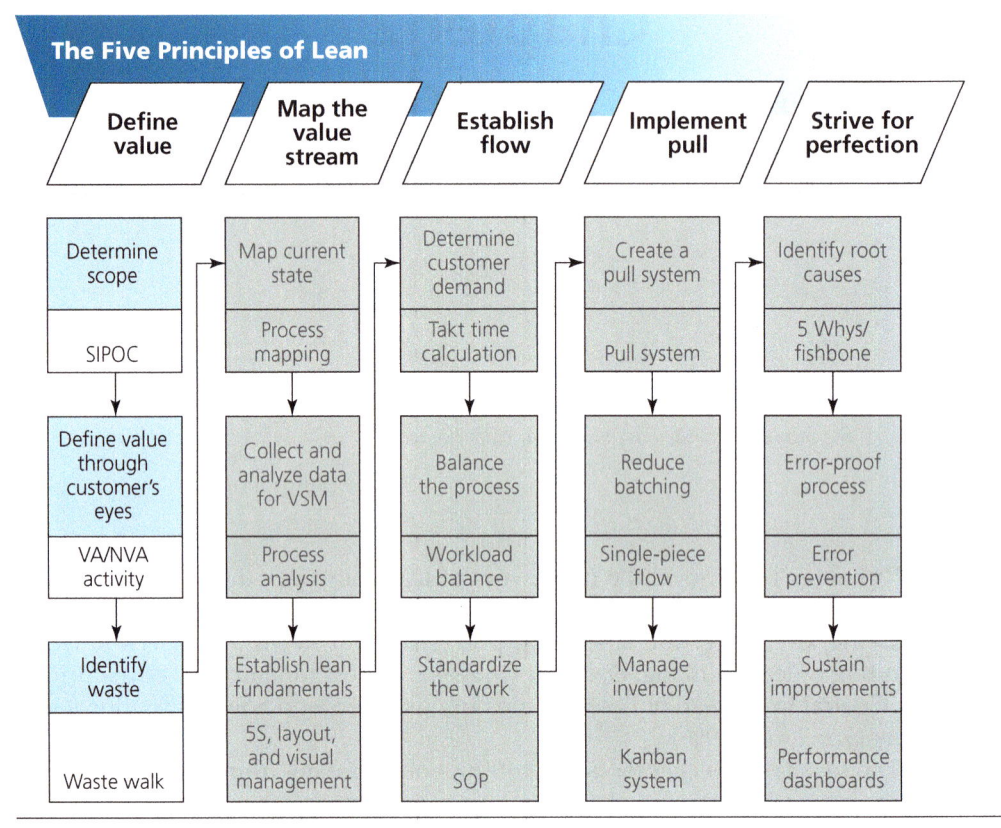

Figure 2.1 Roadmap: Define value.

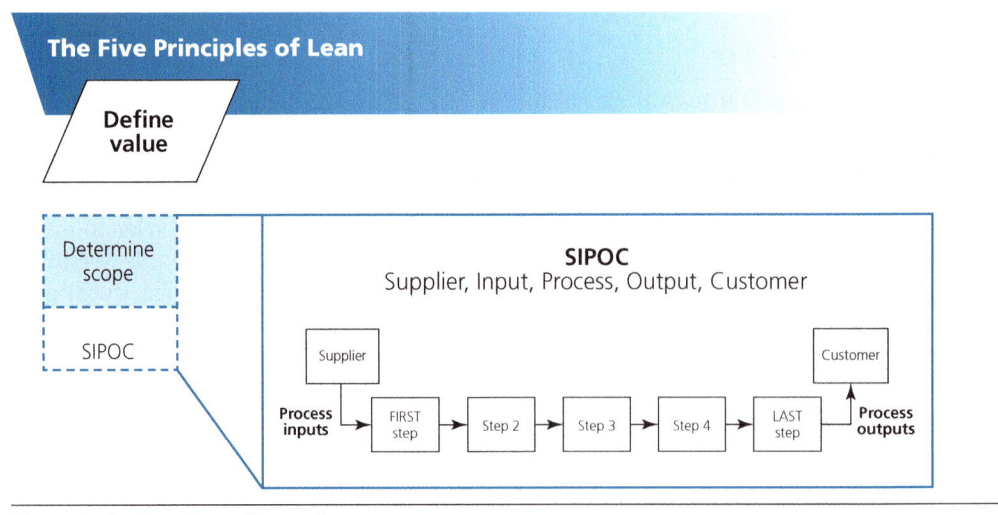

Figure 2.2 Roadmap: Determine scope.

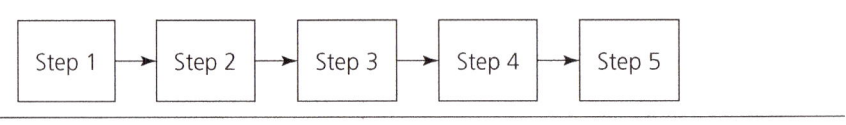

Figure 2.3 Process map structure.

```
┌──────┐   ┌──────┐   ┌──────┐   ┌──────┐   ┌──────┐
│FIRST │──▶│Step 2│──▶│Step 3│──▶│Step 4│──▶│ LAST │
│ step │   │      │   │      │   │      │   │ step │
└──────┘   └──────┘   └──────┘   └──────┘   └──────┘
```

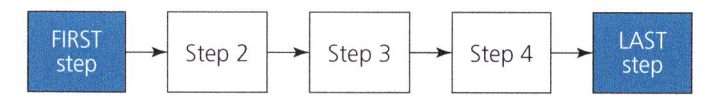

Figure 2.4 Process scoping.

Determining the scope begins with identifying the first and last steps of the process (Figure 2.4). Everything upstream (before the first step) and downstream (after the last step) is out of scope. This is a crucial concept. Many projects fail due to a poorly defined scope or an ever-expanding scope (also known as scope creep).

> *"Don't boil the ocean." Always remember this expression—it will make you an effective leader and problem solver. If you can scope a problem appropriately, you will achieve your desired outcomes and objectives. Too small and the impact is barely noticeable. Too big and nothing gets accomplished. The goal is to find the scope that is just right.*

A common tool used to create a high-level process map is the SIPOC (pronounced *sy-pock*) diagram. SIPOC stands for Supplier, Input, Process, Output, and Customer:

- *Supplier*—Provides inputs to initiate the process (e.g., person, department, organization)
- *Input*—Materials, resources, and/or information required to execute the process (e.g., order, equipment, form)
- *Process*—Series of steps or activities to convert inputs to outputs
- *Output*—Product, service, or outcome resulting from the process
- *Customer*—Receives the outputs of the process

Building the SIPOC is a straightforward activity. It is important to remember to keep the initial map high-level. Depict the process from a 30,000-foot view, and do not get lost in details early in the assessment phase. The SIPOC diagram provides a process overview and is the foundation for improvement.

Building a SIPOC (Figure 2.5)

1. Determine the start and end process steps
2. Identify the inputs and outputs
3. Identify the supplier and the customer
4. Indicate high-level steps in between (process) (30,000-foot view)

Figure 2.6 is an example of a SIPOC for the clinical lab. The process scope is the time from when a specimen arrives at the lab to the time the results are completed. The supplier and the customer are the test-ordering physicians. The physicians are sending the specimen (input) and receiving the test results (output).

Figure 2.7 is another example of a SIPOC for the sterile processing department. This department is responsible for decontaminating, cleaning, sterilizing, packing,

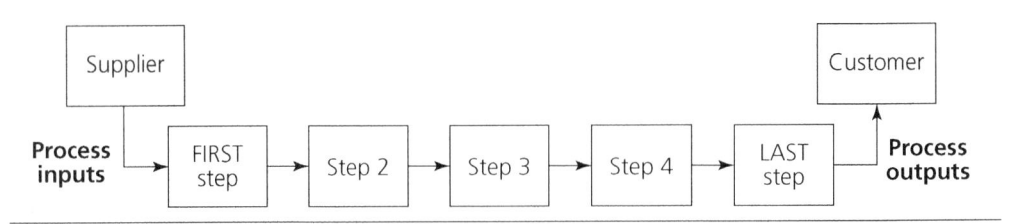

Figure 2.5 SIPOC diagram.

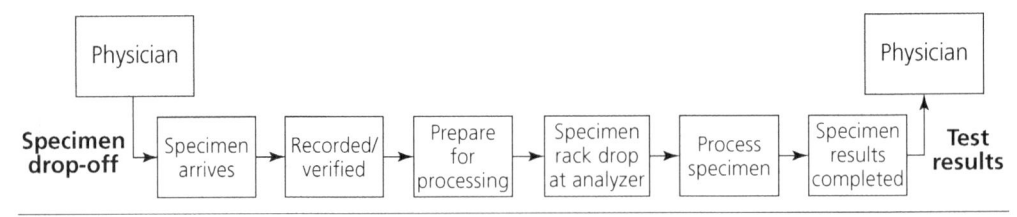

Figure 2.6 Lab receiving process SIPOC.

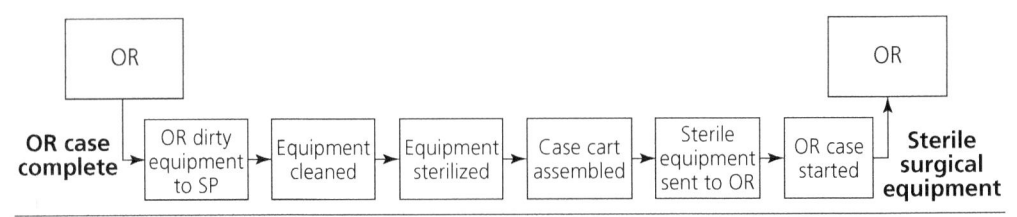

Figure 2.7 Sterile processing SIPOC.

and distributing surgical equipment and supplies to the operating rooms. This process highlights the steps from the time the operating room case is complete to the time the subsequent case using the surgical equipment begins.

DEFINE VALUE THROUGH CUSTOMER'S EYES

After the scope has been determined, value is defined through the customer's eyes (Figure 2.8). For lean thinkers, the focus is identification and reduction of waste. Costs are viewed as an end result, once quality issues are addressed and improved (Berwick, Nolan, & Whittington, 2008). The ultimate goal of a process is to provide the customer value—what the customer wants, when the customer wants it, and in the correct amount (Chalice, 2007).

The lean thinking philosophy targets and eliminates the "firefighting" mentality. Often staff think the value they contribute to their company is their ability to chase down problems and fight fires (Graban, 2012). For example, if information on a form is missing, an employee might make several phone calls and send multiple e-mails in order to gather everything. All of this effort, though well intentioned, is waste. Fighting fires is not a systematic approach to preventing and anticipating problems; it is reactive and inefficient. The reality is that firefighting is not a core competency or desired skill, but rather an unnecessary workaround to poor system and process design.

The Five Principles of Lean

Define value

- Determine scope
  - SIPOC
- Define value through customer's eyes
  - VA/NVA activity

Value-adding (VA) activity:
1. Something the customer is willing to pay for
2. Physically changes the product, good, or service
3. Done correctly the first time (no rework)

Non-value-adding (NVA) activity = waste

Non-value-adding but a regulatory requirement (NVA-R)

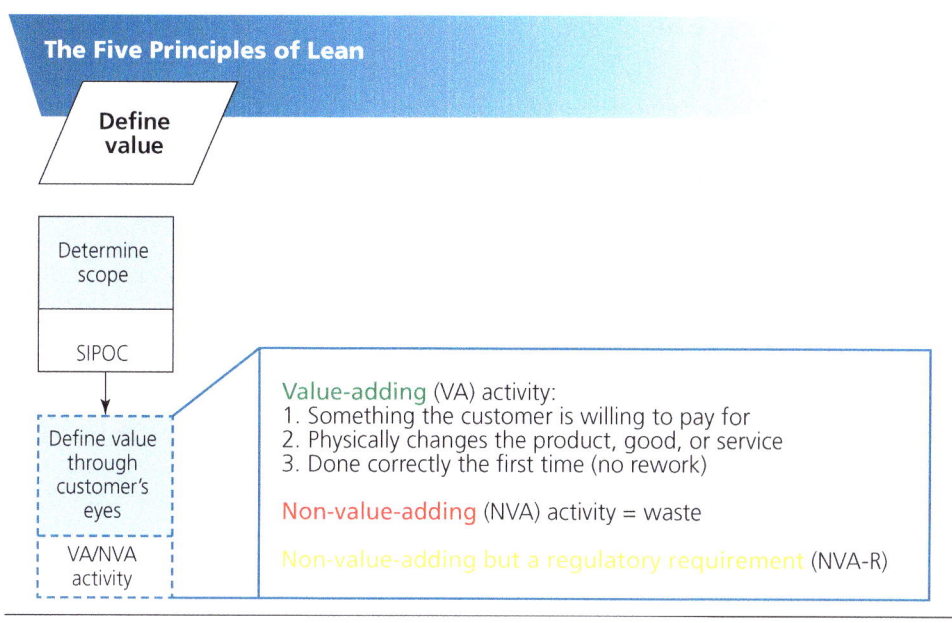

Figure 2.8 Roadmap: Define value through customer's eyes.

Employees want to do their best, but sometimes the system or process does not position them to be successful. At times, it can be difficult for employees to see the forest for the trees. Sometimes they cannot see past the mounds of work at hand. This is why lean thinking shifts the viewpoint from a worker-centric vantage to the eyes of the customer. The customer's perspective enables us to understand not only where we might be standing in the forest but also how to navigate through it.

Using the firefighting analogy, it is important to develop a systematic approach toward risk assessment, prevention, and anticipation of issues. Sprinkler systems demonstrate a higher level of problem solving. To truly innovate, the focus should be on eliminating the likelihood of fires starting in the first place, a concept discussed more in Chapter 7 ("Strive for Perfection").

Who Defines Value?

Value can only be defined by the ultimate customer.

—Womack & Jones, 1996

At the forefront of lean thinking is asking, "Who are your customers?" All concepts, tools, and strategies rely on the identification of customers and their value definition. There is an ultimate customer in a process (e.g., patient, clinician, another department), but there are also many internal customers along the way, from process step to process step. Without understanding the internal customer needs, employees could be passing along defects or unnecessary work and information without even knowing it. Differentiation between internal and external customers is important. The ultimate customer of the process is the main focus and the starting point for defining value. Three criteria define value-adding (VA) activity (Graban, 2012):

1. Something the customer is willing to pay for
2. Physically changes the product, good, or service
3. Done correctly the first time (no rework)

> *Some activities are NVA but are unavoidable (e.g., excessive transportation due to geography or layout constraints).*

The activity under review is waste or non-value-adding (NVA) if all three VA criteria are not met. Activities required by regulatory agencies such as the Department of Health or Joint Commission are considered NVA but are a *regulatory* requirement (NVA-R). These activities must be done, whether or not they meet the three VA criteria. Verifying a patient's identity using his or her name and date of birth before administering any medication is an example of NVA-R. NVA-R steps are infrequent and should be left alone since they cannot be removed. The focus is on differentiating VA and NVA steps and removing the waste. Table 2.1 lists examples of each type of activity category.

It is not always clear whether an activity is VA or NVA. In these scenarios, ask if the step can be eliminated or if there is a better way of doing the step. The point is not to have complete agreement on the classification but rather to look for the removable waste within the process. Identifying waste leads to improvement.

Example: Physician's Office Visit

You have been tasked with improving the patient flow process for a typical physician's office visit. After scoping the project from "Enter the office" to "Check out," you document all the steps that occur in between (Table 2.2).

Table 2.1 Examples of VA, NVA, and NVA-R activities.

Value-adding examples	Non-value-adding examples	Non-value-adding but regulatory requirement examples
Processing lab specimens	Searching for e-mails, documents, or other information	Asking patient to verify name and date of birth
Performing surgery on a patient	Patient walking from registration to waiting area to exam room	Documenting information in multiple areas of medical chart
Doing diagnostic scans (e.g., MRI, X-ray)	Employee waiting for information to perform a task	Double-checking medications prior to administration
Interviewing an individual for a potential job	Calling physician's office to collect missing information	Storing medical charts in a records warehouse for years
Preparing/mixing medications in pharmacy	Nurse toggling between computer systems to document	Performing internal process audits (e.g., financial)

Table 2.2 Physician's office visit example.

List of process steps: Before	List of process steps: After
1. Enter the office	1. Enter the office
2. Sign in	2. Sign in
3. Sit down in waiting area	3. Sit down in waiting area
4. Called back, walk into clinical space	4. Called back, walk into clinical space
5. Get vitals taken	5. Get vitals taken
6. Walk to exam room	6. Walk to exam room
7. Nurse interview	7. Nurse interview
8. Wait for physician	8. Wait for physician
9. Physician exam	9. Physician exam
10. Wait for prescription script	10. Wait for prescription script
11. Receive script	11. Receive script
12. Walk to checkout area	12. Walk to checkout area
13. Check out	13. Check out

The customer in this example is the patient. From the patient's perspective, you determine VA and NVA steps. Using the three criteria, you define the following:

VA steps: 1, 5, 7, 9, 11

NVA steps: 3, 4, 6, 8, 10, 12, 13

The initial process evaluation shows that the patient's office visit was 82 minutes (Figure 2.9). Of that time, 62 minutes (77.5%) was attributed to NVA activities

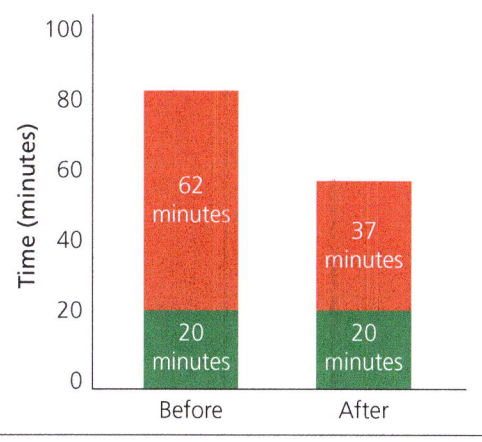

Figure 2.9 VA versus NVA time for the physician's office visit.

(steps 3, 4, 6, 8, 10, 12, and 13) and only 20 minutes (24.4%) was VA time (steps 1, 5, 7, 9, and 11). Through identification and elimination of NVA activities, the "after" office-visit process is 57 minutes. Now, only 37 minutes (64.9%) is NVA time, while the VA time remains the same at 20 minutes (35.1%). However, you can see that the VA percentage increased from 24% to 35% as a result of reducing the NVA time.

Remember, the goal with lean is to identify and reduce/eliminate the NVA activities (Bicheno & Holweg, 2004; Chalice, 2007). Some NVA activity in this example is unavoidable (e.g., walk to exam room), while other steps are pure waste (e.g., wait for physician). Differentiating process steps into VA and NVA steps enables identification of opportunities for improvement. Chapter 3 ("Map the Value Stream") will dive into more detail on ways to analyze and prioritize opportunities based on quality and time-related issues.

Case Study: Presurgery Patient Flow

Patient flow in the operating room was inefficient. The patient traveled to multiple areas: from the registration office to check-in, to the short procedure unit for surgical preparation, to the holding area for IV insertion, and ultimately to the operating room. Delays and coordination issues made the front-end process disorganized. An analysis of the current state revealed that the process from patient check-in at admissions until being ready for transport to the holding area took 70 minutes. More than half of this time was NVA. The lean team assigned to this project targeted reducing the NVA activities, which yielded a 17-minute reduction in throughput (Figure 2.10). Notice how the team did not affect the VA time for surgical prep. This reinforces the approach to identify and reduce NVA activities.

Before improvements

Check in at admissions	Arrive at short-procedure unit	Prep for surgery	Wait for transportation
7 mins	8 mins	25 mins	30 mins

Total time: 70 minutes
54% NVA
36% VA

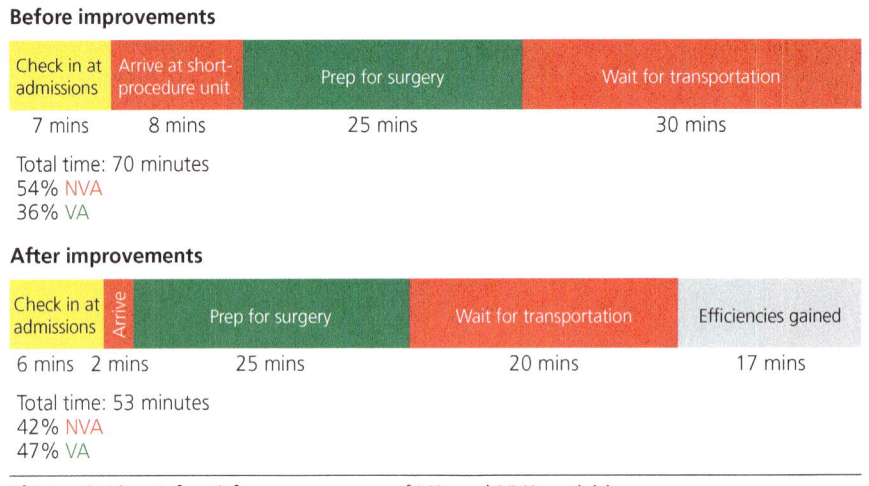

After improvements

Check in at admissions	Arrive	Prep for surgery	Wait for transportation	Efficiencies gained
6 mins	2 mins	25 mins	20 mins	17 mins

Total time: 53 minutes
42% NVA
47% VA

Figure 2.10 Before/after assessment of VA and NVA activities.

Before the improvement, the NVA activity accounted for 54% of the total processing time, whereas VA time made up only 36%. With the reduced NVA time, the patient experienced a shift in proportion of time between VA and NVA. Though the VA time remained at 25 minutes, the reduction in NVA yielded an increase in proportion of VA time within the process from 36% to 47%. From the patient's perspective, more of the processing time was VA and the overall process took less time.

> **Caution about NVA:** *NVA activity is not to be mistaken for a value judgment of individuals or specific roles. Waste tends to be driven by the system and the design (or lack thereof) of processes. The presence of waste does not indicate that an employee is bad or not working hard (Graban, 2012).*

IDENTIFY WASTE

Waste is synonymous with NVA activity (Figure 2.11). Waste exists in all work processes. Identification and elimination of waste is the central focus of a lean system and leads to solution development (Institute for Healthcare Improvement, 2005; Womack, 2011). Effective lean practitioners are able to differentiate between VA and NVA activities within any process (Womack & Jones, 1996).

The DOWNTIME acronym (Defects, Overproduction, Waiting, Nonutilized skill or intellect, Transportation, Inventory, Motion, Extra processing) categorizes waste. Table 2.3 details each waste based on its definition, examples, potential causes, questions to ask to help identify it, and countermeasures for reduction/elimination.

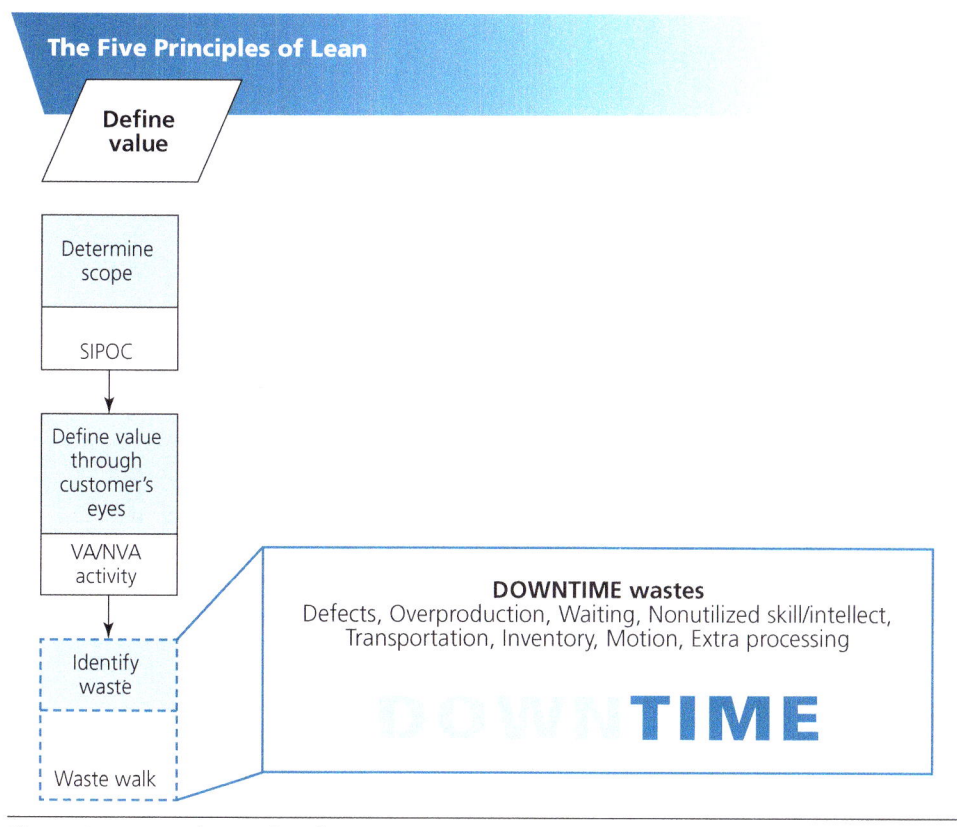

Figure 2.11 Roadmap: Identify waste.

Table 2.3 DOWNTIME waste matrix.

Waste	Definition	Examples	Potential causes	Questions to ask	Countermeasures
Defects	Rework, errors, incomplete or incorrect information	• Medication errors • Process step not performed correctly • Missing information	• Lack of understanding of what "defect-free" means • Insufficient training	• Are tasks clearly defined (who, what, when, how)? • Are errors dealt with directly and promptly or passed along?	• 5S • Visual management • Standard work • Error-proofing
Overproduction	Producing more than what is currently needed (too much or too soon)	• Medications administered early to accommodate start schedule • Printing extra copies of information just in case	• No clear understanding of what is needed, when, in what quantity • Poor communication • Inconsistent process	• Are there more supplies prepared than needed? • Is the demand known?	• Workload balancing • Standard work • Checklists • Pull systems
Waiting	Delays, waiting for anything (people, paper, equipment, information)	• Delays in bed assignments • Delays in receiving information or communication • Waiting for next process steps to begin	• Poor understanding of time required to complete a task • No visual cues to indicate next step in the process • Delays compounding one another	• Are there bottlenecks/delays in the process due to obtaining information, supplies, etc.? • Are there clear expectations for how long process steps should take?	• VSM • Swimlane map • 5S • Workload balancing • Cross-train staff
Nonutilized skill/intellect	Nonutilizing staff skills or knowledge, poor workload balance	• No cross-training • Nurses transporting patients • Physician drawing labs	• Lack of well-defined process • Unclear or undefined roles and responsibilities	• Are employees cross-trained? • Are employees encouraged to suggest/implement improvements?	• Swimlane map • Workload balancing • Standard work

Transportation	Unnecessary movement of something being processed (e.g., forms, patient, specimen, equipment)	• Placing stretcher in hall and constantly having to move it • Transporting forms from building to building or electronically to several areas	• Poor physical layout • Poor system/process design	• Are forms, patients, or materials moved to temporary locations? • Is technology being leveraged to limit physical handoffs?	• 5S • Physical layout • Visual management • Standard work
Inventory	Excessive supplies, batch processing, work-in-process	• Extra/outdated manuals • Obsolete equipment	• Supply/demand not well understood • Outdated supplies/equipment not discarded • Disorganized area, unclear what is necessary/unnecessary	• Is there extra equipment/supplies lying around? • Do forms, supplies, or patients wait in groups/batches?	• 5S • Visual management • Standard work • Pull systems
Motion	Any excess movement of the employee	• Searching for anything (e.g., information, supplies, equipment, patients) • Hand-carrying paperwork to another area	• Poor physical layout • Poor system/process design	• How does the current layout impede the process flow? • Can walking be reduced by repositioning equipment, people, and/or supplies?	• 5S • Physical layout • Visual management • Standard work
Extra processing	Extra or unnecessary steps performed that do not add value to the process	• Ordering more tests than the diagnosis warrants • Entering repetitive/duplicative information	• Complex or multiple forms • Ineffective policies and procedures	• Is there more information available than what needs to be processed?	• VSM • Visual management • Workload balancing • Standard work

Defects

Rework is the result of doing something incorrectly the first time (a core element of defining value). The effort that goes into gathering missing information or correcting errors is waste. The consequence of defects could be significant (e.g., medication error). One of the major causes of defects is that the employee may not know what it means to be defect-free. In other words, the employee does not know that what he or she is doing is not correct. It is leadership's responsibility to provide this valuable feedback (on good performance as well as opportunities for improvement) and coach or train staff appropriately.

Overproduction

Both overproduction and excess inventory are by-products of ineffective forecasting or not knowing actual demand. Overproduction means producing things in excess, too soon, or faster than the customer, employee, or process requires. Presence of this waste tends to indicate poor cross-functional communication and inconsistent processes between supplier and customer. Overproduction is a misuse of resources that does not meet the customer's needs.

Waiting

Waiting is usually the most pervasive waste in any system (Zidel, 2012). In between each process step there is usually a period of waiting. Sometimes it is brief (seconds), but it can span hours or even days. Waiting results from many process inefficiencies, including lack of standardized tasks, poor communication between steps, and no visual management or cues to indicate work that needs to be accomplished. To make matters worse, waiting can have a compounding effect on the process and system, leading to massive bottlenecks. Waiting inhibits flow and the ability to deliver what the customer wants when they want it.

Nonutilized Skill/Intellect

Nonutilized skill or intellect addresses employee engagement and human resource management. Unengaged employees are working below their level of knowledge/certification or are unchallenged. Likewise, an imbalance in workload (too much or too little) can lead to subutilization of staff. There are budgetary implications with nonutilized skill/intellect. Organizations that underutilize highly paid staff are not cost-effective. Cross-training is an effective approach to address nonutilized skill or intellect as well as workload balancing. Additionally, cross-training challenges staff to do different tasks, which can promote buy-in and engagement.

Transportation

Transportation represents movement of the item in the process. In healthcare, examples include patients, lab specimens, equipment, medication, and forms, among others. Any movement is NVA activity if it does not transform the good, product, or service. Though traveling from one location to another might be unavoidable due to geographic constraints, it does not make it VA. The presence of transportation indicates a worker-centric process design rather than a customer-centric one. Many processes within the delivery system (probably most) are not designed as patient-centric models and thus patients have to do most of the work (i.e., travel, navigate documentation) (Teich & Faddoul, 2013).

Inventory

Inventory includes physical items and supplies in stock as well as electronic information and work-in-process (WIP). Supplies can take up valuable physical space and tie up cash. Additionally, there is a risk for expiration with certain perishable supplies like medications. WIP describes the backlog of items in between process steps. WIP develops when processes are not evenly balanced and standardized. Patients sitting in a waiting room are a form of WIP.

Motion

Motion represents the movement of the worker. It is different from transportation (movement of item being processed). Just because an employee looks busy and constantly moves around does not mean he or she is doing VA tasks. Do not confuse movement and activity with productivity and efficiency. Motion is an NVA activity if it takes up unnecessary time and energy in between VA steps. When it comes to process design, it is better to observe more motion than transportation. This is indicative of a process that brings the work to the customer, not the other way around.

Extra Processing

Extra processing defines any extraneous processes or tasks that do not add value. These tasks are not necessary to produce the end product or service. In other words, they are tasks or outputs that the customer does not require or want. Extra processing is the result of poor process knowledge and understanding of customer needs (similar to overproduction). The end product is variable, leading to other wastes (inventory, rework, etc.).

The moral of the story is that VA, NVA, and NVA-R are not black and white, which is why we use red, green, and yellow. There are a lot of cases in which steps fit both categories. In those instances it is best to ask:

- How long does the step take? If it is not long, do not worry about it. If it is significant, break it into smaller components to differentiate between VA and NVA activities.
- Can we live without doing the step? If yes, then eliminate it.

Understanding waste includes acknowledgment of the elements and factors of the surrounding environment. No process or system operates in isolation. Changes in one process or step can affect the efficiency of another elsewhere. Understanding the interplay of processes and drivers of waste will lead to effective problem solving. All employees should learn and develop the ability to differentiate VA and NVA activities. Waste recognition is an integral skill set for effective lean thinkers.

Figure 2.12 shows a preliminary waste diagnostic tool that provides another way to depict the presence and impact of waste on process flow. Evaluate wastes along a continuum from low to high impact. The example shows waiting and defects as high drivers of inefficiency along with transportation and motion. Use this simple diagnostic tool during gemba walks.

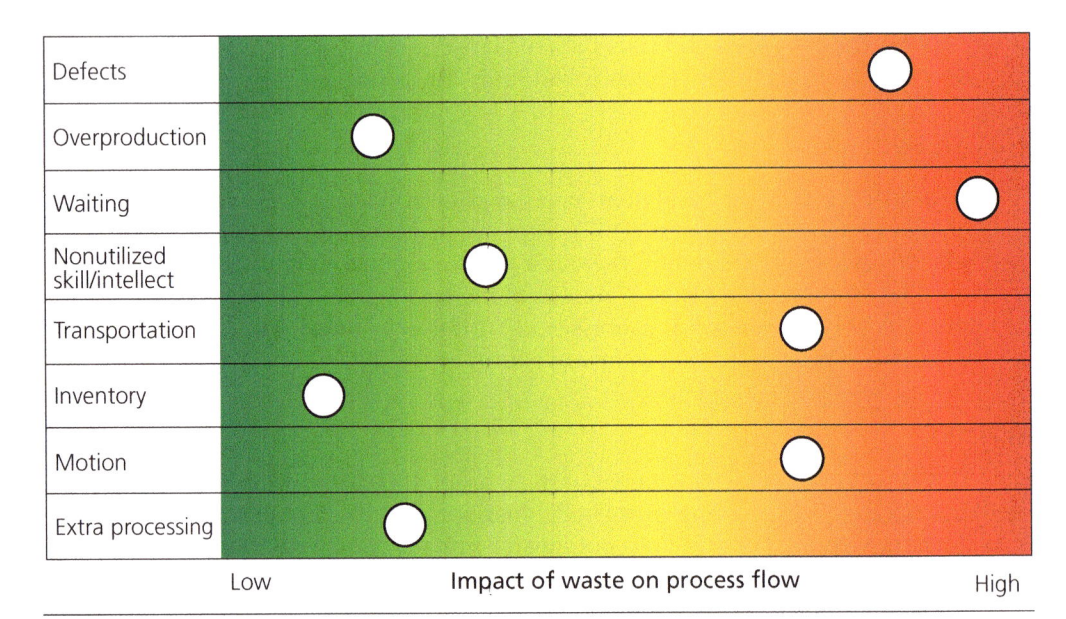

Figure 2.12 Preliminary waste diagnostic tool.

The lean thinking process asks four basic questions:

1. Who is the customer?
2. How does the customer define *value*?
   - Something the customer is willing to pay for
   - Physically changes the product, good, or service
   - Done correctly the first time (no rework)
3. If a step is determined to be NVA, what kind of *waste* is it?
   - DOWNTIME
4. Based on the type of waste, what is the best countermeasure to implement?
   - Refer to DOWNTIME matrix for countermeasures

Figure 2.13 shows the logical progression that leads to solution development.

The following are examples of process analyses from various Jefferson lean projects. Each of the pie charts shows distributions of VA and NVA activities. The NVA is broken down into the DOWNTIME wastes. This categorization enables lean teams to target improvement strategies. The process value analysis, a Microsoft Excel tool, produces this analysis (detailed tool review in Chapter 3).

Figure 2.14, the operating room (OR) turnover process, is over 80% NVA activities. The largest portion of waste is waiting (45%). Patients wait to be transported out of the OR while staff break down surgical equipment, wipe surfaces, and complete documentation. Transportation (movement of the patient) and motion (movement of the OR staff) make up the remaining 37% of NVA activities.

The surgical equipment sterilization process (Figure 2.15) shows a process that is predominantly VA (66%). A large portion of VA time is equipment sterilization. Again, waiting is the most prominent waste at 19%.

Principle #1: Define Value

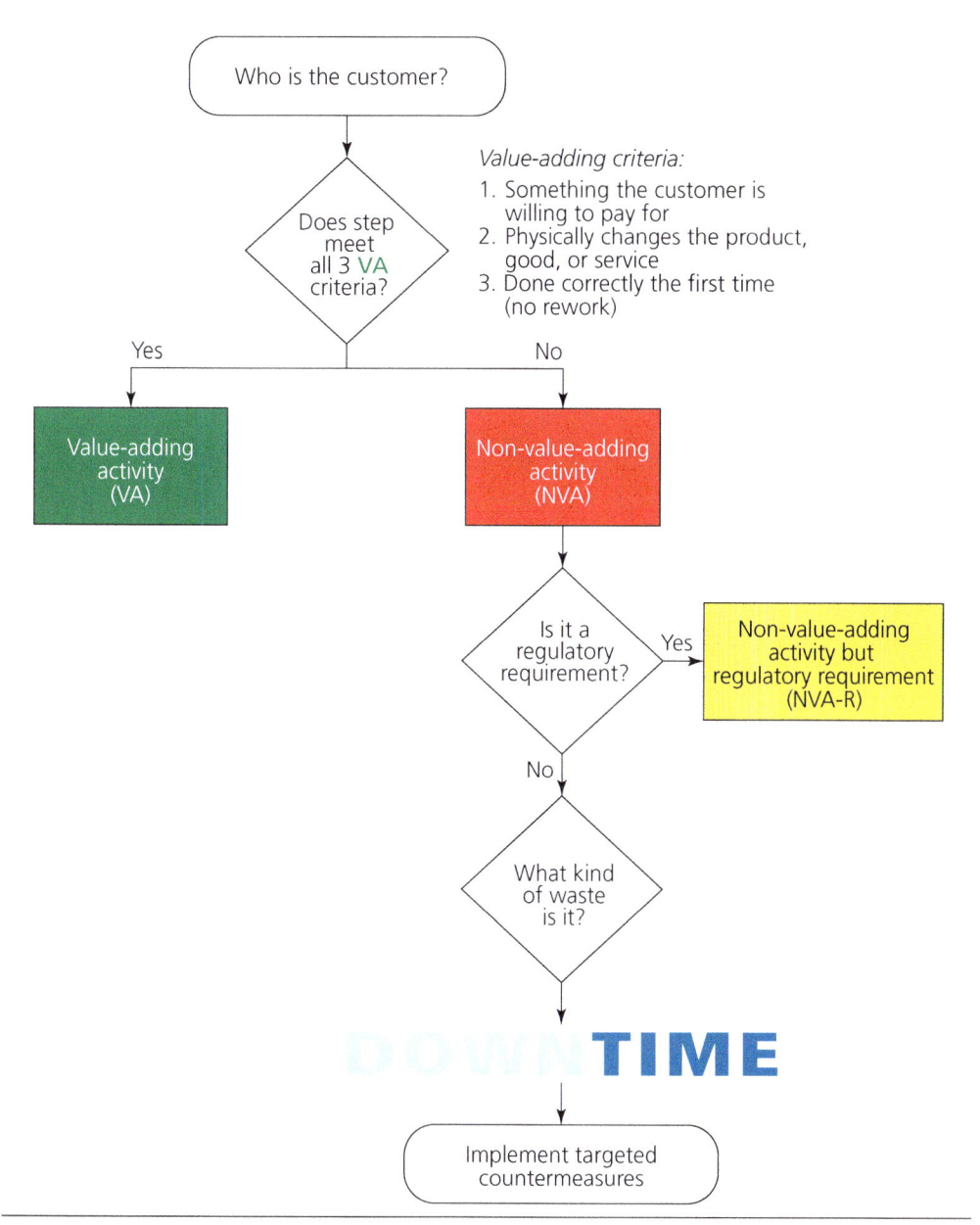

Figure 2.13 Lean thinking process.

Patient flow is a common process evaluated through a lean thinking lens. In the oncology infusion center, patients were experiencing delays in receiving care due to several administrative steps and logistical barriers. Patients had a cumbersome check-in process that resulted in a significant amount of waiting (48%) (Figure 2.16). Employee workflow was suboptimal, leading to communication challenges, workarounds, and delays in receiving and disseminating information. As a result, two-thirds of the process was NVA through the eyes of the patients.

24 Chapter Two

Value analysis—DOWNTIME breakdown

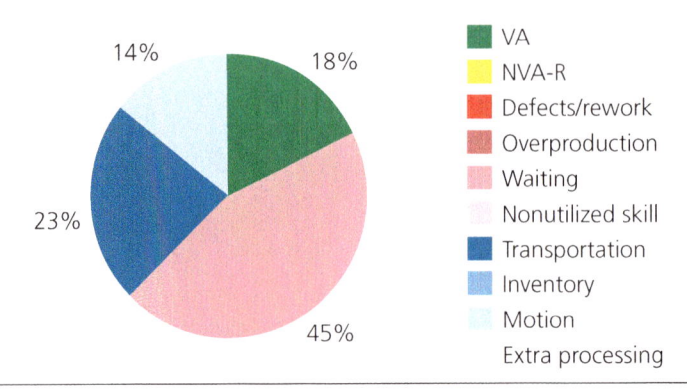

- VA: 18%
- Waiting: 45%
- Transportation: 23%
- Motion: 14%

Legend: VA, NVA-R, Defects/rework, Overproduction, Waiting, Nonutilized skill, Transportation, Inventory, Motion, Extra processing

Figure 2.14 Operating room turnover (wheels out to wheels in) value analysis.

Value analysis—DOWNTIME breakdown

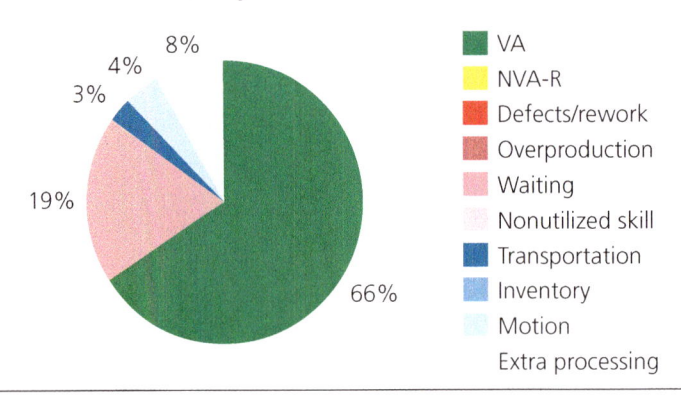

- VA: 66%
- Waiting: 19%
- Transportation: 3%
- Inventory: 4%
- Motion: 8%

Legend: VA, NVA-R, Defects/rework, Overproduction, Waiting, Nonutilized skill, Transportation, Inventory, Motion, Extra processing

Figure 2.15 Surgical equipment sterilization value analysis.

Value analysis—DOWNTIME breakdown

- VA: 37%
- Defects/rework: 5%
- Waiting: 48%
- Transportation: 6%
- Motion: 4%

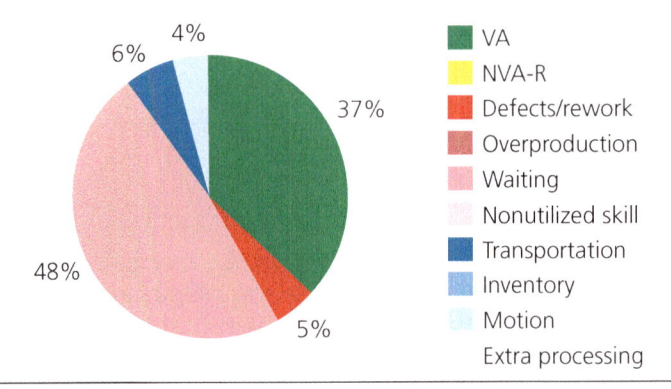

Legend: VA, NVA-R, Defects/rework, Overproduction, Waiting, Nonutilized skill, Transportation, Inventory, Motion, Extra processing

Figure 2.16 Oncology infusion center patient flow value analysis.

PRINCIPLE #1: DEFINE VALUE   25

Case Study: Clinical Lab Workflow

The clinical lab was experiencing delays in processing lab requests. A lean team helped the lab analyze workflows and facilitate an improvement effort to ensure optimal turnaround times of lab specimen results.

Delays in results reporting can inhibit the clinical team's ability to make timely decisions regarding a patient's plan of care. Such delays impact quality indicators as well as operational capabilities. This lean project focused on improving the efficiency of lab processes from order entry to result reporting.

The lean team conducted several process value analysis time studies to evaluate the specimen flow from receipt within the clinical lab to the results. The lean leaders walked through the process from the perspective of the specimen and documented all related tasks and wastes (Figure 2.17). Employees from the lab described their responsibilities, discussed common barriers and issues, and offered suggestions for process improvement.

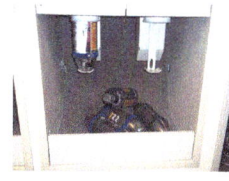

1. Specimens arrive via a tube system
2. Technician takes specimens and lab test orders out of the tube
3. Specimens and tests are time-stamped
4. Specimens are registered in information system
5. Technician distributes specimens for processing
6. Specimens are loaded onto processing rack
7. Technician loads specimens onto analyzer

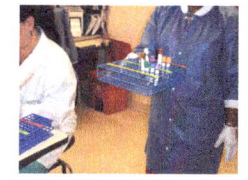

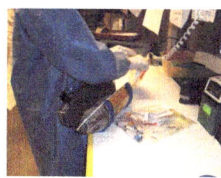

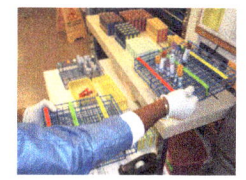

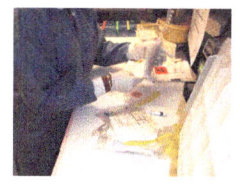

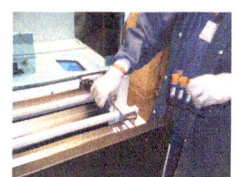

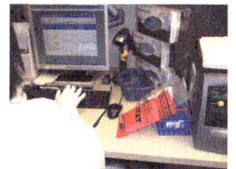

Figure 2.17   Clinical lab workflow process.

Through observations and data collection, the lean leaders identified opportunities for improvement within the front end of the process. The pie chart (Figure 2.18) displays the proportion of NVA activity that leads to delays in timely resulting. The process consisted of only 25% VA activities but 75% NVA activities. Upon further evaluation, the team identified transportation as the main waste (49%).

(continued)

Value analysis—DOWNTIME breakdown

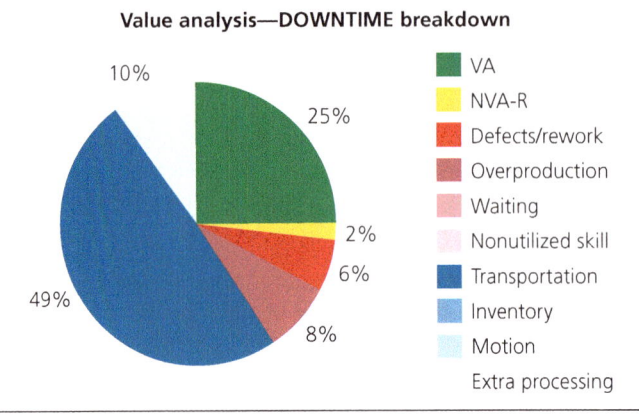

- VA: 25%
- NVA-R: 2%
- Defects/rework: 6%
- Overproduction
- Waiting: 8%
- Nonutilized skill
- Transportation: 49%
- Inventory
- Motion: 10%
- Extra processing

Figure 2.18 Clinical lab receiving process for specimen throughput value analysis.

Workflow and layout issues resulted in unnecessary movement of the lab technician. The technician bounced from bench to bench like a pinball, without a sense of organization or flow. After following the lab technician through her work, the lean leaders calculated that 74% of the tech's time was motion. Chapter 3 presents the workflow value analysis tool used for this analysis. The technician had to move throughout the receiving and processing area to move specimens from station to station. The lab processing area is very small; therefore, it was a lot of movement in a tight space, which created a sense of chaos. Figure 2.19 shows the results of the analysis.

Workflow value analysis

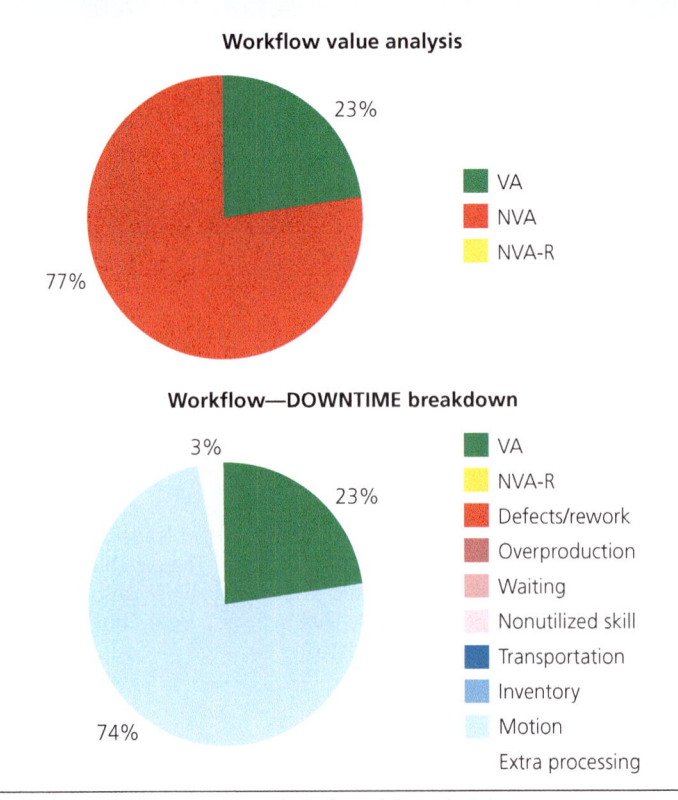

- VA: 23%
- NVA: 77%
- NVA-R

Workflow—DOWNTIME breakdown

- VA: 23%
- NVA-R
- Defects/rework
- Overproduction
- Waiting
- Nonutilized skill
- Transportation
- Inventory
- Motion: 74%
- Extra processing: 3%

Figure 2.19 Workflow value analysis for a lab technician.

In order to effect change, the lean team conducted a rapid improvement event (discussed in detail in Chapters 8 and 9) with process experts within the lab. The lean leaders shared their analysis and observations with the improvement team. It was clear that the layout needed to be improved in order to promote efficiency. Bench assignments (where other technicians processed the specimens and prepared them for analysis) were organized in a single-piece flow to establish smoother production. The specimens could move down the line without requiring an individual to transport them by foot. A floater position helped handle add-ons, problem specimens, triage, specimen tracking, and processor loading. This new role enabled the process to run smoothly and address problems as they occurred.

Changes were developed through gemba walks and brainstorming activities. The improvement team reviewed proposed solutions with staff prior to piloting (Figure 2.20).

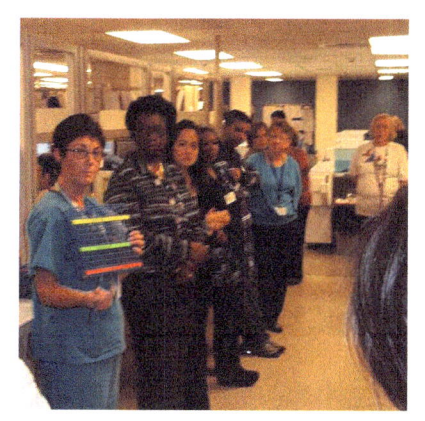

Improvement team participants (lab personnel) explain the new pilot process to their colleagues.

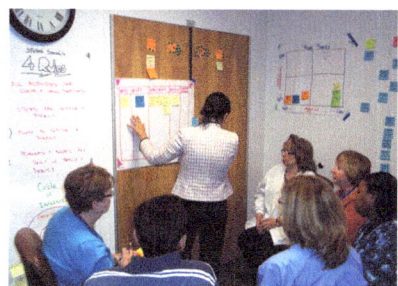

Lean leaders facilitate action plan development with the improvement team.

Figure 2.20 Rapid improvement event pictures of the clinical lab project.

As a result of the change, the lab saw meaningful improvements in turnaround times (Figure 2.21). The lab KPIs included overall tests as well as tests from the emergency department (ED). Every test has a defined goal for the turnaround time based on best practices. The percentage of time that STAT tests achieved their targeted turnaround time for all tests rose from a pre-intervention mean of 73% to a post-intervention mean of 82% (95% confidence interval of 79.76%–84.52%, standard deviation of 0.0413, $p = .008$). ED STAT processing improved from a pre-intervention mean of 76% to a post-intervention mean of 86% (95% confidence interval of 83.875%–87.985%, standard deviation of 0.0356, $p = .004$).

(continued)

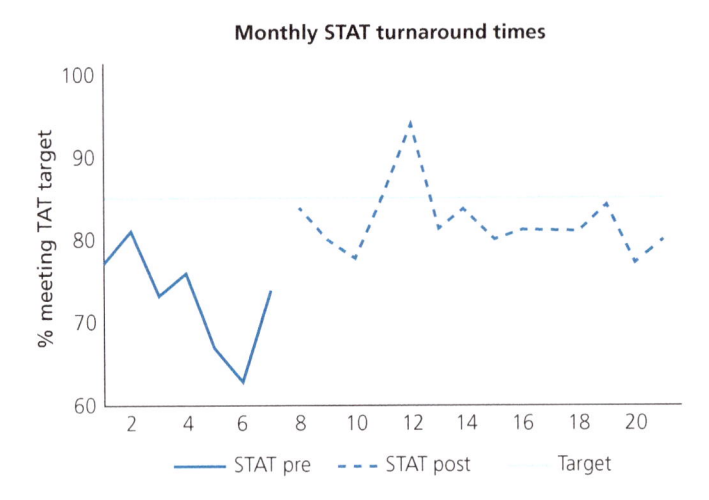

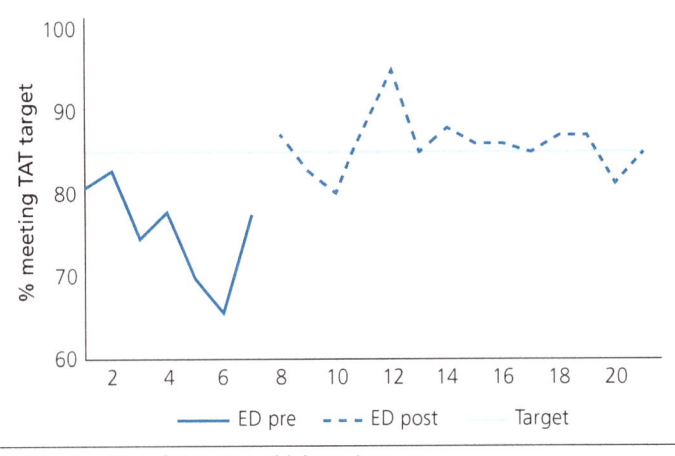

Figure 2.21 Results of the clinical lab project.

Remember, NVA activity is not to be mistaken for a value judgment of individuals or specific roles. Waste tends to be driven by the system and the design (or lack thereof) of processes. The lab technician in this example spent three-fourths of her time doing NVA activities as a result of the poor layout. The technician worked tirelessly to keep the process running despite the inefficient layout. Lean thinking helps objectively identify the wastes and systematically pilot and sustain appropriate countermeasures.

CHAPTER CHALLENGE

Identify a problem you can investigate by going to the place of action (gemba). Perform a waste walk and document examples of each DOWNTIME waste. Conduct informal staff interviews to learn about their barriers and concerns.

QUESTIONS

1. What happens when the scope is too broad or too narrow?
2. What is the significance behind the statement "Don't boil the ocean"?
3. What is the difference between internal and external customers? Why does the differentiation matter?
4. How come some NVA activities are unavoidable? How do you address them?
5. What is the impact of a process step not performed correctly the first time?
6. What are examples of VA, NVA, and NVA-R activities in your work area?
7. What waste is the most prevalent in your own workflow?

Chapter 3
Principle #2: Map the Value Stream

The best way to predict your future is to create it.

—Thomas Jefferson

The previous chapter stressed the importance of asking "Who are our customers?" in order to define value. In addition, the eight DOWNTIME wastes provide the basis for categorizing all NVA activity. This chapter guides further process analysis utilizing a core lean tool known as the value stream map (Figure 3.1). To improve, we must first understand where we are (current state)

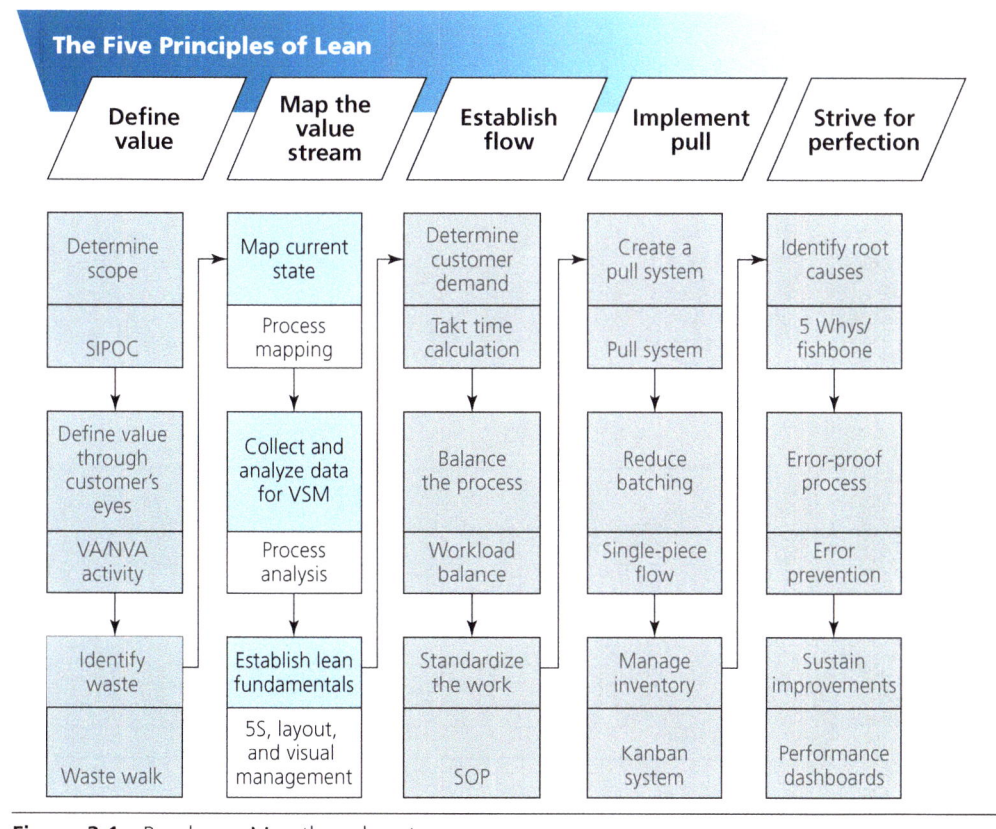

The Five Principles of Lean

Define value	Map the value stream	Establish flow	Implement pull	Strive for perfection
Determine scope	Map current state	Determine customer demand	Create a pull system	Identify root causes
SIPOC	Process mapping	Takt time calculation	Pull system	5 Whys/ fishbone
Define value through customer's eyes	Collect and analyze data for VSM	Balance the process	Reduce batching	Error-proof process
VA/NVA activity	Process analysis	Workload balance	Single-piece flow	Error prevention
Identify waste	Establish lean fundamentals	Standardize the work	Manage inventory	Sustain improvements
Waste walk	5S, layout, and visual management	SOP	Kanban system	Performance dashboards

Figure 3.1 Roadmap: Map the value stream.

and then determine where we should be (future state). This becomes our path of incremental improvement.

MAP THE CURRENT STATE

The current state is how the work actually happens, not how it should or could be done (Jimmerson, 2010). The current process baseline provides the foundation for improvement. The future state, defined as what could or should be done, becomes the goal. Lean thinking promotes working backward from the future state (Bicheno & Holweg, 2004).

There are many forms of process maps (Figure 3.2). An important consideration is the level of detail to document. Process maps can be segmented and refined, showing layers of detail. The starting point, as described in "Determine Scope" in the previous chapter, is the high-level map. The high-level map documents the major steps (30,000-foot view of a process). The midlevel map includes more detailed steps in between the high-level steps (Figure 3.3).

The most effective way to build a process map is to walk the process. Follow the flow of the patient, specimen, form, and so forth, from start to finish and evaluate the work from the customer's eyes (Womack, 2011). The following is an example of process mapping using the physician's office visit from Chapter 2.

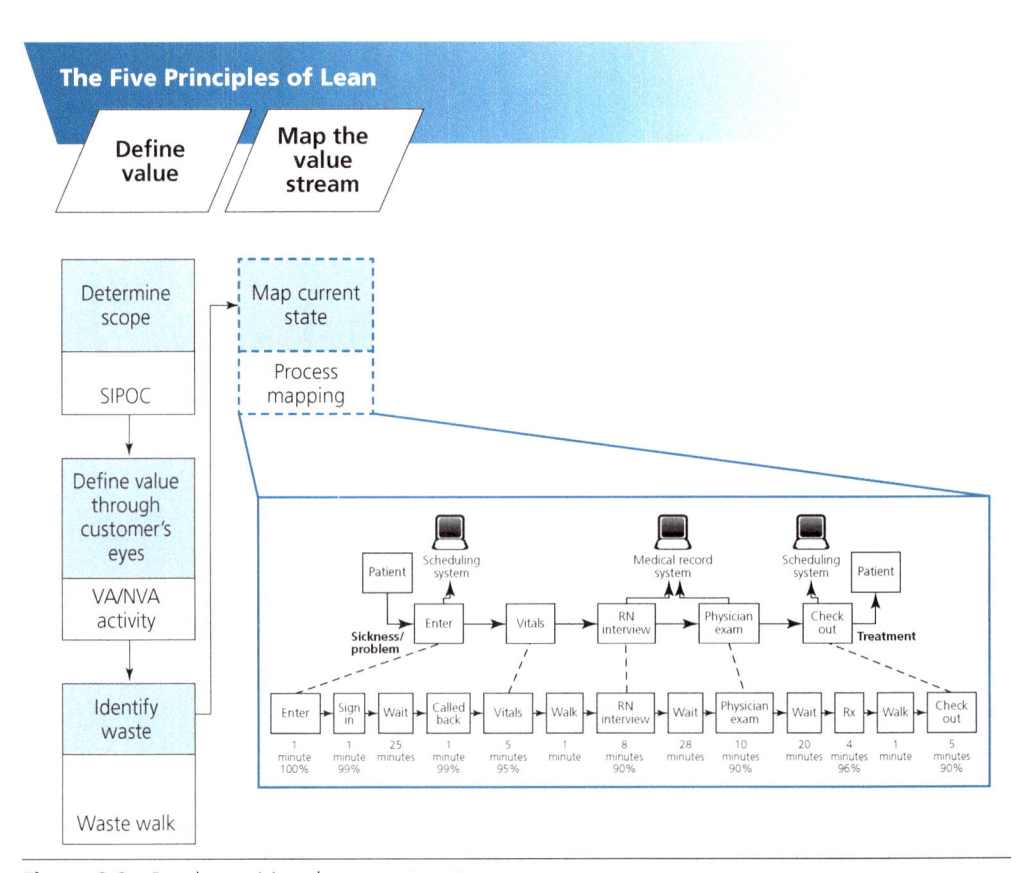

Figure 3.2 Roadmap: Map the current state.

High-level process map

```
Step A → Step D → Step G → Step J → Step L
```

Midlevel process map

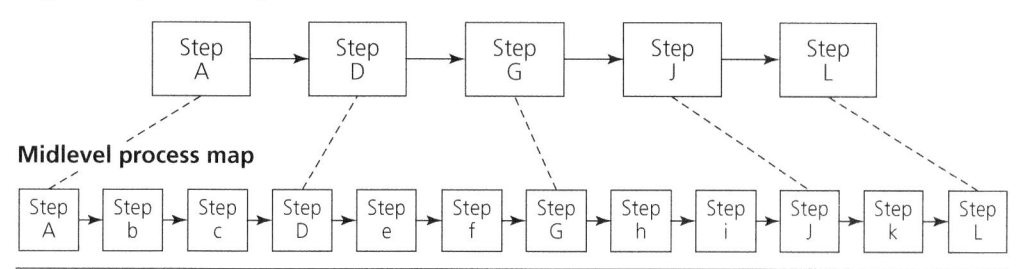

```
Step A → Step b → Step c → Step D → Step e → Step f → Step G → Step h → Step i → Step J → Step k → Step L
```

Figure 3.3 High- and midlevel process maps.

Example: Physician's Office

Step 1: Start by documenting all steps (it is OK to start granular here) (Figure 3.4, on page 34)

List of Process Steps

1. Enter the office
2. Sign in
3. Sit down in waiting area
4. Called back, walk into clinical space
5. Get vitals taken
6. Walk to exam room
7. Nurse interview
8. Wait for physician
9. Physician exam
10. Wait for prescription script
11. Receive script
12. Walk to checkout area
13. Check out

Step 2: Identify five to eight key high-level steps (30,000-foot view) (Figure 3.5)

Step 3: Fill in midlevel steps (Figure 3.6)

Step 4: Estimate/calculate processing times for each midlevel step (Figure 3.7)

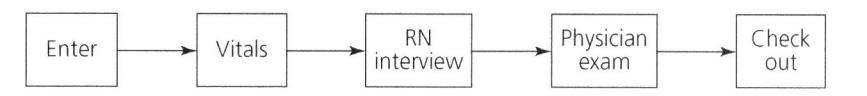

```
Enter → Vitals → RN interview → Physician exam → Check out
```

Figure 3.5 High-level process steps for physician's office visit.

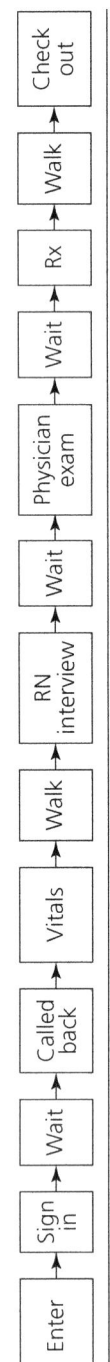

Enter → Sign in → Wait → Called back → Vitals → Walk → RN interview → Wait → Physician exam → Wait → Rx → Walk → Check out

Figure 3.4 Process map of physician's office visit.

High-level process map

Enter → Vitals → RN interview → Physician exam → Check out

Midlevel process map

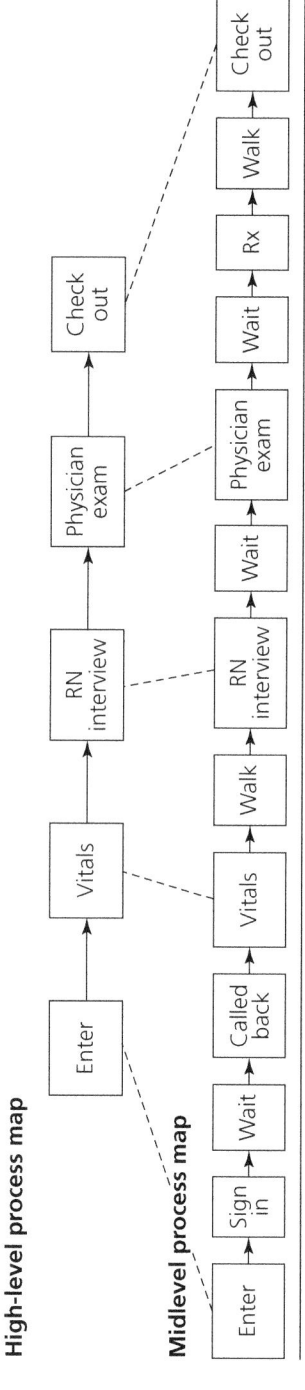

Enter → Sign in → Wait → Called back → Vitals → Walk → RN interview → Wait → Physician exam → Wait → Rx → Walk → Check out

Figure 3.6 High- and midlevel process steps for physician's office visit.

High-level process map

Enter → Sign in (1 minute) → Wait (25 minutes) → Called back (1 minute) → Vitals → RN interview → Physician exam → Check out

Midlevel process map

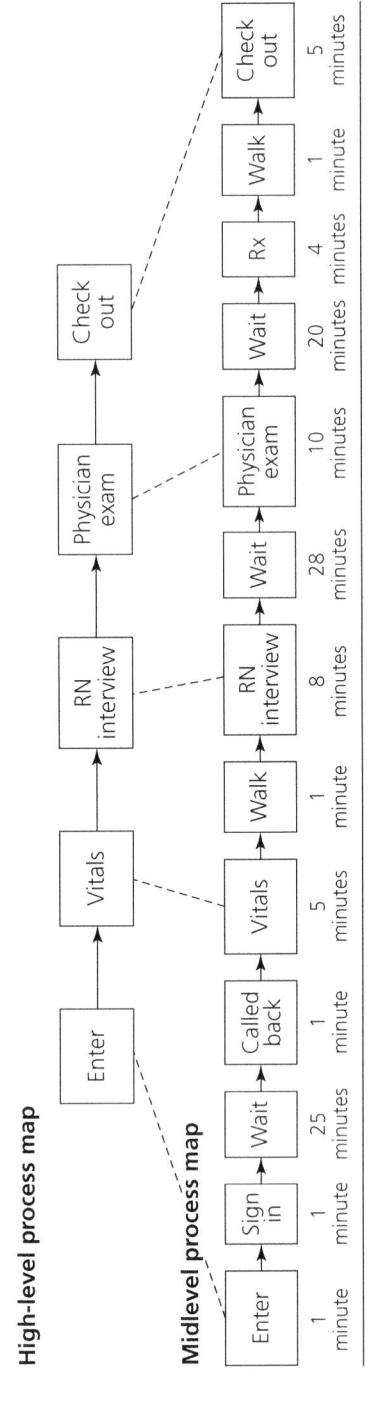

Enter (1 minute) → Sign in (1 minute) → Wait (25 minutes) → Called back (1 minute) → Vitals (5 minutes) → Walk (1 minute) → RN interview (8 minutes) → Wait (28 minutes) → Physician exam (10 minutes) → Wait (20 minutes) → Rx (4 minutes) → Walk (1 minute) → Check out (5 minutes)

Figure 3.7 Cycle times for physician's office visit.

Principle #2: Map the Value Stream

> **First-Pass Yield (FPY):** *The percentage of time a process is done correctly the first time. If data are not available, ask the people who do the work (process experts) to estimate the FPY. Calculate the overall FPY by multiplying the FPY for every process step. The resulting number is the percentage of time the process will work without an error occurring. The goal is to have every process step at or close to 100% (Figure 3.8).*

A process can have a lot of complicated steps. The first-pass yield (FPY) estimates the percentage of time a process step is performed correctly the first time. Each subsequent step relies on the quality, validity, and reliability of the previous one. If a process step is not performed correctly, whether it takes someone 10 minutes or 1 hour, the end result is the same—rework. Rework often comes at a higher cost, too. As the saying goes, a dollar of prevention is worth $100 of intervention. Think about that saying. Usually when a mistake occurs, it goes to the supervisor, who might have to take it to his or her boss. This could result in meetings/discussions held with other leaders, a work group could form, and so on. All of this costs time, resources, and money, not to mention whatever consequence the error could have on the customer. This is why understanding FPY is so important. We want to design quality into the system, not just work faster.

Lean is about doing better with less, not just being faster and more efficient and producing more output. How do you become better? Fix quality-related issues. First, when evaluating the current state of a process, determine whether any underlying quality issues exist. There is no point in streamlining process steps without addressing quality issues first. Why? If you streamline a process that creates a lot of defects, you just made it faster to create more problems. Always look to improve the FPY before attempting anything else.

Current state

Step 1 (99%) → Step 2 (70%) → Step 3 (99%) → Step 4 (99%)

First-pass yield = (0.99*0.7*0.99*0.99) = 67.92%

Improvement strategies

Improve the first-pass yield

Step 1 (99%) → Step 2 (90%) → Step 3 (99%) → Step 4 (99%)

First-pass yield = (0.99*0.9*0.99*0.99) = 87.32%

Eliminate the step

Step 1 (99%) → Step 3 (99%) → Step 4 (99%)

First-pass yield = (0.99*0.99*0.99) = 97.02%

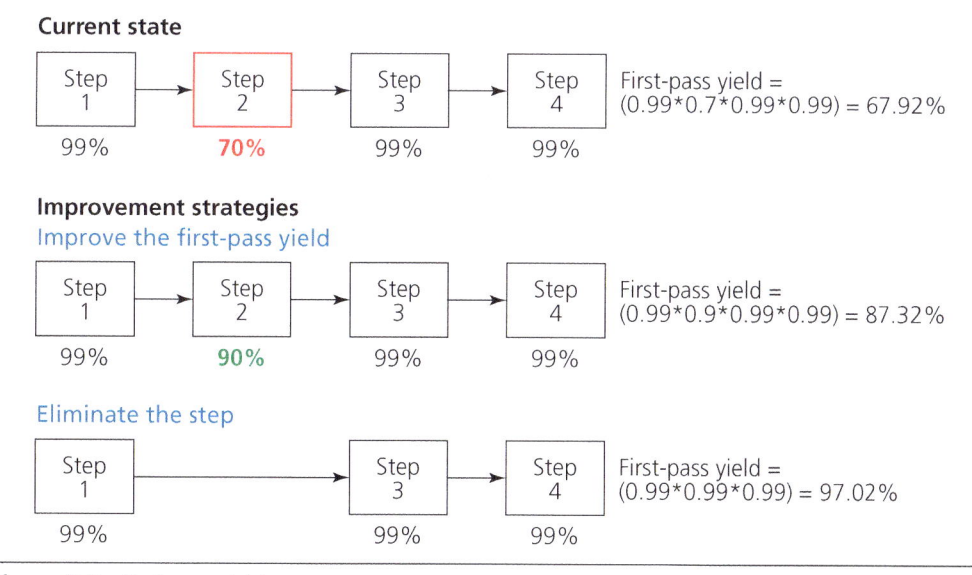

Figure 3.8 First-pass yield.

VALUE STREAM MAPS

A value stream map (VSM) is a process map that documents the sequence of steps from start to finish, using specific information like material, information, and workflow and associated processing and wait times (Jimmerson, 2010; Tapping et al., 2009). The flow of value is horizontal (Womack, 2011). VSMs are effective tools in breaking down silos by looking at processes from a customer-centric perspective (Graban, 2012; Kenney, 2011; Øvretveit, 2005). Without an understanding of the stream of value, decisions and workflow are designed suboptimally, which inevitably leads to building workarounds.

> *In the clinical setting, the complexities and multidisciplinary approach amplify the importance of effective communication and coordination. This is why lean thinking is horizontal rather than vertical. We need to ask the question, how are we communicating key information across the value stream? What is our mechanism for feedback to ensure that our internal and external customers' needs are being met?*

Healthcare processes are complex and multifaceted. Patient flow is impacted by many areas (ED admissions/volume, OR inpatient cases, intensive care unit [ICU] capacity/census, telemetry utilization/census, ability to discharge efficiently, off-unit diagnostics, transportation, etc.). We operate in vertical functional/department silos while work flows horizontally (Ballé & Régnier, 2007; de Souza & Pidd, 2011; Mazur, McCreery, & Rothenberg, 2010). Care coordination across the entire continuum is a major issue in healthcare (Armstrong, Fox, & Chapman, 2013; Neufeld et al., 2013). We are designed to function in silos, which affects the way decisions are made and what work gets done. As a result, the processes are fragmented. The lack of coordination and effectiveness is typically more obvious to customers of the process than to employees working within a silo.

Systems and processes with complex interrelationships between groups, departments, and so forth, require a well-thought-out plan that targets incremental improvement over time. It is vital to narrow the focus to manageable bite-sized chunks. Clinical service lines attempt to use a matrix/hybrid infrastructure to manage "streams" of similar patients (i.e., by procedure, disease) from admissions through outpatient and home care (Kenney, 2011). This is one strategy used to address horizontal flow.

The VSM serves as the primary tool for documenting the baseline (current state) from which to develop a roadmap to improvement (future state). Opportunities or gaps between current and future states mark the jumping-off point for improvement activities.

> **VSM Key Terms**
> - **Cycle time:** time needed to complete a specific process step. *Example: Patient registered*
> - **Lead time:** total process time from start to finish (order to completion). *Example: From patient arrival to discharge*
> - **Current state:** process as it currently stands; what actually takes place, not what should take place
> - **Future state:** how the process could or should be
> - **First-pass yield:** percentage of time process step is performed correctly the first time
> - **Value-adding ratio:** percentage of VA time divided by lead time (total time)

The process of building a VSM is similar to that for the process maps shown earlier. The first four steps are the same. Using the same example, we will continue to build out the map (Figure 3.9).

Process Mapping Steps

1. Start by documenting all steps (it is OK to start granular)
2. Identify five to eight key high-level steps (30,000-foot view)
3. Fill in midlevel steps
4. Estimate/calculate processing times for each step
   – Include time spent waiting in between steps

Note: For the VSM, you can add the supplier/input and customer/output at the high level. This is the SIPOC, as reviewed in Chapter 2.

Building a VSM

Many different approaches, tools, and pieces of information are used in value stream mapping. The following four steps provide simple, straightforward instructions, rather than offering a confusing or complicated approach. Remember that the current state VSM enables you to target potential areas for improvement through waste identification. Once you analyze and determine where the opportunities lie, you can then dive into the details of the tasks and inefficiencies. The next section within this chapter describes process analysis tools.

Steps for Building a VSM (continuing from steps 1–4 of process mapping)

5. Estimate/calculate FPY for each step (identify communication flow where applicable) (Figure 3.10).
6. Evaluate VA versus NVA activity. Evaluate each midlevel step's contribution to customer value (Figure 3.11). Indicate which steps are VA, NVA, or NVA-R using their associated colors.
7. Identify opportunities for improvement based on FPY and NVA activities (Figure 3.12). Look for sections of the VSM with consecutive NVA steps and target long-duration NVA steps. For example, the third midlevel step "Wait" accounts for 25 minutes. The first section identified for improvement is the "Sign in" to "Vitals" component. The first four steps of the process total 28 minutes, of which only 1 minute is VA. The second opportunity identified is waiting from "RN interview" until "Rx." Within this section of the process, waiting accounts for 48 minutes of the total process.
8. Prioritize improvement opportunities and reduce/eliminate NVA activities. Two targeted areas for improvement narrow the focus within the 13-step midlevel physician's office visit. Given the large portion of NVA activity at the front end, it makes the most sense to begin problem solving here. Waiting from "RN interview" until "Rx" is the subsequent opportunity. Front-end efficiencies will not necessarily help downstream flow.

40 Chapter Three

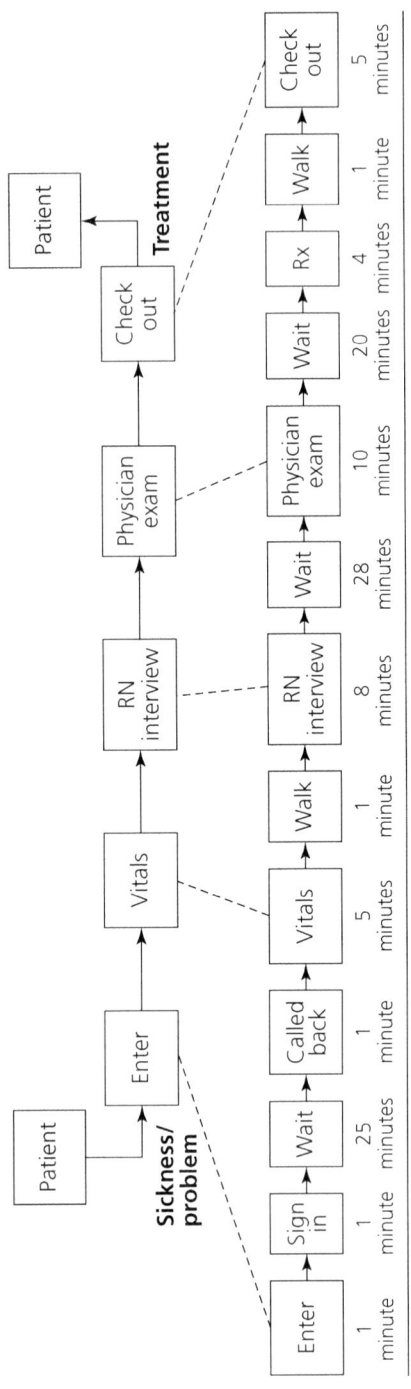

Figure 3.9 Value stream map for physician's office visit.

Principle #2: Map the Value Stream

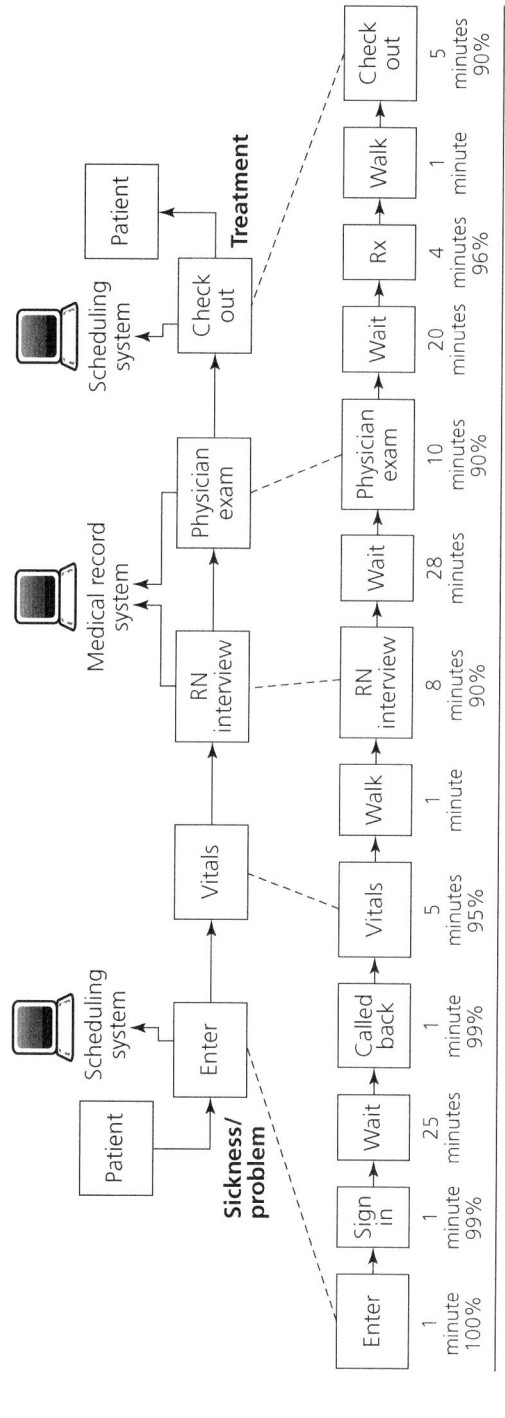

Figure 3.10 First-pass yield for physician's office visit.

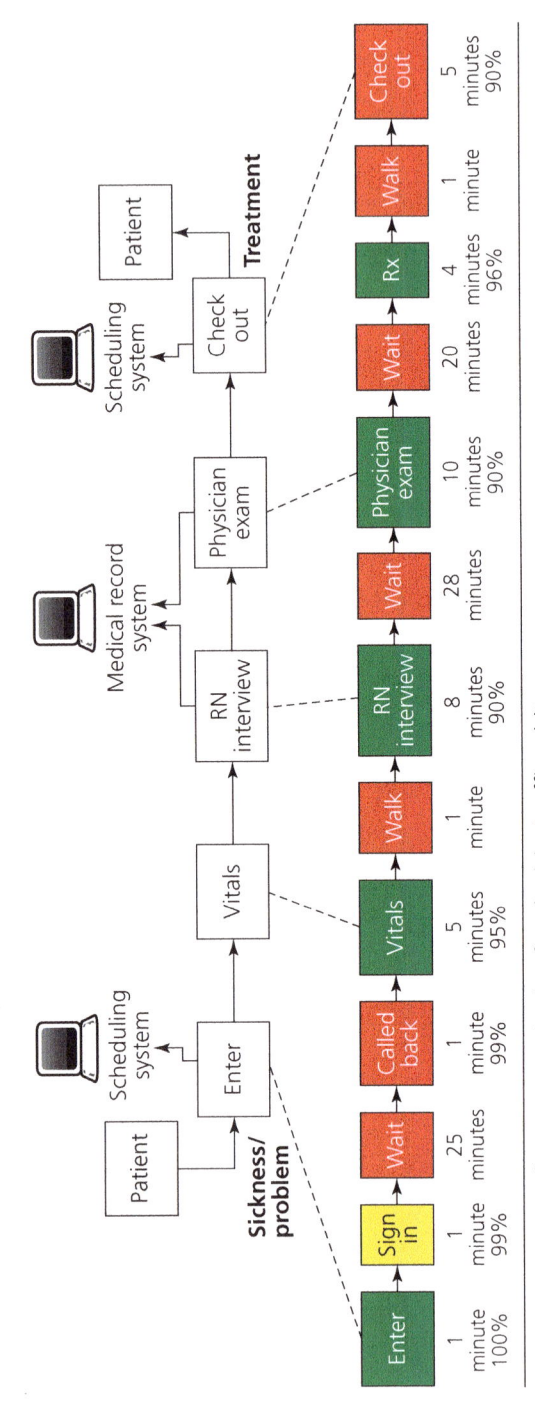

Figure 3.11 VA and NVA categorization for physician's office visit.

PRINCIPLE #2: MAP THE VALUE STREAM   43

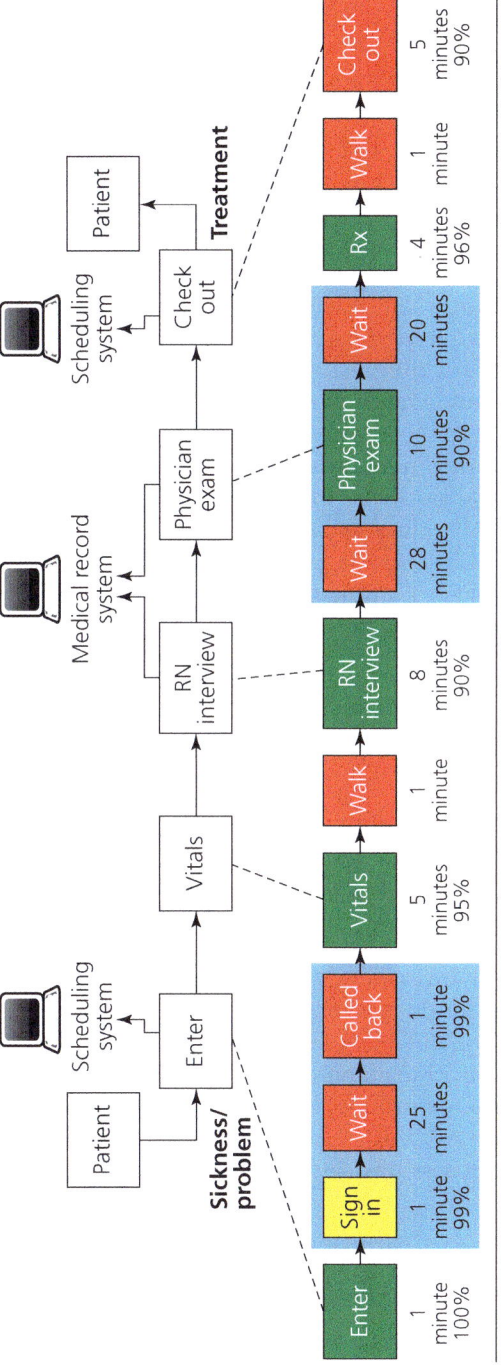

Figure 3.12   Identified opportunities for improvement for physician's office visit.

> **VSM Calculations**
>
> - **Cycle time:** duration of process step (VA plus NVA activity)
> - **Wait time:** duration between process steps
> - **Lead time:** cycle times plus wait times (total time start to finish)
> - **Value-adding ratio:** (VA time)/(Lead time)
> - **First-pass yield:** multiply every process step FPY

Focus on the future state once the current state VSM is constructed. The future state map depicts what the process should or could be (Jimmerson, 2010). It provides the path toward progress, how to get from the current state to the future state through continuous incremental improvement.

Figure 3.13 details the process within the sterile processing department. Using the current state assessment, a lean team identified upstream and downstream opportunities. They prioritized the focus based on the longest time delays and the lowest FPY. Kaizen 1 and kaizen 2 indicate the prioritized improvement approach. *Kaizen* (pronounced *ky-zen*) is a Japanese word representing change for the good. In this example, kaizen 1 and kaizen 2 describe the focus of rapid improvements with lean facilitators and process experts. Figure 3.14 depicts the VSM made by the team before converting it to an electronic document.

> **Tips for Value Stream Mapping**
>
> - Walk the process
> - Talk with staff
> - Listen, observe
> - Write down all wastes that you see

The VSM is not always the appropriate tool to use. Some processes require a different approach for documentation and evaluation. Swimlane maps are useful for processes that contain a lot of handoffs and responsibilities across several roles and/or departments. Swimlane maps help identify work process problems that arise from handoffs, suboptimal sequencing of steps, or other inefficiencies (Joint Commission on the Accreditation of Healthcare Organizations, 2006). The swimlane map depicts process flow by position (Figure 3.15).

How to Construct a Swimlane Map

Using the physician's office visit process, we will review the steps in creating a swimlane map:

Step 1: Document the positions involved in the process (Figure 3.16)

Step 2: Document the patient/chart/specimen flow (Figure 3.17)

Step 3: Document the process steps by position (Figure 3.18)

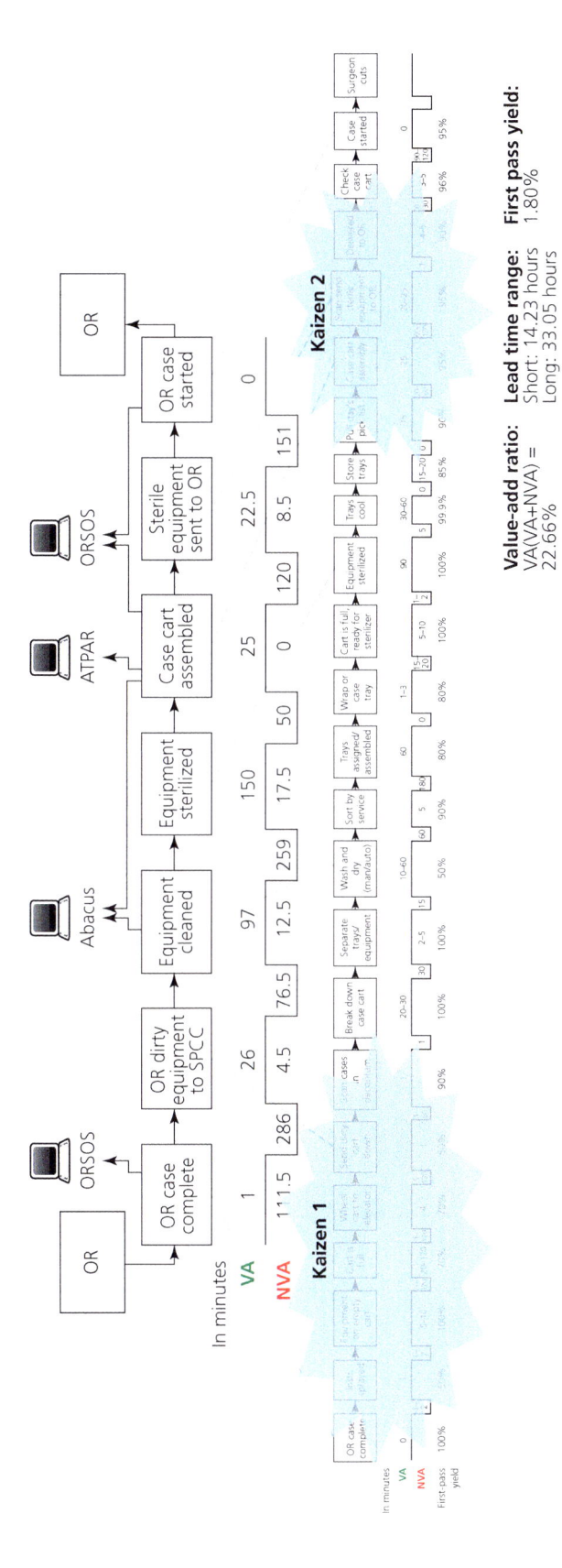

Figure 3.13 Example of VSM with improvement (kaizen) prioritization.

46 *Chapter Three*

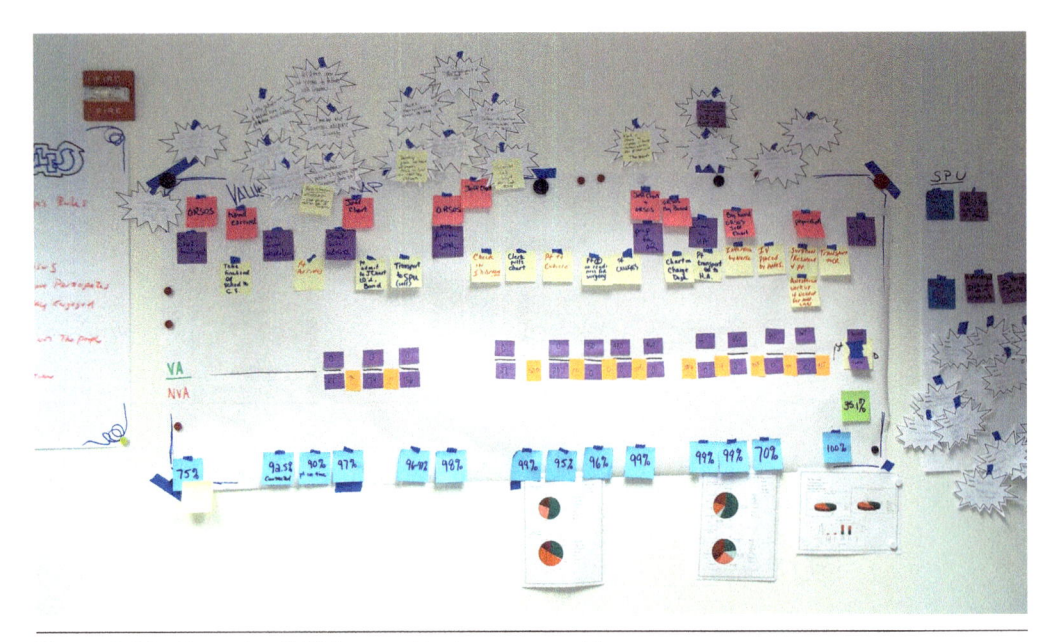

Figure 3.14 Example of VSM created by improvement team.

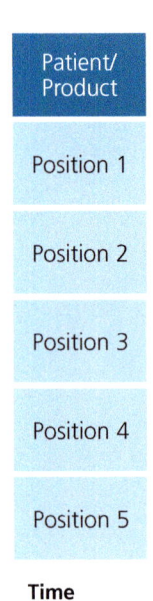

Figure 3.15 Swimlane map template.

PRINCIPLE #2: MAP THE VALUE STREAM   47

| Patient/Product |
| Registrar |
| Technician |
| Nurse |
| Physician |
| Scheduler |

Time

Figure 3.16   Swimlane map example with position.

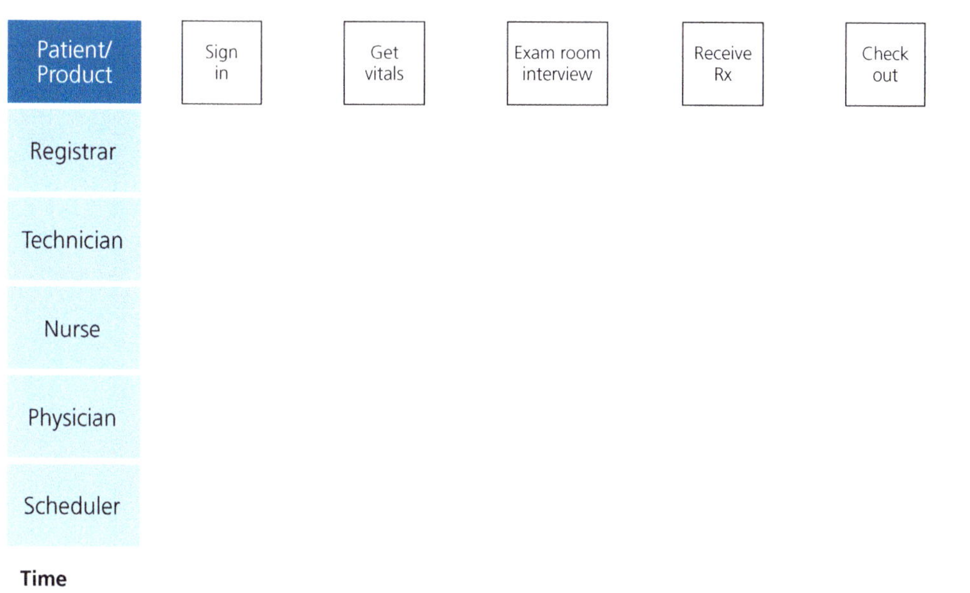

| Patient/Product | Sign in | Get vitals | Exam room interview | Receive Rx | Check out |
| Registrar |
| Technician |
| Nurse |
| Physician |
| Scheduler |

Time

Figure 3.17   Swimlane map example with patient flow process.

48 Chapter Three

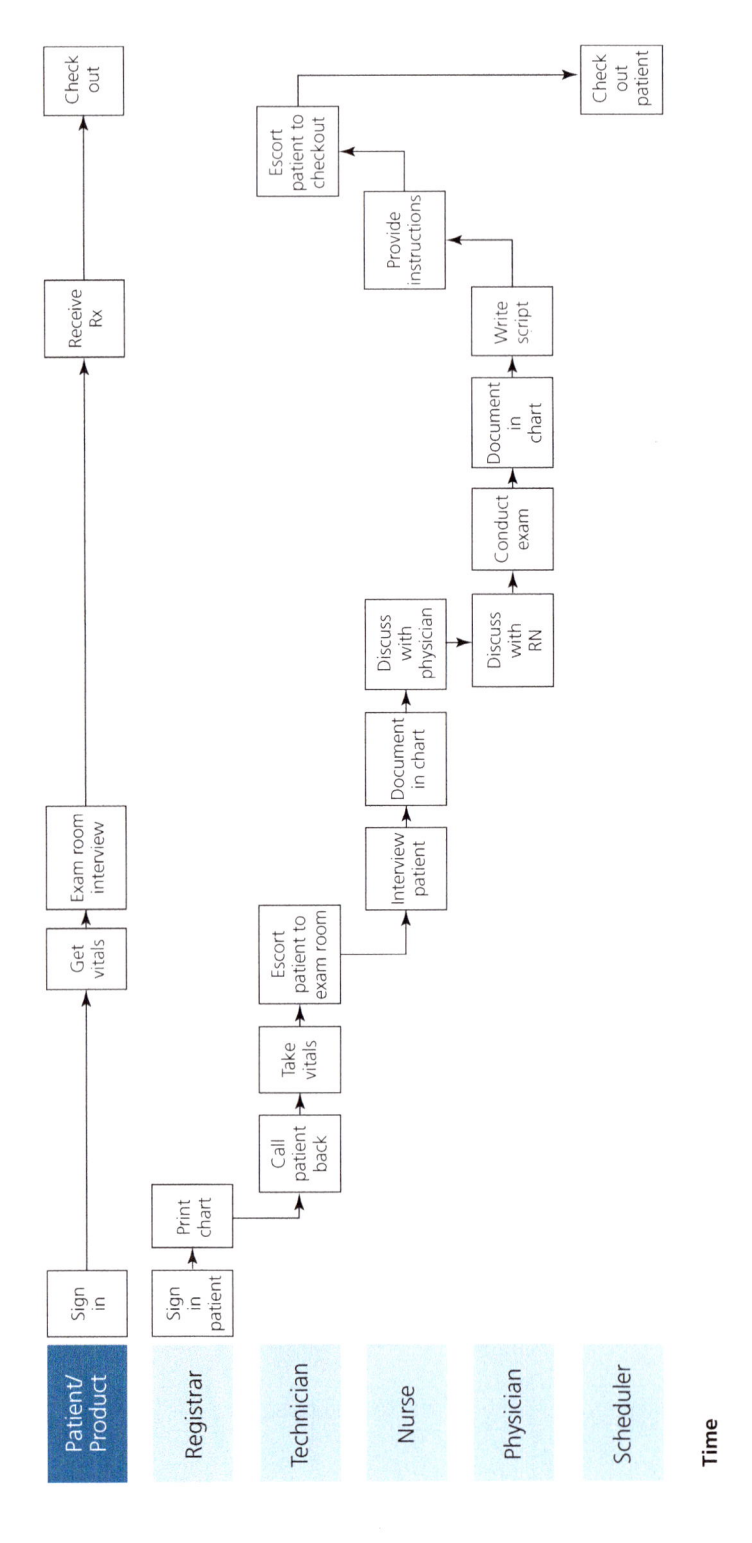

Figure 3.18 Swimlane map example with process steps by position.

PRINCIPLE #2: MAP THE VALUE STREAM   49

The swimlane map shows the sequence of steps by position along the patient flow process. Every arrow that crosses a swimlane indicates a handoff. Handoffs pose potential risks for miscommunication, lack of standardization, and delays in queuing next steps (Jimmerson, Weber, & Sobek, 2005). This mapping tool creates a strong visualization of the process and identifies each position's contribution to value (Figure 3.19).

For a more advanced application of the swimlane map, apply steps 5–8 from value stream mapping. By adding cycle and wait times and FPY, and by categorizing activities as VA or NVA, you can easily identify the opportunities for improvement.

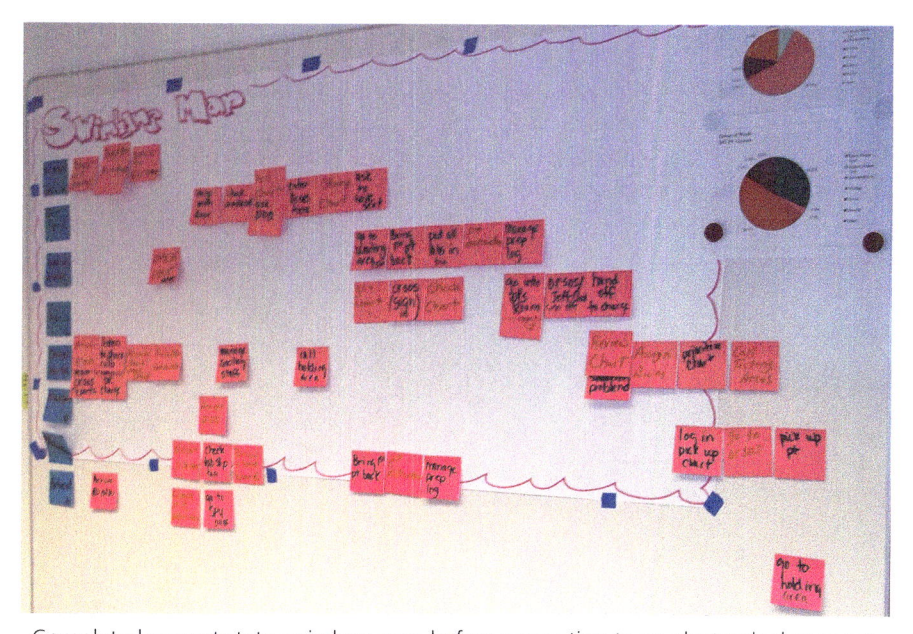

Completed current state swimlane map before converting to an electronic document.

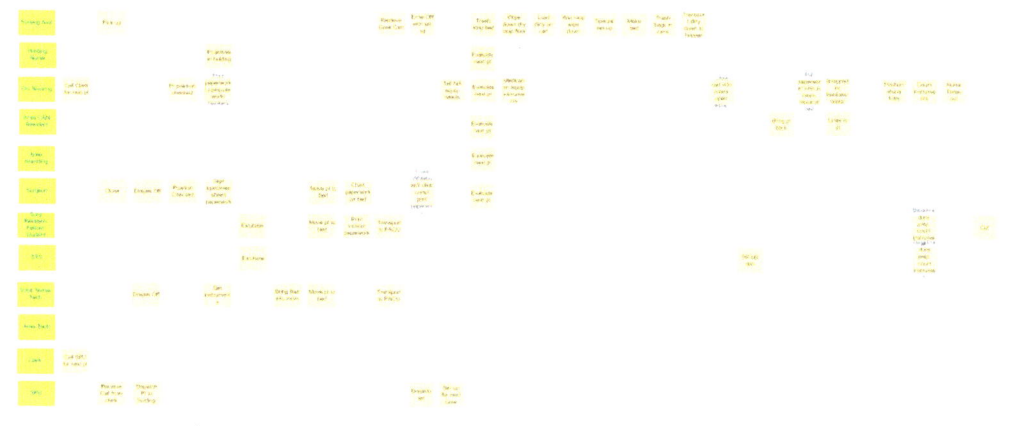

Electronic version of swimlane map for the OR turnover process.

Figure 3.19   Example of swimlane map created by improvement team.

Questions to Ask

- Are there steps/activities that do not add value?
- Can steps run in parallel?
- Are there redundant steps?
- Are there handoffs that can be eliminated?
- Are steps appropriately allocated based on roles/responsibilities?
- Is the workload evenly distributed?

COLLECT AND ANALYZE DATA FOR VSM

Once the VSM or other current state map has been drafted, the next step is to collect and analyze data (Figure 3.20). These tasks are gemba activities (Bicheno & Holweg, 2004). The gemba is where the work takes place (Womack, 2011). Going to the gemba ensures verification of observations. Evaluate the process through the eyes of the customer as well as the employee workflow (Graban, 2012).

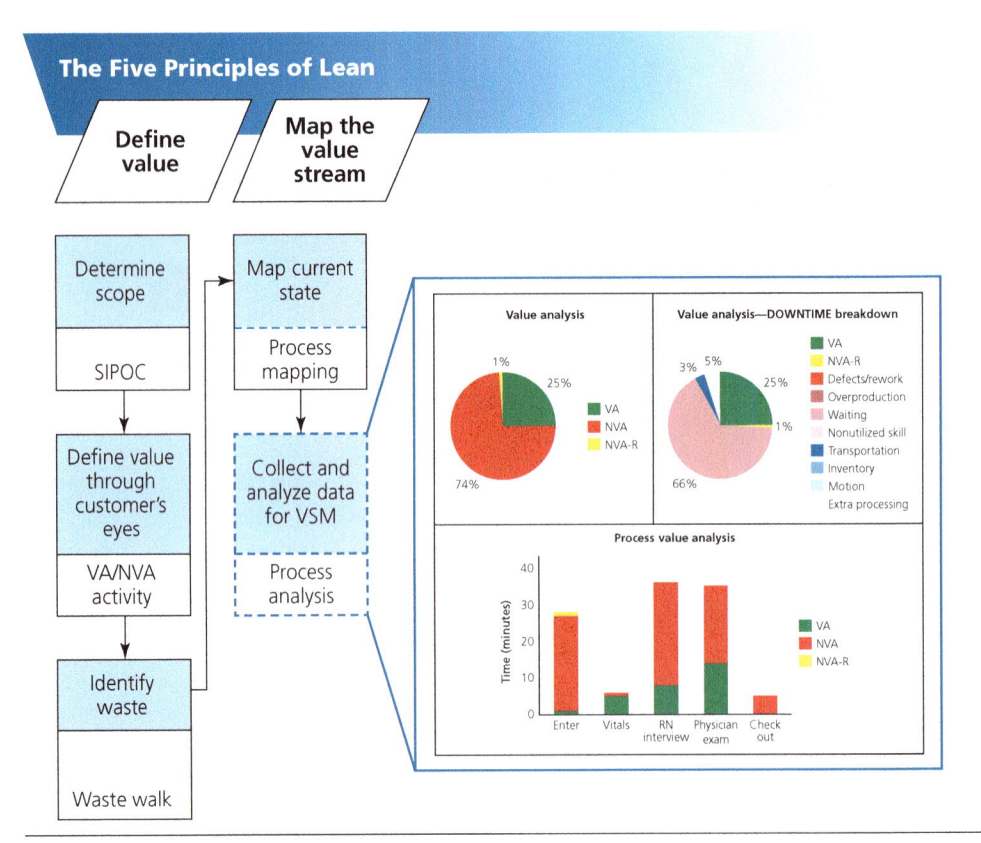

Figure 3.20 Roadmap: Collect and analyze data for VSM.

Process Value Analysis

The process value analysis tool assesses the activity of the product (or patient) (Lighter, 2013). It is one of the most important and effective lean tools for streamlining processes. The tool output consists of pie and bar graphs that display the proportion of VA to NVA activity. This visual tool makes areas of opportunity for improvement obvious.

> *Taking 5–10 cycle time measurements will give you a good sense of the process effectiveness* (not sufficient to infer statistical significance).

Conducting a Process Value Analysis

1. Go to the gemba with stopwatch in hand
2. Shadow a customer/patient, recording every step you observe from their perspective (include waiting times)
   - Identify high-level and midlevel process steps
   - Record waste observed and other general comments
   - Input observation times into the process value analysis tool in Microsoft Excel
3. Assess the results and identify opportunities for improvement (Hint: look for large portions of NVA activity)

The process value analysis tool is a Microsoft Excel–based document (Figure 3.21). The following steps explain how to use the tool:

1. Write in the high-level steps in column B.
   a. There should be five to eight high-level steps.
2. Add midlevel steps in column C.
   a. Repeat the high-level step as the first task in column C. For example, high-level step, row 7 column B "Enter" and midlevel step, row 8 column C "Enter."
   b. There should be no more than six midlevel steps. If you have more than that it might be too granular and detailed for this analysis. Condense process step descriptions.
3. Add observation times for each midlevel step.
   a. Average observed cycle times. Typically 5–10 observations will give you a good, general idea of the capability of the process. The more observations you have during different hours of operation, the more reflective the results will be to the actual current state.
   b. All rows in gray will auto-sum the results. Do not overwrite the formulas.

52 Chapter Three

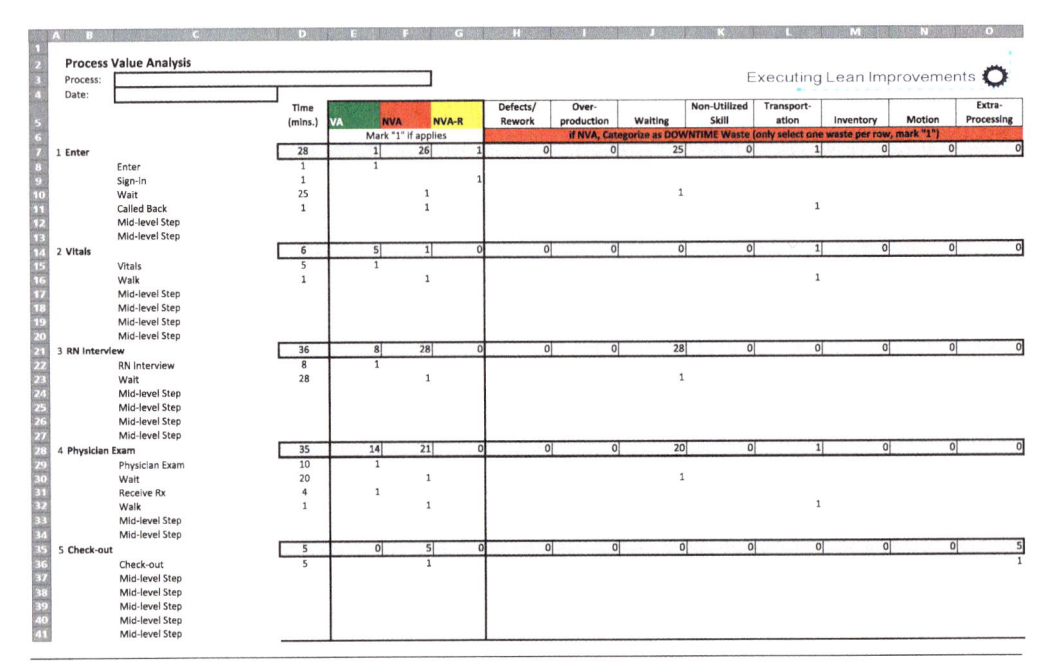

Figure 3.21 Process value analysis screenshot.

4. Determine whether midlevel steps are VA, NVA, or NVA-R.

   a. Indicate category by placing a "1" in column E, F, or G.

   b. Do not place "1" in more than one column. If you do, the template will double count the time and skew the results.

5. If NVA, categorize the activity by type of waste.

   a. Indicate category by placing a "1" in column H through O.

   b. As above, do not place "1" in more than one column.

6. Evaluate process value analysis output. The output of the table is three graphs.

   a. Value analysis—pie chart that depicts proportion of VA, NVA, and NVA-R at a high level.

   b. Value analysis—DOWNTIME breakdown—pie chart segmenting NVA activities by specific DOWNTIME wastes. This chart enables you to effectively diagnose the major process issues.

   c. Process value analysis—bar graph showing proportion of VA, NVA, and NVA-R times per high-level process step. This output is one of the most important components of effective problem identification. The bar graph provides an assessment of opportunity per step and enables targeted lean improvements.

PRINCIPLE #2: MAP THE VALUE STREAM 53

We can use the physician's office visit example to see how the tool works. List the high-level and midlevel process steps. Then add observed cycle times and categorize VA, NVA, and NVA-R with further refinement of DOWNTIME wastes for all NVA steps.

The output of the physician's office visit shows 74% of the process as NVA (Figure 3.22). The DOWNTIME breakdown highlights waiting (66%) as the predominant waste. Extra processing is the second highest at 5%. The process value analysis bar graph shows the distribution of NVA across the patient's visit. Large portions of NVA activity sit atop the VA steps. This graph suggests the best opportunities for improvement lie within the first two steps, "Enter" and "Vitals," with subsequent opportunity between steps 3 and 4.

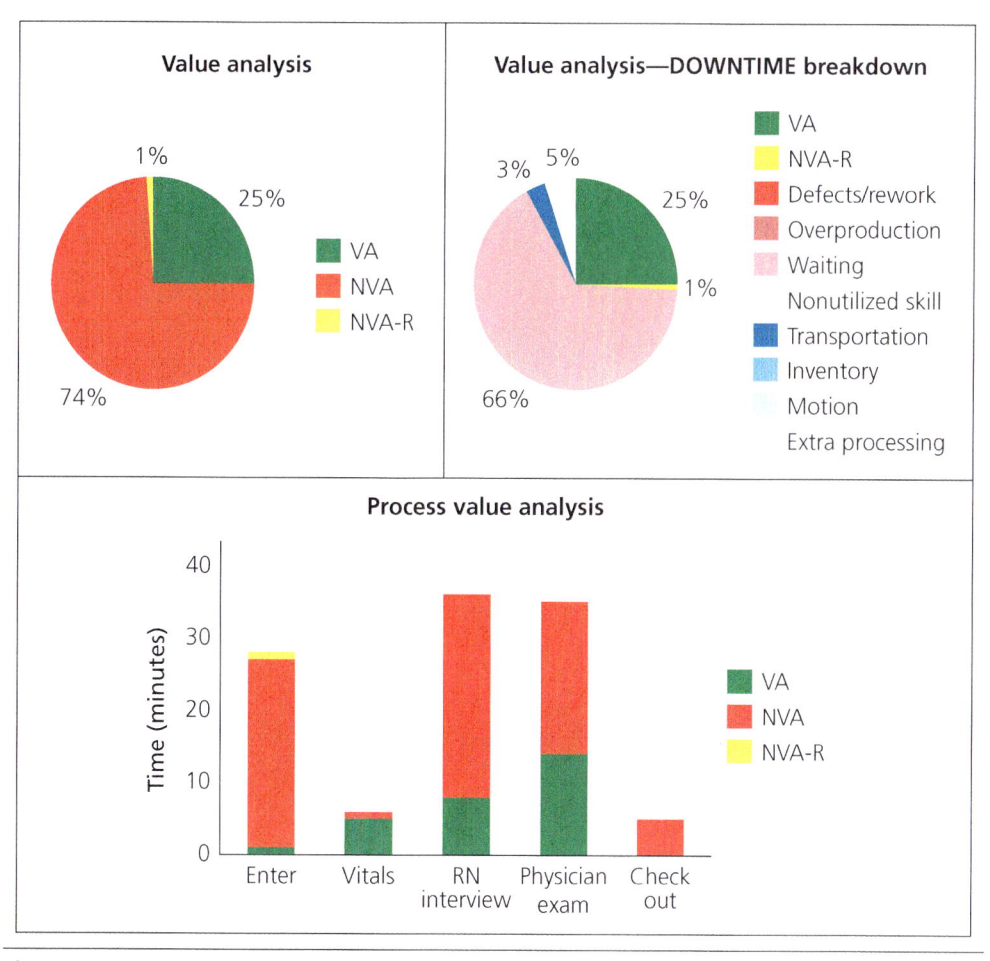

Figure 3.22 Process value analysis output example.

Case Study: Patient Flow in the Patient Testing Center

The patient testing center (PTC) is responsible for presurgical history and physicals, screening, and other tasks. Figure 3.23 shows 56% of the process is NVA. The NVA is broken into the eight DOWNTIME wastes, of which waiting accounts for 39%. Similarly, the bar graph shows the distribution of VA and NVA steps. There is a significant opportunity for improvement within the first three steps since no VA activities take place until step 4 (clinician 1 assessment). This would be the first area of focus for waste elimination.

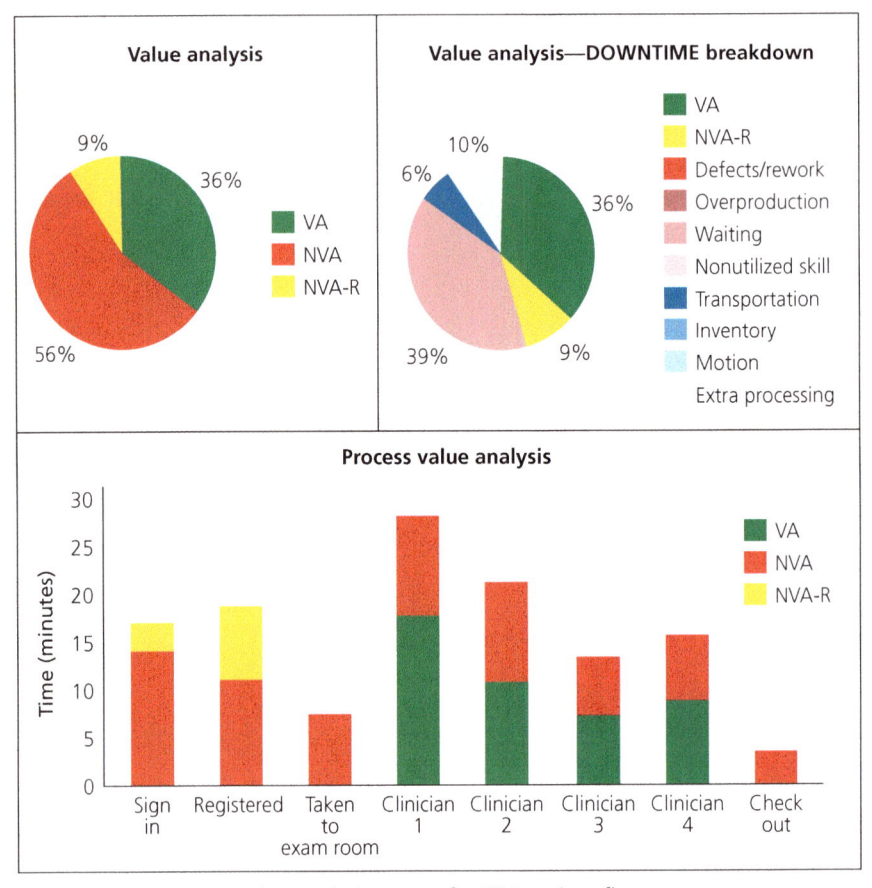

Figure 3.23 Process value analysis output for PTC patient flow.

Workflow Value Analysis

In addition to process value analysis, another way to evaluate processes is through assessing employee workflow. Workflow inefficiencies lead to NVA activities and customer dissatisfaction. A tool called the workflow value analysis evaluates employee workflow.

Conducting a Workflow Value Analysis

1. Go to the gemba with stopwatch in hand
2. Shadow the employee, recording every step you observe (include waiting)
   - Record observed wastes and make notes for other general comments
   - Input observation times into the workflow value analysis tool in Microsoft Excel (Figure 3.24)
3. Assess the results and identify opportunities for improvement (Hint: look for large portions of NVA activity)

The workflow value analysis tool is a Microsoft Excel–based document. The following steps explain how to use the tool:

1. Write in all observed tasks in column C.
   a. When observing employee workflow, it is important to document all tasks, including walking and waiting.
2. Add observation times for each task.
3. Determine whether midlevel steps are VA, NVA, or NVA-R.
   a. Indicate category by placing a "1" in column E, F, or G.
   b. Do not place "1" in more than one column.
4. If NVA, categorize the activity by type of waste.
   a. Indicate category by placing a "1" in column H through O.
   b. As above, do not place "1" in more than one column.

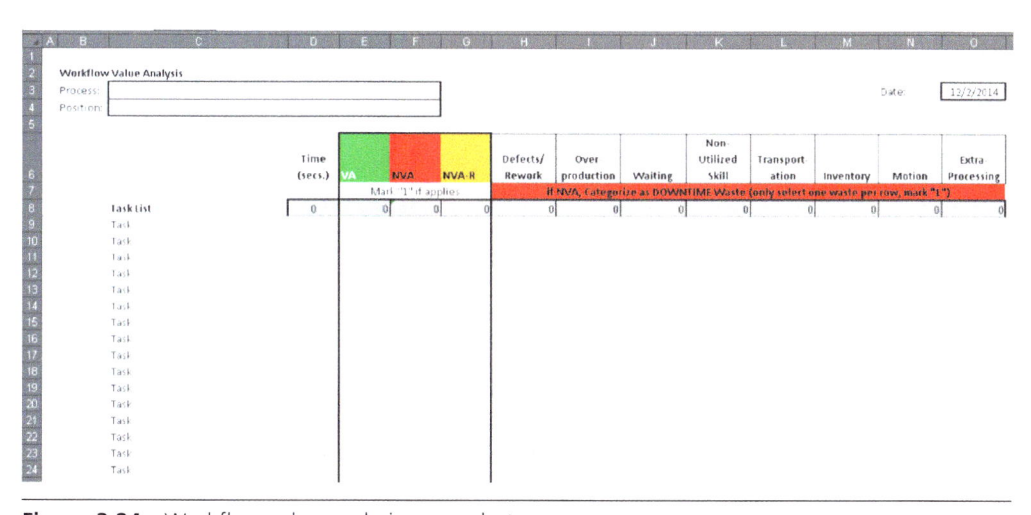

Figure 3.24 Workflow value analysis screenshot.

56 Chapter Three

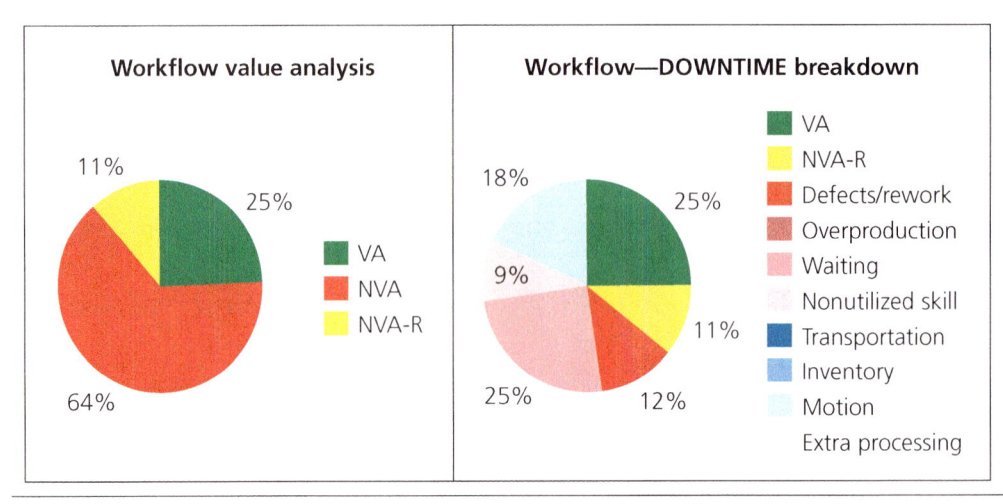

Figure 3.25 Workflow value analysis output example.

5. Evaluate workflow value analysis output. The output of the table is two pie charts.

   a. Workflow value analysis—pie chart that depicts proportion of VA, NVA, and NVA-R at a high level.

   b. Workflow—DOWNTIME breakdown—pie chart segmenting NVA activities by specific wastes. This chart enables you to effectively diagnose the major process issues.

Figure 3.25 displays 64% of the employee's time as NVA activity. The DOWNTIME waste breakdown indicates waiting (25%), motion (18%), and defects (12%) as the primary contributors of NVA. In the subsequent chapters we'll uncover strategies to address these results.

> **Hints for Identifying Opportunities**
>
> *Initially, fix the FPY. If process steps are not performed correctly the first time, the downstream process becomes wasteful in rework and extra processing, among others.*

PUTTING THE PIECES TOGETHER

Once you reach this point, it is time to put all of the pieces together. The diagnostic tools, from value stream mapping to process analysis, tell a story about the process under review. Each tool helps assess and isolate areas of opportunity.

Case Study: OR/SPCC Value Stream Mapping Event

As part of the perioperative department's strategic plan, a team of lean leaders was assigned to analyze and improve the sterile processing and case cart (SPCC) workflow process (Delisle, 2013). Through data analysis and voice of the customer, it was determined that surgical equipment was not turning over efficiently, causing delays throughout the system. The lean leaders facilitated a value stream mapping event. The event focused on identifying and prioritizing key improvement initiatives within the value stream. Delays in SPCC cause bottlenecks and workflow inefficiencies and negatively impact both patient and staff satisfaction (Farrokhi et al., 2013).

The objective of the value stream mapping event was to identify the first and subsequent improvement areas of focus. The SIPOC starts with the operating room (OR) sending the dirty equipment to sterile processing (SP) (Figure 3.26). The last step is the subsequent OR case starting with sterile surgical equipment.

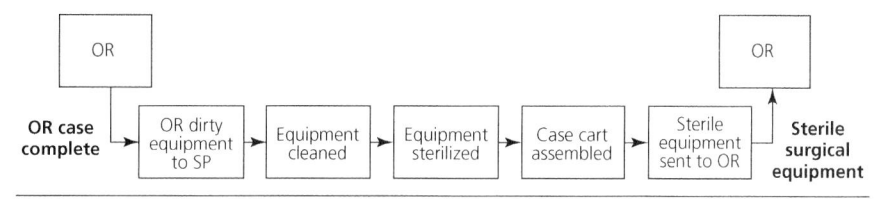

Figure 3.26 Sterile processing SIPOC.

The lean team worked with process experts to conduct observations and document midlevel steps. The VSM includes wait times between processing steps (Figure 3.27).

The process value analysis indicated that 73% of the process was NVA (Figure 3.28). The DOWNTIME waste breakdown revealed that waiting (59%) was the largest component, while extra processing was the second largest (10%). The bar graph shows the distribution of VA and NVA activities. Waiting was pervasive due to missing items and poor communication between the SP department and the OR. The majority of issues began upstream and caused subsequent bottlenecks and inefficiencies. As a result, the lean team recommended that the first improvement project scope address the time from when the OR case is completed to the time the equipment is cleaned. The objective of this initial effort was to ensure that all of the surgical equipment was sent down on the appropriate trays, sorted correctly, and cleaned in a timely manner. Following the standard guidelines would limit the likelihood of missing equipment and delays caused by waiting on parts or rework.

(continued)

Chapter Three

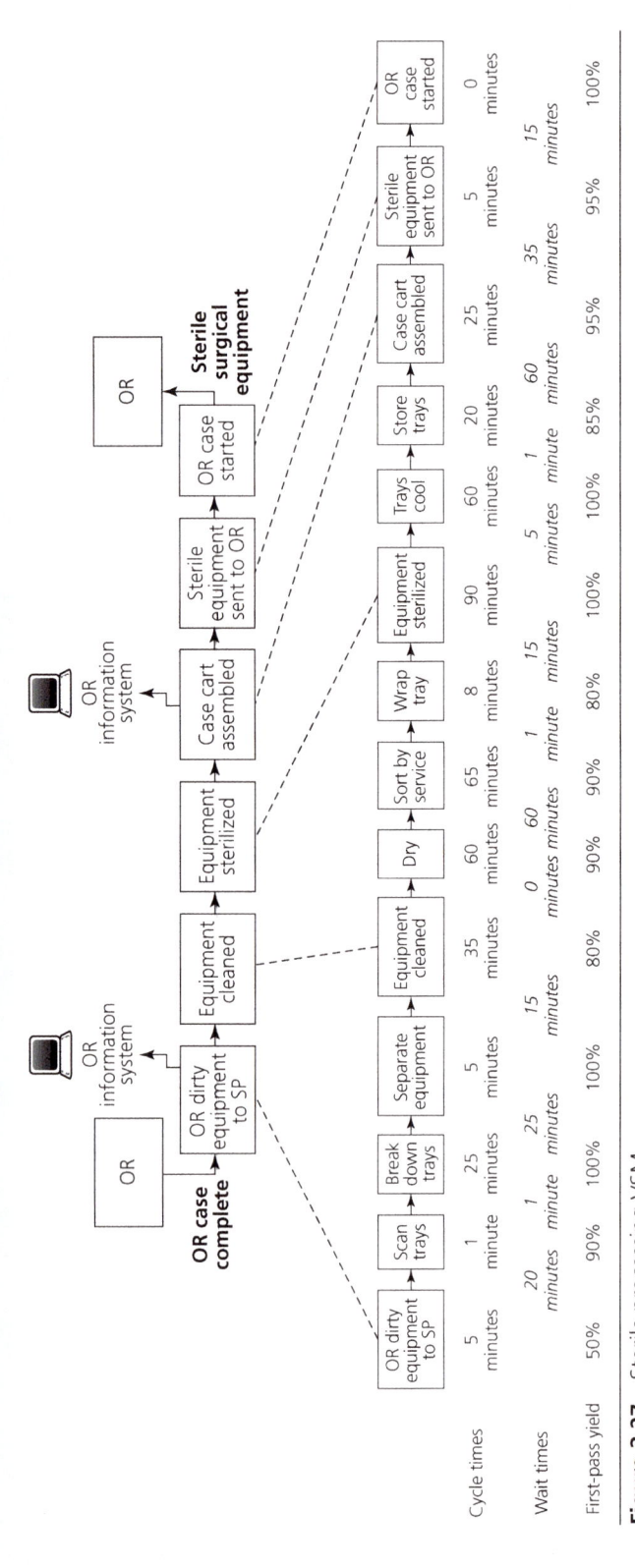

Figure 3.27 Sterile processing VSM.

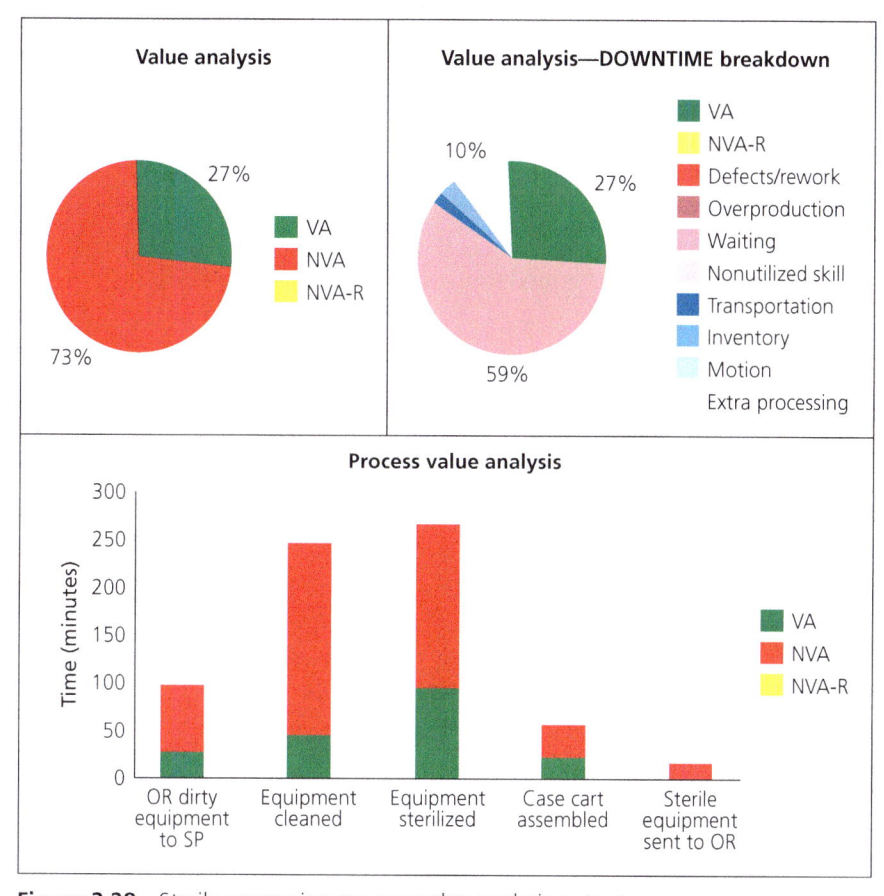

Figure 3.28 Sterile processing process value analysis output.

CHAPTER CHALLENGE

Identify a process that has quality-related issues. Go to the gemba and talk with staff. Discuss the problem/issue and ask what percentage of time the process step is done correctly the first time. What is the reaction you got? Was it expected? Why or why not?

QUESTIONS

1. Why is it easier to start by documenting all of the steps first when building a process map?

2. What is the difference between high-level and midlevel steps? What is the purpose of drilling down to lower-level steps?

3. How can the FPY affect a process?
4. What are the best strategies to improve the FPY?
5. How do VSMs differ from process maps?
6. Why do you need to prioritize improvement opportunities on the VSM?
7. What information does a swimlane map provide? When is it most effective to use?
8. Why do the process analyses tools need to be performed at the gemba? What information do these tools produce?
9. Why is the process value analysis considered one of the most effective lean diagnostic tools?
10. What are the main considerations for conducting the workflow value analysis?

Chapter 4
Establish the Lean Fundamentals

Nothing worth doing stays done forever without diligence, discipline, and hard work.

—David Mann

The lean fundamentals are central to creating lean processes (Figure 4.1). Lean improvements do not just happen; they require ready and willing individuals as well as an efficient and organized work setting. The lean

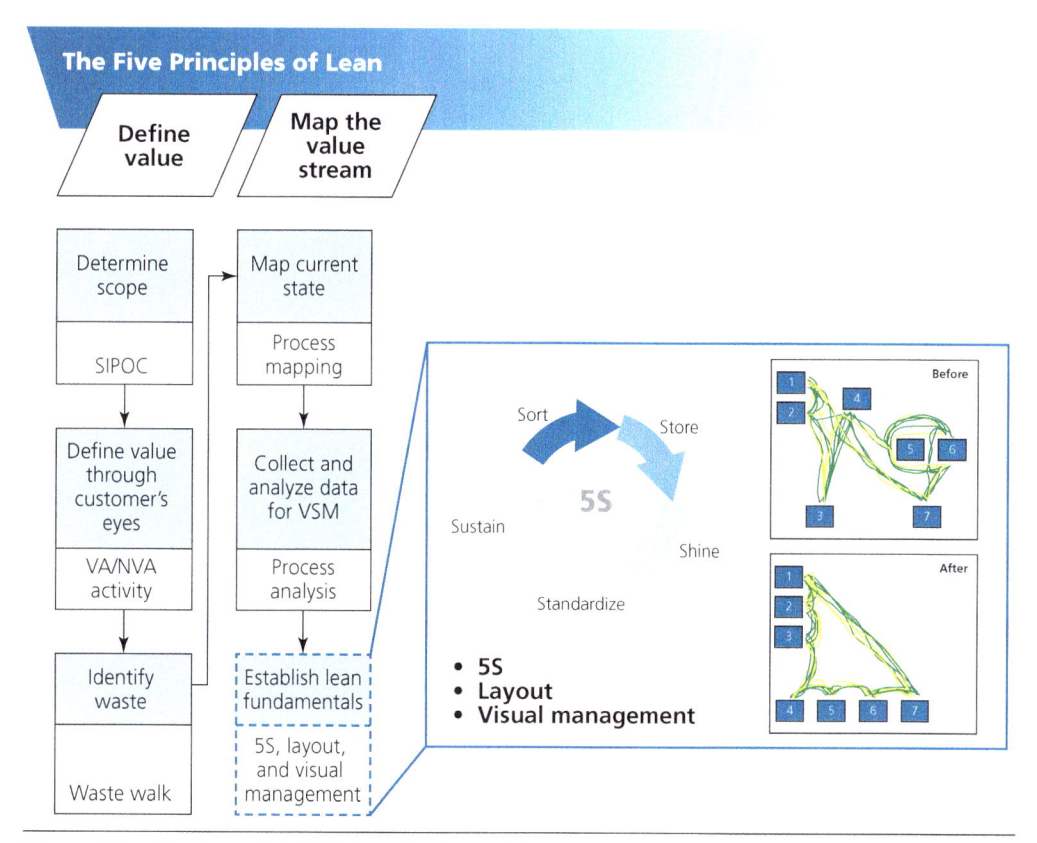

Figure 4.1 Roadmap: Establish lean fundamentals.

61

Table 4.1 Lean fundamentals.

Fundamental	Description
5S	Prepare the workplace to enable improvements to be effective and implemented efficiently
Layout	Arrange the physical space to enable flow and provide improved communication and quality
Visual management	Provide an immediate understanding of a situation or condition

fundamentals focus on the preparation and facilitation of efficient processes. The fundamentals serve as the starting block for lean improvements. If the fundamentals are not in place, a process will not achieve optimal results. Each fundamental is effective on its own, but when combined, they serve as a powerful tool set (Table 4.1).

5S*

5S was first introduced in the late 1980's and early 1990's (Nakajima, 1988; Takahashi & Osada, 1990). The 5S framework (Table 4.2) supplies a logical, user-friendly approach towards the assessment, design, and implementation of improvements to systems and processes as well as developing standardized tasks to improve quality and patient safety (Graban, 2012). Traditionally, 5S organizes physical space and items (i.e., workspace, desk, charts, department) (Tapping et al., 2009). The 5S approach eliminates waste, provides visual control, and prepares the workplace to enable improvements to be effective and implemented efficiently. 5S does this in distinct phases: (1) sort; (2) store; (3) shine; (4) standardize; and (5) sustain (Graban, 2012). This framework is not unfamiliar. Professional organizers take the same steps to help people de-clutter their homes (e.g., TV shows *Hoarders* and *Hoarding: Buried Alive*). As stated in the law of entropy, over time organized systems move toward increasing states of disorganization (Mann, 2010). Hard work, discipline, and structure are required to fight against this natural tendency (Zidel, 2012).

> *Sorting is critical in just about everything you do. In process improvement or life in general, the ability to sort the necessary from the unnecessary is an essential skill.*

The potential of 5S remains largely untapped due to its narrow application typically only on physical space and organization. 5S has tremendous opportunity

---

*Content of this section is modified from "Everything Is 5S: A Simple yet Powerful Lean Improvement Approach Applied in a Preadmission Testing Center" (Delisle & Freiberg, 2014).

Table 4.2 5S approach for organizing physical space and systems/processes.

Phase	Description for organizing physical space	Description for organizing systems/processes
Sort	Sort the necessary from the unnecessary. Remove items and supplies that do not belong in that area.	Sort the necessary steps/components from the unnecessary. Remove activities that do not add value.
Store	Store the needed items in the appropriate location based on frequency of use, keeping the things used most often in easily accessible areas.	Store the necessary steps/components in the appropriate order based on sequence and timing.
Shine	Shine the space. Keeping areas clean and clear of clutter enables easy location of items and aids in the identification of missing or misplaced things.	Shine or streamline the step. Refine processes (e.g., cycle times) to further reduce the impact of NVA activities.
Standardize	Standardize the organizing approach to all applicable areas. Label drawers and shelves with the same nomenclature. Stock storage areas the same way. Consistent, standard approaches reduce wasted time searching.	Standardize the system/process to all applicable areas (e.g., standard operating procedures) to ensure every step is done the same way, every time, by everyone.
Sustain	Sustain the improvement through discipline and follow-up. Monitor storage to assure everything is in its proper place.	Sustain the improvement through discipline and follow-up. Monitor key performance indicators to track outcomes and employ audits to ensure compliance.

to also enhance system/process design and improvement. Figure 4.2 illustrates a hypothetical example of applying 5S to a process. The first row is a current state process map. The current state is a display of how the process actually functions prior to any improvements, with an overall processing time of 95 minutes. The first task in 5S is to sort and evaluate items/steps based on need. Though seemingly simple, this is profound. Most processes have NVA steps that delay throughput and consume resources. During the sort phase (rows 2 and 3) steps 2 and 6 were determined to be NVA and removed from the process.

Process sequence evaluation occurs during the Store phase (row 4). Step 4 shifts ahead of step 3 in an effort to increase efficiency and productivity. Row 5, streamlining steps 4, 3, and 5, shaves off additional processing time. The overall time is now 57 minutes. Standard work for steps 4, 5, and 7 ensures consistent productivity (row 6). The new process will undergo sustainability measures to maintain processing times around 48 minutes. Core to sustainability is hardwiring a performance assessment and feedback loop to staff. Effective approaches include regularly posting process outcomes on run charts, daily huddles to discuss barriers and issues, and periodic brainstorming sessions to determine further refinements. Row 7 demonstrates sustainability of results achieved through rows 1–6.

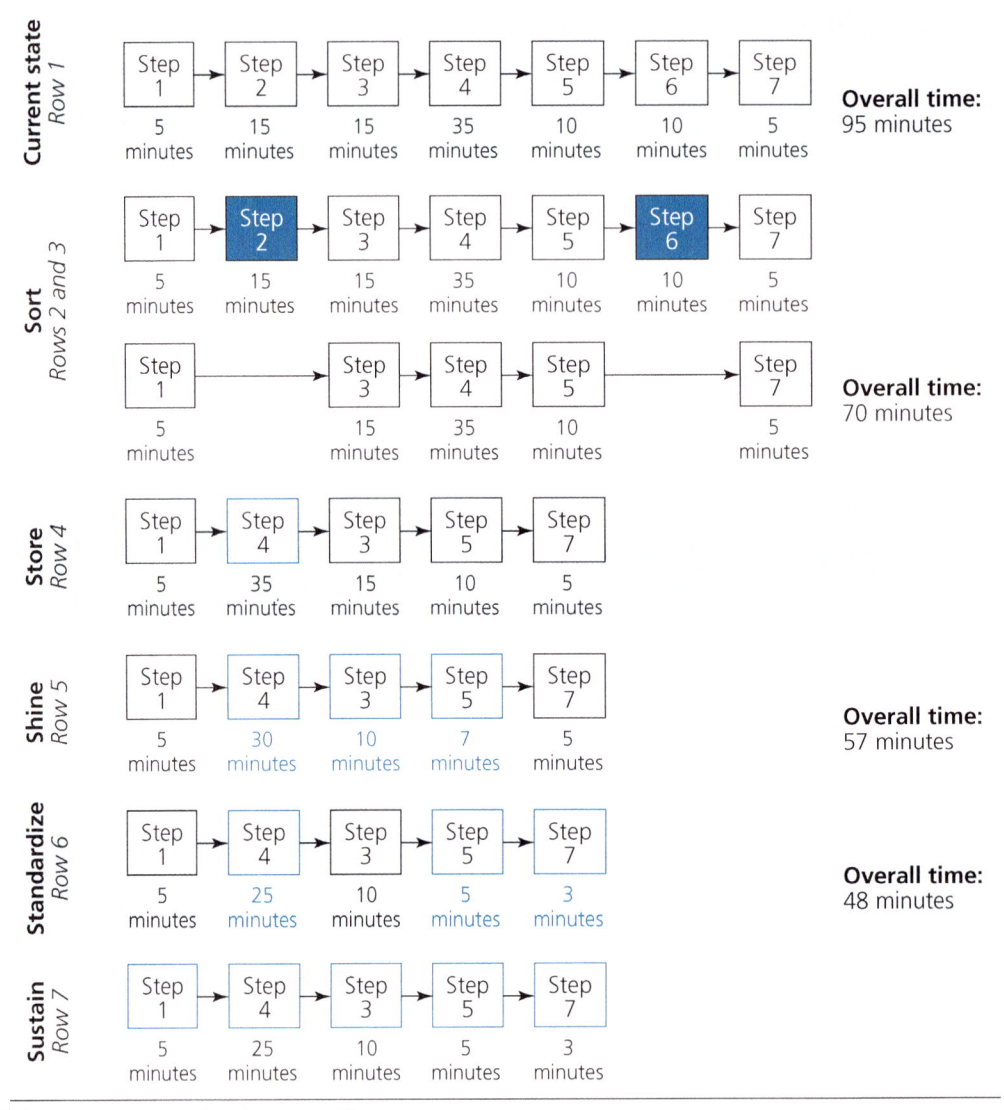

Figure 4.2 Example of process 5S.
Source: Delisle & Freiberg 2014.

5S Audit Tool

To assess the physical organization of a workspace you can apply the Excel-based 5S audit tool, a representation of which is shown in Figure 4.3. The tool enables workspace evaluation through each "S" based on defined questions. For each item that applies, enter "1" to indicate YES. The radar map provides an output that highlights the strengths and opportunities within an area. The tool is an objective assessment of the work area.

	Area: _____ Date: _____	
	Criteria	**1 if "yes"**
Sort	Is the floor/workspace clutter-free?	0
	Are unnecessary equipment and supplies removed?	0
	Are items stored in appropriate locations?	0
	Is there an appropriate amount of equipment and supplies as needed?	0
Store	Do all equipment, supplies, and personnel have a dedicated location?	0
	Do storage areas and floor indicate where to or not to place things?	0
	Are workstations organized?	0
	Are there designated storage areas for temporary items?	0
Shine	Is the work environment conducive to productivity (well lit, clean)?	0
	Are the floors clean?	0
	Is equipment clean and well maintained?	0
	Are workstations free of clutter?	0
Standardize	Are staff trained on the 5S approach?	0
	Is visual management appropriately used?	0
	Are workstations set up similarly?	0
	Are issues/problems made readily apparent?	0
Sustain	Are checklists used to detail tasks and expectations?	0
	Is the area periodically audited for 5S elements?	0
	Are visual cues or pictures used to highlight expectations?	0
	Are staff maintaining progress and identifying other areas for 5S?	0

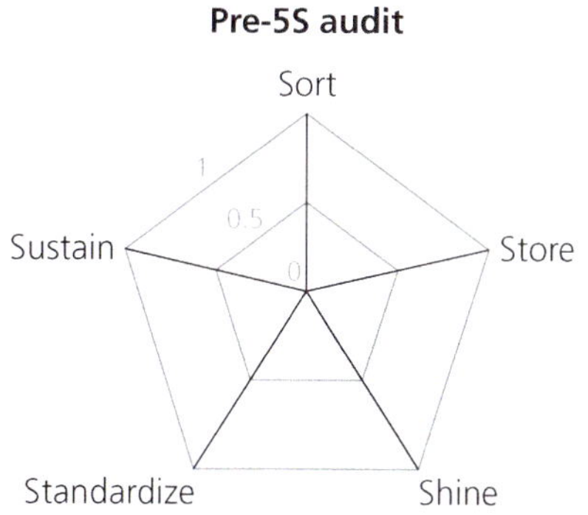

Pre-5S audit

Figure 4.3 5S audit tool for physical space and layout assessment.

After improving an area, the post 5S-audit illustrates progress in each of the five components, a representation of which is shown in Figure 4.4. The radar chart indicates if the work area aligns to promote efficiency.

> *The power of 5S exceeds application in the workspace. 5S can be applied to your personal life and home, as well as your e-mails!*

Pre/post-5S audits

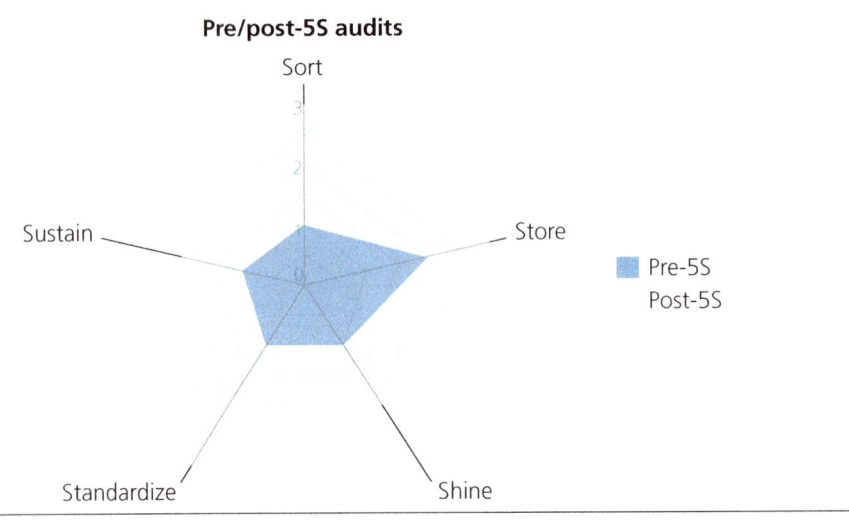

Figure 4.4 5S audit tool output (radar chart).

5S Applied to E-mails and Electronic Information

The balance with storing things electronically is the ability to do so in an organized way. The challenge with physical space is that it is limited. There is only so much room for "stuff." In the electronic environment, storage is almost limitless. Space is not the issue. The issue becomes can you find what you saved? This is why 5S is a fundamental of lean. Without an effective and sustainable 5S approach to process design and physical space, you will perpetuate waste (especially motion, nonutilized skill, transportation, and inventory).

Electronic storage, especially for e-mails, can make you more productive. Use folders to sort and store e-mails accordingly. It becomes very easy to sustain once you get through the initial phases. Try using an e-mail triaging system (folder categories below) with a goal of having an inbox with zero e-mails. Take the approach that if you open it, do something with it: respond, file, or delete.

1. Read: any interesting e-mail/attachment/article that is not time sensitive.

2. Needs response: any e-mail that requires a response from you.

3. Urgent: should always be empty if used correctly. If it is urgent, what are you waiting for?

4. To do: anything that requires you to do something/follow-up on an action/request.

5. Awaiting response: a personal favorite, e-mails from you to other people go directly into this folder when asking someone to do something (i.e., project follow-up, response). By the end of the week you can review this folder and see what is still outstanding. When the appropriate time passes, forward that e-mail back to the person as a friendly reminder. This is highly effective and makes your life easier so you do not have to try and remember who owes you what, by when.

Searching for information is a major issue that pervades most areas. Remember with the lean fundamentals, the goal is to organize things in a way that promotes efficiency and quality. This is not limited to the physical organization of "stuff." It includes the virtual/electronic organization of documentation, files, etc. as well as the design/redesign of systems and processes. The most valuable step in 5S is the first one, sort. Remove the necessary from the unnecessary, de-clutter. Sorting (like in the e-mail example) is an ongoing process that does not end. Sorting closely links to standardization and sustainability.

LAYOUT

Layout, the second lean fundamental, focuses on work area design. The goal of layout is to enable flow of the things processed (e.g., patient, specimen) (Liker, 2004). Efficient layouts make it easier to accomplish work by reducing the wastes of motion, transportation, and waiting. Figure 4.5 depicts a process in which the layout redesign reduces the amount of required travel from one step to the next. Additionally, due to the improved layout, there is more free space in the "After" scenario. Layout is an intuitive improvement solution.

Assessing Layout with the Spaghetti Diagram

The best way to assess layout is to create a visual representation of the actual flow. The spaghetti diagram illustrates the wastes of transportation (item) and motion (worker). The tool is simple to use.

Step 1: Draw a scaled diagram of the layout (Figure 4.6).

Step 2: Mark processing areas and indicate who does which tasks at each location (Figure 4.7).

Step 3: Walk the process. Use different colors for different parts/staff if applicable or necessary (Figure 4.8).

Step 4: Document travel time/distance. Do a before and after to assess improvement (Figure 4.9).

The before and after layouts depict improvements in workflow and reductions in motion and transportation (Figure 4.10). The new layout releases previously used floor space for other purposes.

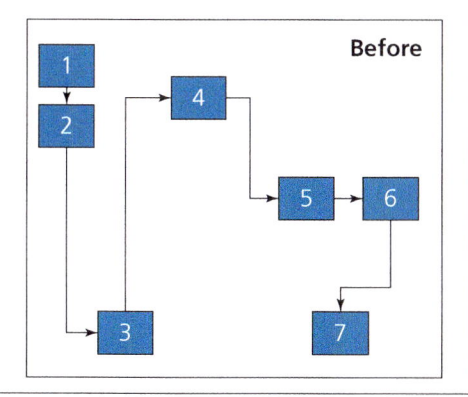

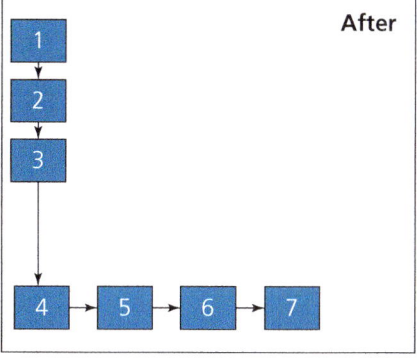

Figure 4.5 Layout example.

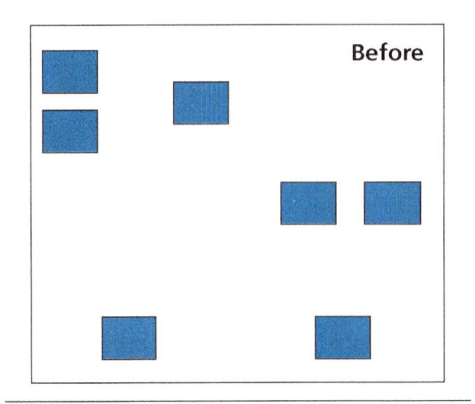

Figure 4.6 Example of current state layout.

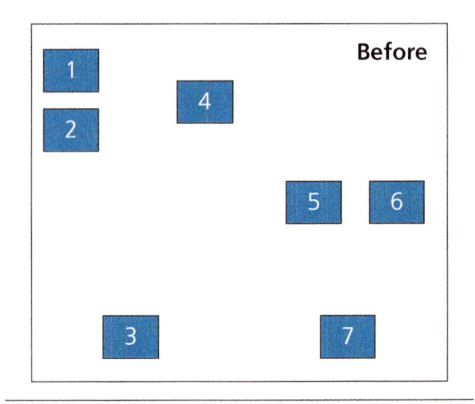

Figure 4.7 Example of current state layout with labeled processing areas.

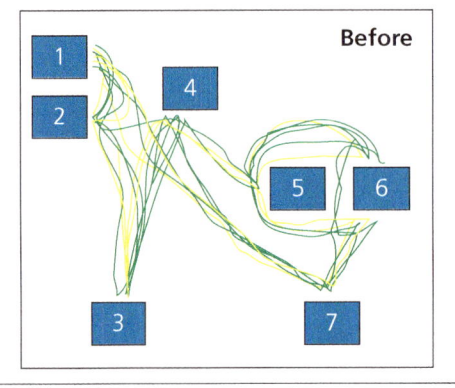

Figure 4.8 Example of spaghetti diagram of current state.

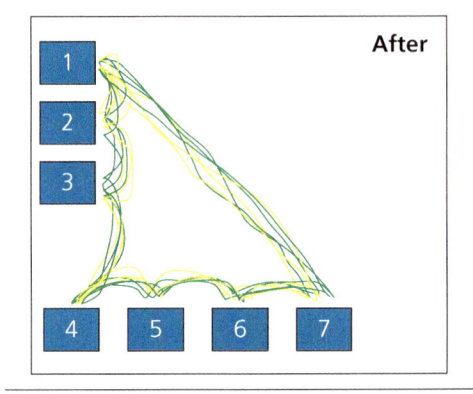

Figure 4.9 Example of spaghetti diagram of improved state.

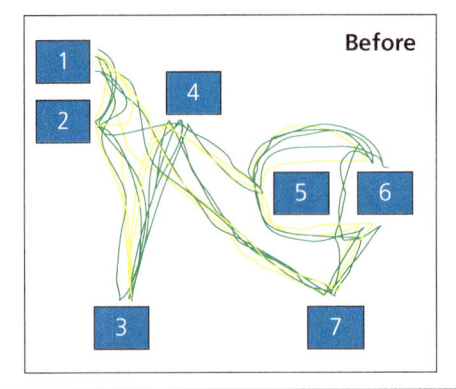

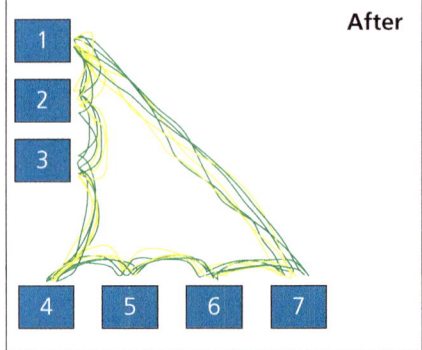

Figure 4.10 Comparison of spaghetti diagrams before and after improvement.

There are several ways in which layout can improve flow. Figures 4.11–4.13 compare traditional configurations with improved layouts. Figure 4.11 shows how to achieve workload balancing by sharing the workspace and increasing access to each employee rather than working in isolated silos. Similarly, Figure 4.12 depicts employees working independently versus collaboratively. Finally, Figure 4.13 compares straight-line flow with the U-shaped orientation. U-shaped orientations allow employees to evenly distribute workflow and reallocate effort to ensure flow.

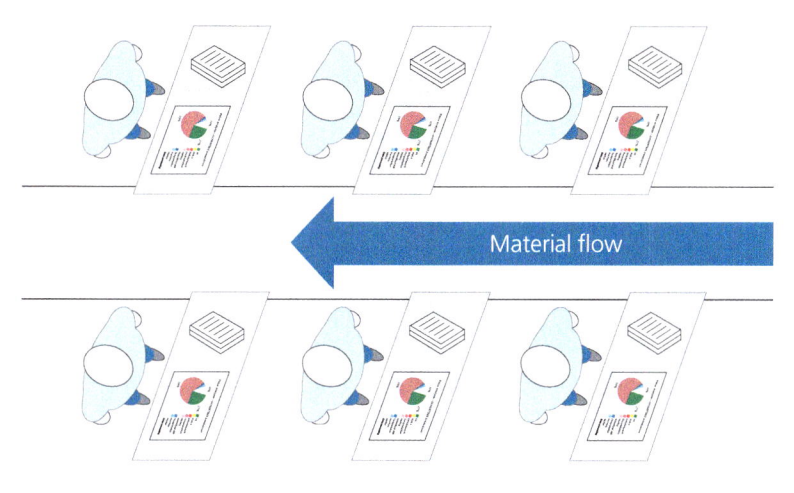

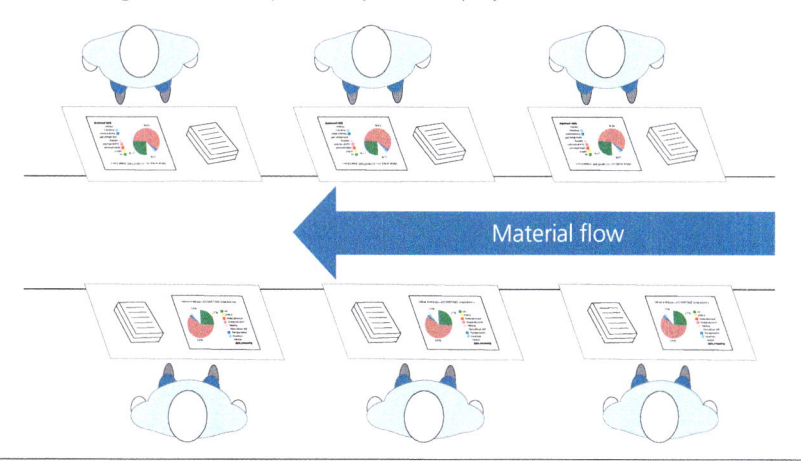

Figure 4.11 Layout improvement 1 of 3.
Source: Adapted from Jacobs & Chase, 2008.

Configuration 1: Bad layout—employees are working in isolation.

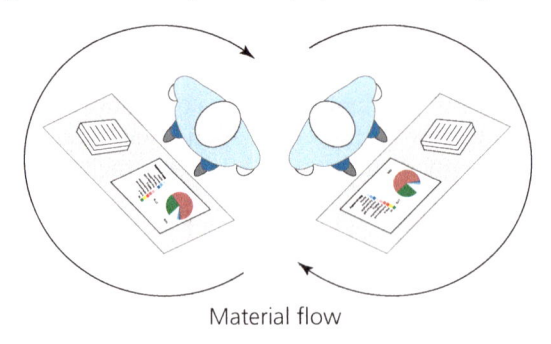

Material flow

Configuration 2: Improved layout—employees can help each other.

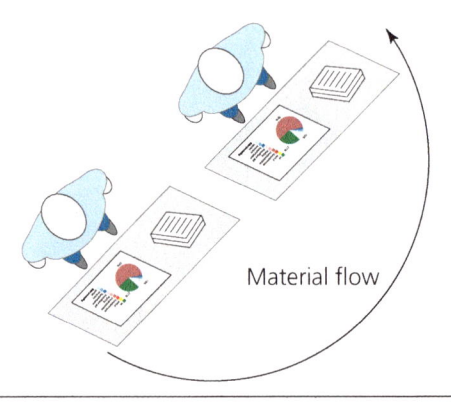

Material flow

Figure 4.12 Layout improvement 2 of 3.
Source: Adapted from Jacobs & Chase, 2008.

VISUAL MANAGEMENT

Visual management, the final component of the lean fundamentals, is a set of strategies that creates a productive work environment that reduces the likelihood of errors and delays in information (Bicheno & Holweg, 2004). Visual management focuses on the ability to communicate important information to anyone without requiring a verbal exchange between two parties. In areas with strong visual management you should be able to scan the workspace in a brief amount of time and understand the current state, including issues to address.

Visual management aims to provide an immediate understanding of a situation or condition and make waste, problems, and abnormal conditions readily apparent (Graban, 2012). There are many benefits, including to:

- Reduce confusion in completing a task
- Reduce opportunities for error and defects
- Assist in adhering to a process standard

Configuration 1: Bad layout—employees are working in a straight line, which makes it difficult to balance the workload.

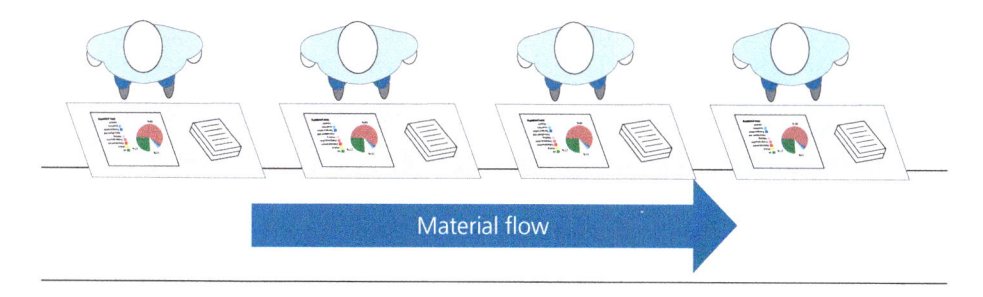

Configuration 2: Improved layout—employees are organized in a U shape, which enables them to share work and enhances flow.

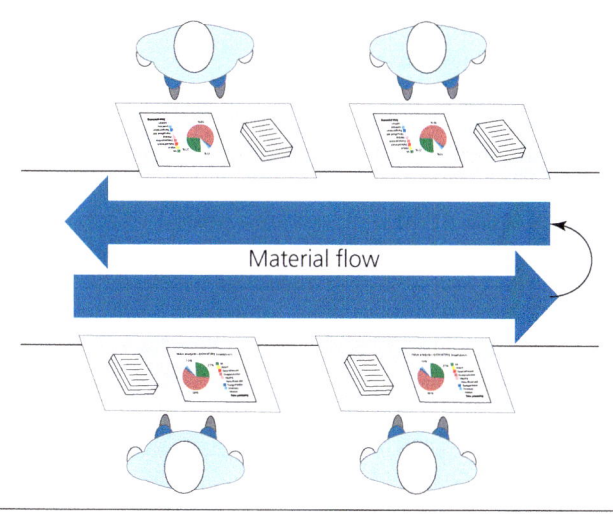

Figure 4.13 Layout improvement 3 of 3.
Source: Adapted from Jacobs & Chase, 2008.

- Improve productivity
- Improve staff/customer satisfaction

In order to create effective visual management cues (Breakthrough Management Group International):

1. Define information that needs to be available
2. Select the appropriate mechanism to communicate the information (e.g., picture, checklist, sound)
3. Determine the prompt that creates a "call to action"
4. Create the visual signal that produces the "call to action" alert

Be cautious of overutilization of visual cues. For example, alerts are a form of visual management used to communicate information without requiring a verbal exchange between individuals. The alert might mean something is wrong, a warning, or approval for something is needed. Too many alerts creates alert fatigue; people start ignoring them. This also happens with posters, flyers, signs, or other mechanisms. Too many visual cues leads to "noise" that ultimately blends into the work setting.

In workspaces without visual management, staff tends to ask a lot of questions. Some of the questions repeated throughout the course of the workday suggest required information is consistently unavailable. Examples of such questions include the following (Graban, 2012):

- Does the patient have any more tests, or can he or she go home?
- Have these medications been double-checked?
- Which patient should be brought back next?
- Who is the physician for this patient?
- Is this room available?

The Clinical Lab utilized visual management to communicate the status of lab specimens (Figure 4.14). Tubes placed in the red section are STAT or urgent, tubes in the green section are normal/no rush, and tubes in the yellow row require more information before processing. This simple approach taken by the lab enables the employees to prioritize work as it arrives and reduces the need to look up every tube specimen to determine its status as either STAT, normal, or requires additional information.

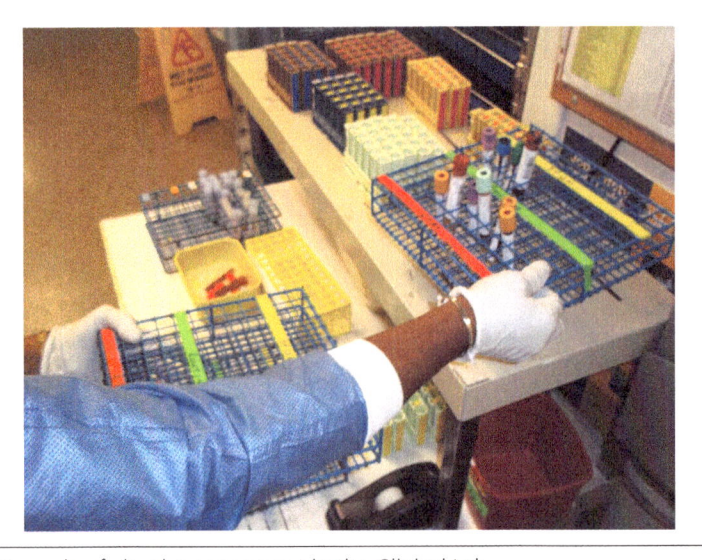

Figure 4.14 Example of visual management in the Clinical Lab.

Case Study: Patient Flow in the Patient Testing Center

The application of 5S for process improvement was tested as a case study. A team of lean leaders was assigned a project to analyze and improve the pre-admission testing (PAT) processes. PAT is a vital part in perioperative flow, responsible for screening scheduled patients prior to surgery. Patient evaluation includes registration, chart preparation, evaluation by a nurse practitioner and anesthesiologist, blood draws, electrocardiogram, and an occasional chest X-ray.

Delays in PAT patient processing cause bottlenecks and workflow inefficiencies. Streamlining patient throughput enables the PAT to effectively manage variation in its daily schedule while delivering efficient, patient-focused service. The wide degree of variation in patient flow was erratic, resulting in long delays for both patients and providers (i.e., nurse practitioners, anesthesiologists). The project objective was to improve the overall mean length of stay (LOS) by 39 minutes (from 141 minutes to 102 minutes).

On average, the PAT services nearly 60 patients every day from 7 a.m. to 4 p.m. The scope of the initiative was from patient arrival at PAT until checkout. The study design was a pre-/post-intervention assessment utilizing the 5S framework. The primary outcome measure was patient LOS.

Implementing 5S

Sort: Sort the Necessary Step Components From the Unnecessary. Remove Those Things That Do Not Add Value.

The lean team conducted several voice of customer (VOC) interviews from representatives of all roles (technicians, registrars, administration, nurse practitioners, anesthesiologists, etc.). Salient issues that came out of the VOC interviews included: (1) lack of patient and staff flow coordination; (2) insufficient cross-training; (3) duplication of effort; (4) scheduling—both how it is done and patient compliance to arriving at set time; and (5) low staff morale.

Next, the team analyzed the process utilizing multiple lean tools including the SIPOC. The process begins when a patient arrives at the PAT and ends when he/she leaves the department. The patient checks in at the front desk then sits in a waiting room. The registration clerk calls for the patient, registers him/her, then the patient returns back to the waiting room. When an exam room is available, an employee escorts the patient to the clinical area and the patient waits for an available nurse practitioner (NP) to conduct the history and physical. Then, the patient waits for the anesthesiologist interview, laboratory technician blood draw, and EKG. Upon completion of testing, the patient awaits discharge. In the process map, Clinician 1–4 indicates interactions with EKG/lab technicians, NPs, and anesthesiologists (which happen in no particular order).

A second tool used to evaluate the process in more detail is the current state swim-lane map (Figure 4.15). Through swimlane map analysis, the team identified several steps that occurred prior to the patient seeing the first clinician. Data were gathered through time study observations, in addition to collection from the information system. Each process step was evaluated and categorized as VA or NVA. After review, the PAT patient flow process VA ratio (the total VA time divided by total time) was 36%. This means nearly two-thirds of the process was NVA time for the patient.

To evaluate the distribution of NVA time, the team used the process value analysis. The result of the tool is a bar graph depicting the distribution of VA to NVA per step (Figure 4.16). The opportunity clearly lies within the first three process steps, as they are purely NVA activities (waiting accounted for nearly 50% of all NVA).

(continued)

74 Chapter Four

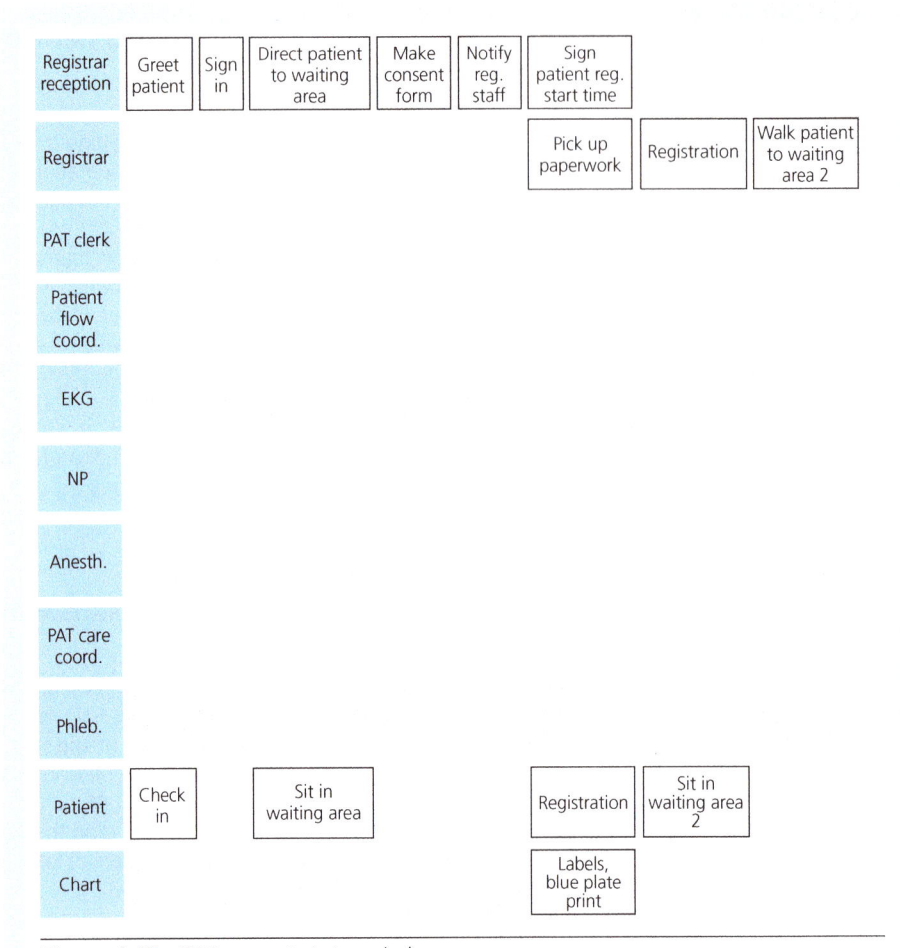

Registrar reception	Greet patient → Sign in → Direct patient to waiting area → Make consent form → Notify reg. staff → Sign patient reg. start time
Registrar	Pick up paperwork → Registration → Walk patient to waiting area 2
PAT clerk	
Patient flow coord.	
EKG	
NP	
Anesth.	
PAT care coord.	
Phleb.	
Patient	Check in → Sit in waiting area → Registration → Sit in waiting area 2
Chart	Labels, blue plate print

Figure 4.15 PTC current state swimlane map.

Data analysis shows patient volume peaking before 11 a.m., which leads to bottlenecks between 12–2 p.m. Nearly 50% of all patients arrive by 10 a.m. (first three hours of the day). Initial delays lead to subsequent bottlenecks. Additional factors reducing PAT efficiency included poor visual management throughout the clinical area. The lack of visual information reduces the ability of staff and the PAT flow coordinator to appropriately assess the current situation and allocate resources as needed.

Store: Store the Necessary Steps/Components in the Appropriate Order Based on Sequence and Timing.

The intervention component (store/shine/standardize) of the project was a team-based, three-day rapid improvement event (RIE). The RIE focused on identifying critical issues and barriers then developing and piloting high-impact solutions. The team reconstructed the current state swimlane map and identified opportunities to streamline duplicative efforts and remove NVA activities. Issues were prioritized based on impact on the primary metric of LOS. Solutions were prioritized based on impact with the aim to identify those actions that produce the highest payoff with relatively low degree of effort.

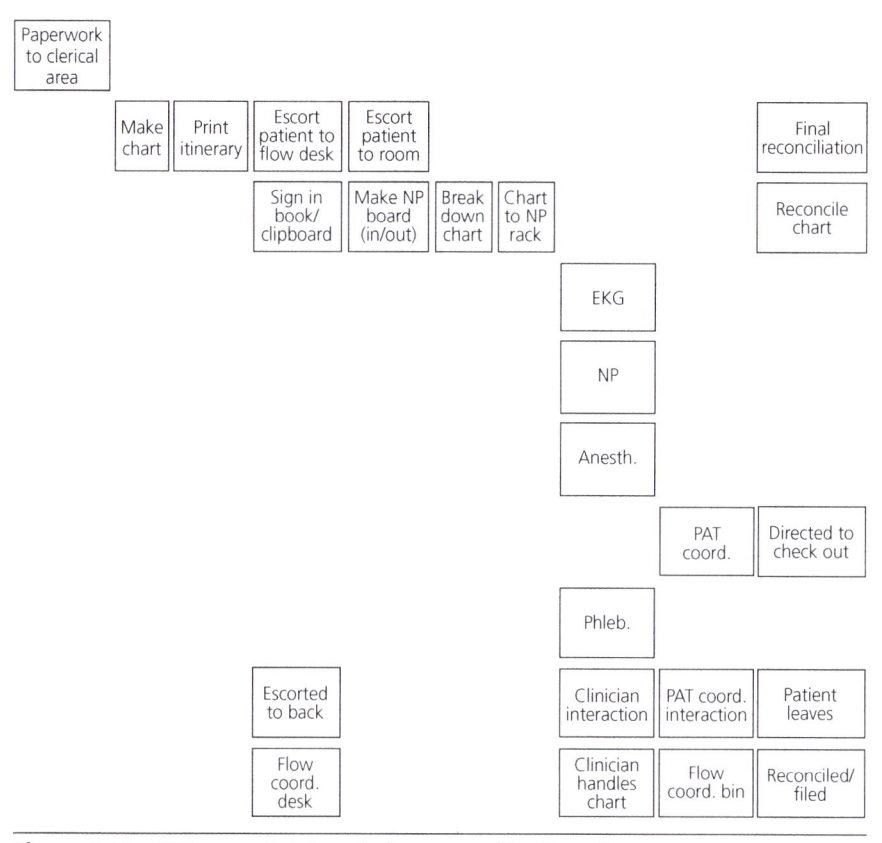

Figure 4.15 PTC current state swimlane map. *(Continued)*

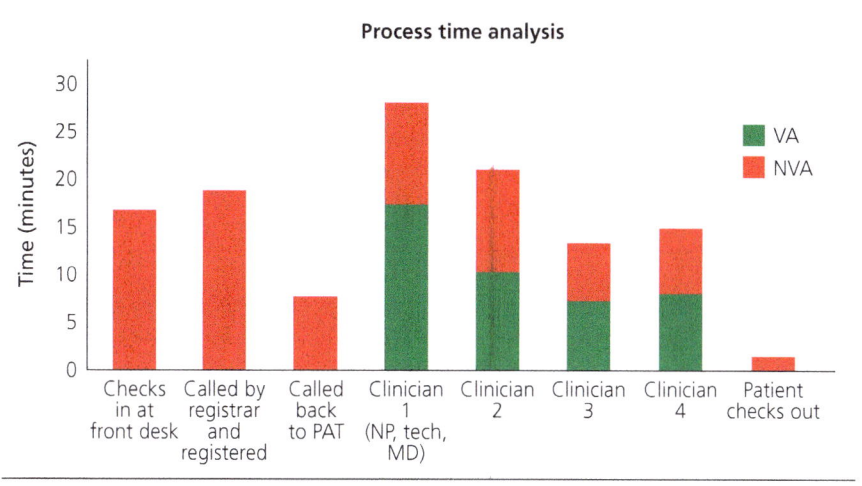

Figure 4.16 PTC current state process value analysis.

(continued)

The process was redesigned (store) using the swimlane mapping approach. The team conducted several observations of the process prior to redesigning the flow. Based on the prioritized issues and solutions, the team determined that there were opportunities to run tasks in parallel and eliminate NVA activities. As a result, the newly designed process was simulated with "mock" patients (members of the team) to assess efficacy and effectiveness.

Shine: Shine or Streamline the Step. Refine Processes (for example, Cycle Times) to Further Reduce the Impact of Non-Value-Adding Activities).

Evaluation of mock patients led to refinement of the new changes. The end process contains a reduced number of steps, bringing the patient back upon arrival, and better utilizing staff by cross-training and multi-tasking. Table 4.3 compares pre-/post-intervention processes.

Table 4.3 Pre-/post-intervention process.

Pre-intervention	Post-intervention
Patients would check in, wait in registration area, get registered, wait in PAT waiting area, and then get called to exam room.	Patient checks in, then PAT clerk escorts patient directly to exam room. This improvement eliminates two waiting rooms and brings the service to the patient, not the other way around.
Registration was completed "out front" right after check-in.	Registration takes place in the exam room. This change puts the patient in process immediately rather than waiting 10–20 minutes prior to entering the exam room. This reduces the waste of transportation as well as motion for staff.
NP only did patient history and physical, then patient waited for EKG tech and/or lab tech.	NPs do workup (including EKGs and labs). This change enables better flow of work, as patients are no longer waiting for techs to do EKG and/or lab. In addition, this better utilizes the NPs.
No visualization of PAT room/patient status.	Added whiteboard for status indicator of patient progress and staffing for PAT flow coordinator. This improvement idea alleviates the lack of visual management throughout the area. The PAT flow coordinator is better equipped to manage and coordinate resources throughout the day.
Patient checks out at front desk after examination.	Patient discharged in exam room. This further reduces waiting. In order to cue the work of staff, "registration" and "discharge" tags were added to exam room doors.

Standardize: Standardize the System/Process to all Applicable Areas (for example, Standard Operating Procedures) to Ensure Every Step Is Done the Same Way, Every Time, by Everyone.

After the RIE, final process changes were documented, along with a new swimlane map depicting new responsibilities (Figure 4.17). All employees were educated on the new process, and weekly follow-up meetings are held to evaluate progress, troubleshoot issues, and further refine improvements.

Establish the Lean Fundamentals 77

Figure 4.17 Redesigned process swimlane map.

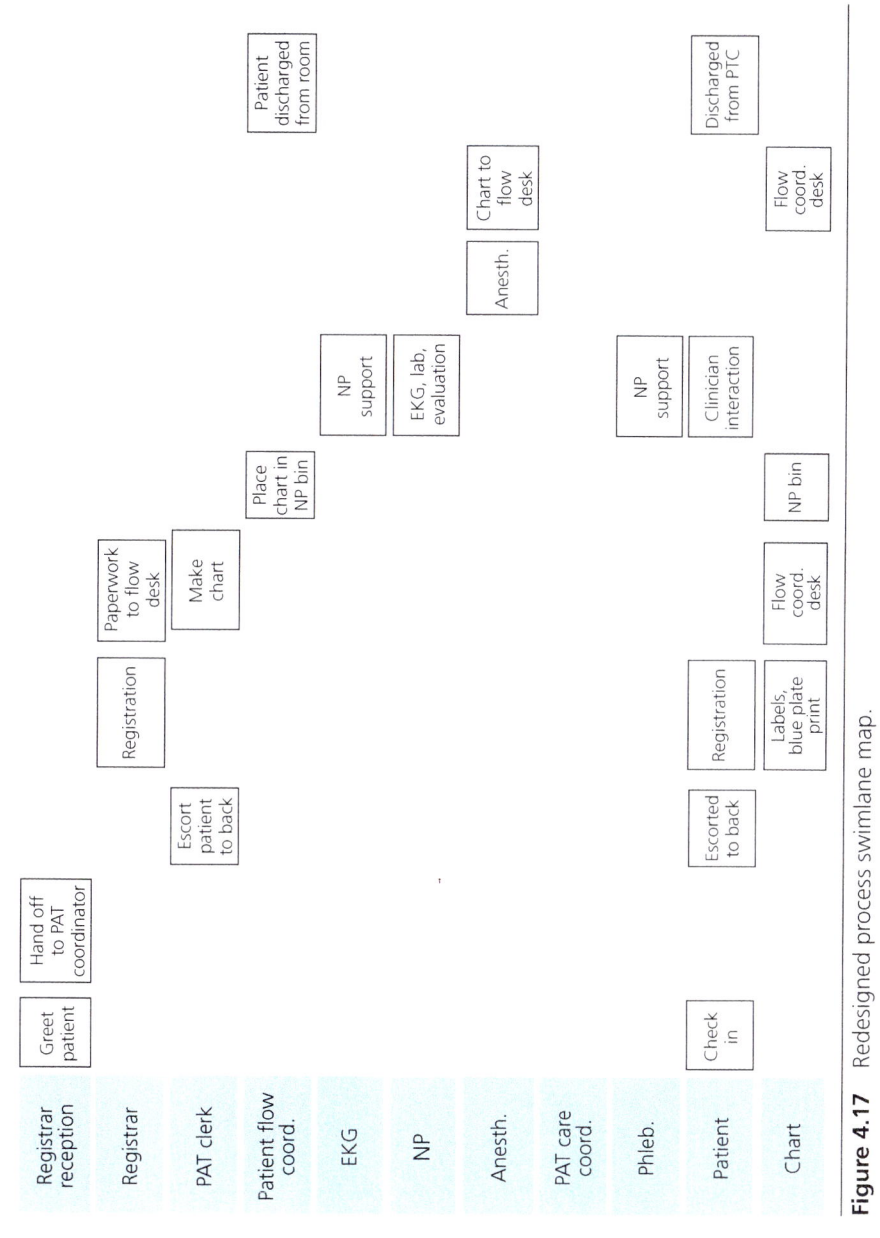

(continued)

78 Chapter Four

Sustain: Sustain the Improvement Through Discipline and Follow-Up. Monitor Key Performance Indicators to Track Outcomes and Employ Audits to Ensure Compliance.

In order to assure sustainability, LOS data continue to be monitored and the PAT process will undergo re-evaluation and iterative improvements every few months.

Results

Reducing or eliminating steps that do not add value lessens the time patients spend in the process. Figure 4.18 depicts the weekly length of stay pre-/post-intervention. During the pre-intervention time period, the PAT achieved its daily target of a 90-minute average LOS 4.29% of the time. Post-intervention, the target was exceeded 35.0% of the time, marking a 715.9% improvement ($p < 0.000$).

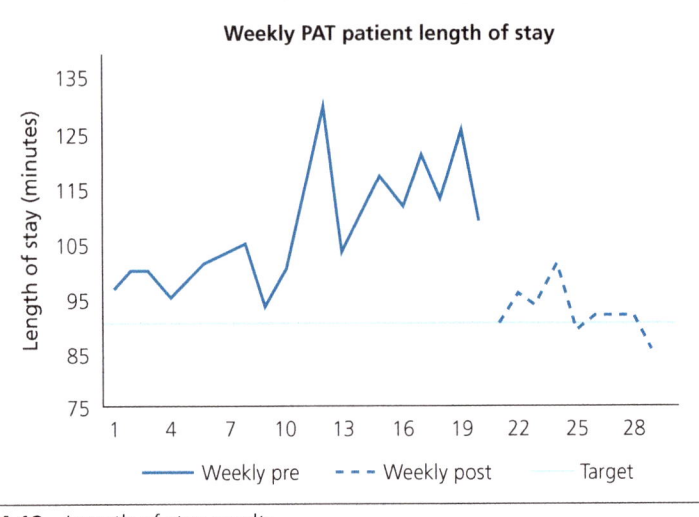

Figure 4.18 Length of stay results.

LOS by hour shows a dramatic reduction at every time interval (Figure 4.19). The new process design reduces overall process variation (pre-intervention range 36.5 minutes, standard deviation of 10.23; post-intervention range 17.02 minutes, standard deviation 4.7). A correlation analysis of volume to LOS confirms this assertion. The pre-intervention Pearson correlation of LOS and volume was 0.474 ($p = 0.000$), indicating a moderately positive relationship. Post-intervention, however, yields a Pearson correlation of 0.085 ($p = 0.604$). There is no statistically significant correlation of volume to LOS since the process is stable. Throughout the course of the day, changes in volume do not have the same impact on LOS midday in the post-intervention data. Since PAT is able to process patients more efficiently, the bottlenecks are limited.

Delays in PAT patient processing led to compounding workflow interruptions, creating inefficiencies and negatively impacting patient satisfaction. Through the use of lean thinking and the 5S framework, the team of lean leaders and PAT staff streamlined patient throughput (Figure 4.20). The result was the ability for PAT to effectively manage arrival and volume variation in its daily schedule.

Crucial to successful implementation of the 5S framework was the inclusion of process experts from PAT. The multidisciplinary team led the store phase of the project (solution development and subsequent pilots). Their active involvement enabled the entire team to garner support from PAT staff not directly participating in the RIE. Staff buy-in is an

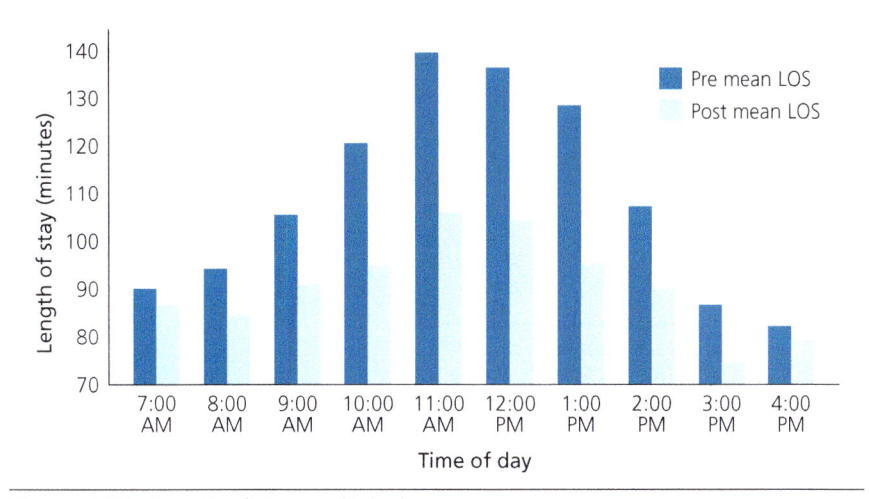

Figure 4.19 Length of stay results by hour.

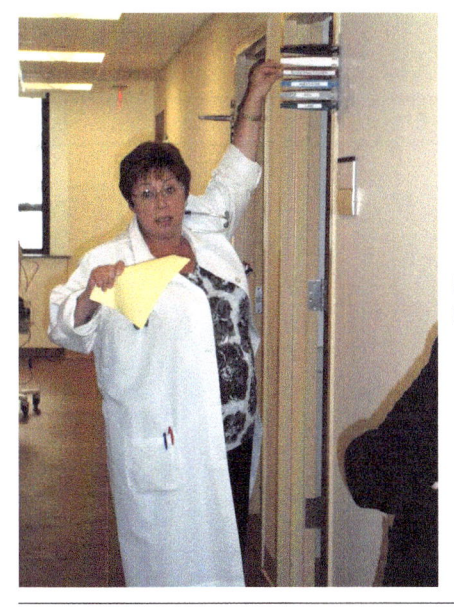

Example of visual clues implemented to notify physicians of exam room/patient status.

Figure 4.20 PTC visual management example.

essential element to success. Consistent two-way communication by the lean team and PAT leadership before, during, and after the intervention increased employee engagement through solicitation of ideas and discussions regarding challenges.

The improvement ideas developed over the three-day effort were not earth-shattering innovations. The application of lean thinking in process assessment and use of 5S as a framework for improvement generally lead to straightforward solutions. Despite the relative simplicity of countermeasures, their impact is significant.

Source: Modified from "Everything Is 5S: A Simple yet Powerful Lean Improvement Approach Applied in a Preadmission Testing Center" (Delisle & Freiberg, 2014)

80 Chapter Four

By following a systematic lean approach and applying it to healthcare processes, improvement teams can realize dramatic results in a relatively short period of time (Figure 4.21). The lean fundamentals serve as the foundation for improvement. The DOWNTIME waste matrix provides the corresponding countermeasures for the specific wastes. For many of the wastes, 5S, layout, and visual management are ways to remediate or eliminate them.

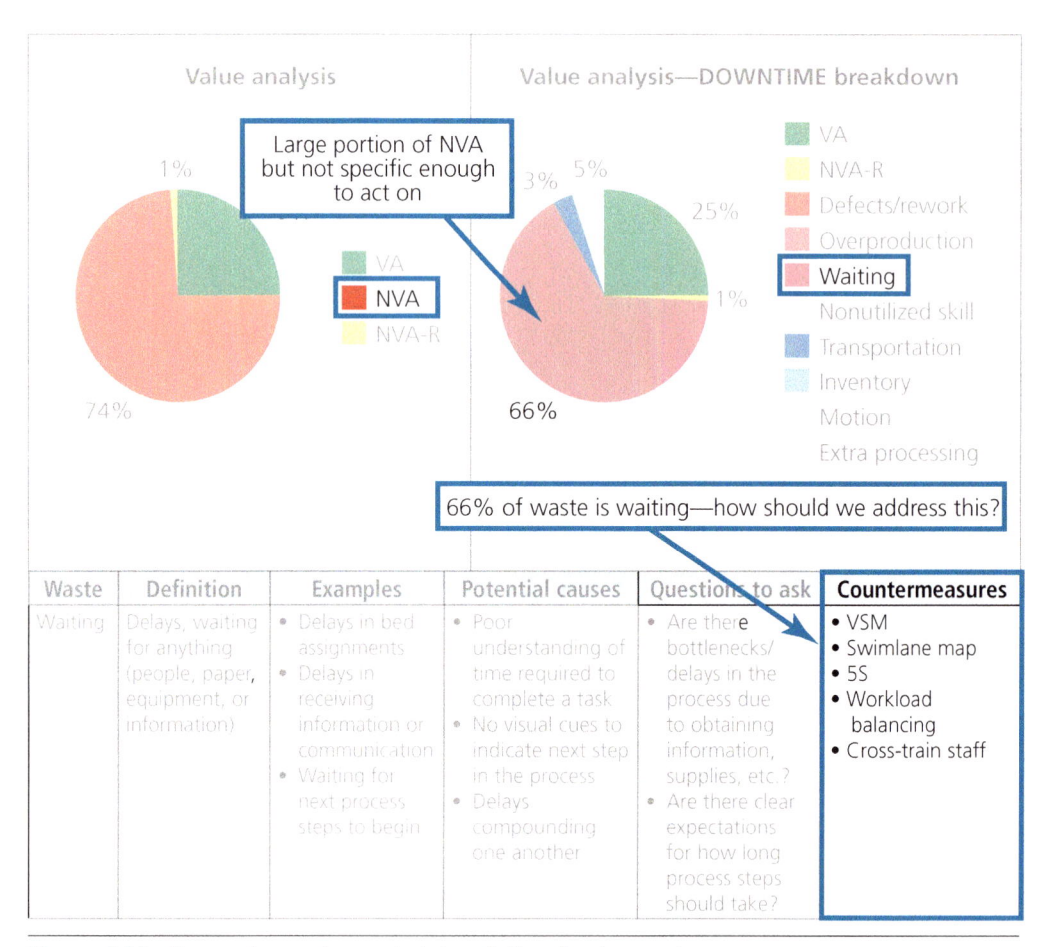

Waste	Definition	Examples	Potential causes	Questions to ask	Countermeasures
Waiting	Delays, waiting for anything (people, paper, equipment, or information)	• Delays in bed assignments • Delays in receiving information or communication • Waiting for next process steps to begin	• Poor understanding of time required to complete a task • No visual cues to indicate next step in the process • Delays compounding one another	• Are there bottlenecks/delays in the process due to obtaining information, supplies, etc.? • Are there clear expectations for how long process steps should take?	• VSM • Swimlane map • 5S • Workload balancing • Cross-train staff

Figure 4.21 Process from value analysis to solution development.

CHAPTER CHALLENGE

Identify a process or physical area in which to apply the lean fundamentals. Work with staff through the 5S framework. What were the main barriers or reasons for the disorganization? What were the main improvements made? Is the change sustainable? Why or why not?

BONUS CHALLENGE

5S your work e-mail using the triage process provided.

QUESTIONS

1. Why are 5S, layout, and visual management considered fundamental?
2. Why is "Everything 5S"? What are examples of areas/processes where you can apply the 5S approach?
3. What is the potential impact of unorganized electronic information (e.g., e-mail, computer hard drive)?
4. How does layout contribute to process flow?
5. What happens in an area with limited or no visual management?
6. What are common questions you hear or ask in your area on a daily basis? Would visual management address these questions?
7. What visual management tools exist in your work setting?

Chapter 5
Principle #3: Establish Flow

The fastest way around is through.

—Dennis R. Delisle

The third principle of lean is establishing flow (Figure 5.1). The goal is to reduce disruption of VA activity by identifying and eliminating waste and sources of unevenness. The three components of flow (determine customer demand, balance the process, and standardize the work) provide a stable,

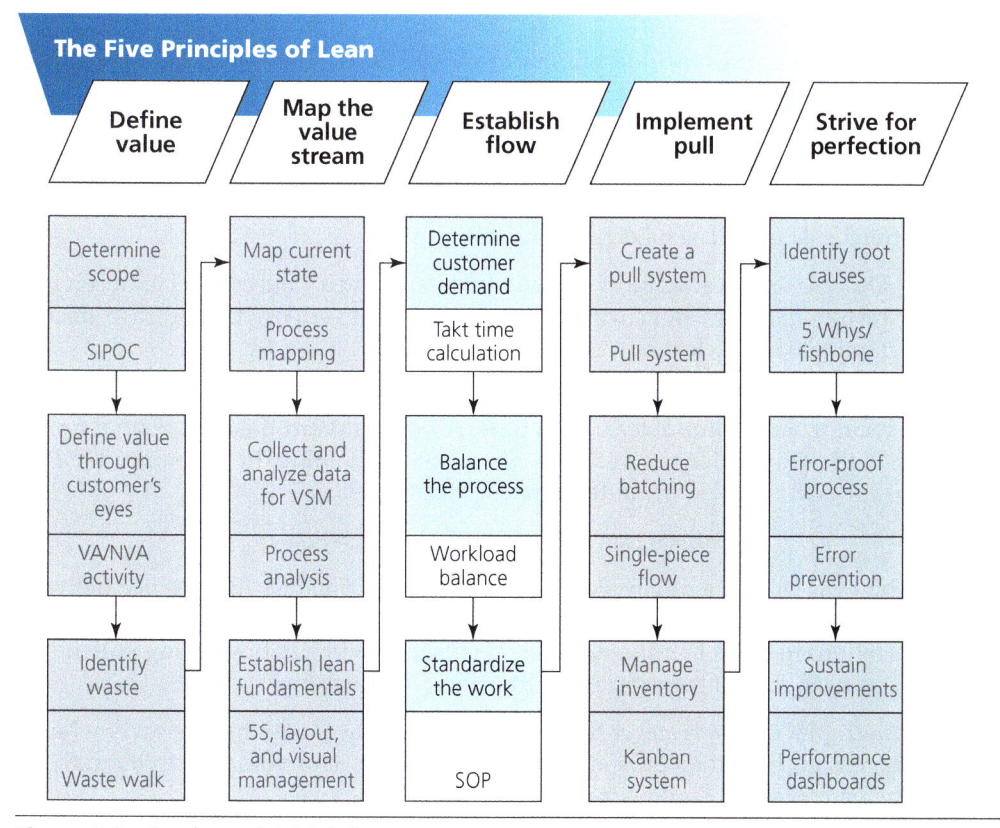

Figure 5.1 Roadmap: Establish flow.

predictable process. Flow is a critical lean management approach, highlighting the significance of doing things correctly the first time. This concept is something most managers do not recognize or promote (Womack, 2011). Unevenness and overburdening of processes create excessive waste throughout the system. Variation in processing times, customer demand, and work responsibilities leads to an unstable process filled with NVA activity.

Continuous flow results in more VA than NVA activity (Liker, 2004). In continuous flow, the people, products, and information move along the process with limited waiting and interruptions. The concept of flow derived from the Ford River Rogue Plant, where the assembly line was famously started (Chalice, 2007). In healthcare, there are many different types of flow, for example (Graban, 2012):

1. *Patients:* The patient's journey spans the care continuum from outpatient to acute to post-discharge care. Flow is internal within an organization (e.g., ED to ICU) or external between organizations (e.g., transfer from community hospital to academic medical center).

   – Other examples include patient flow in the ED, OR, outpatient physician office, and oncology infusion center.

2. *Staff:* Employees move within and across departments as part of their workflow.

3. *Information:* Whether verbal, electronic, or hard copy, information flows among people, departments, and organizations.

   – Other examples include human resources transactions, finance department processes, and information systems processes.

4. *Supplies/equipment:* The components needed to perform the workflow throughout a department and organization. The flow of supplies and equipment can include medications, lab specimens, and wheelchairs and stretchers, as well as medical/surgical supplies.

   – Other examples include clinical labs (specimen collection, lab receiving, result reporting) and surgical equipment (sterilized, used in OR case, decontaminated and cleaned).

Waiting is reduced as a result of establishing flow. From the customer's perspective, waiting is nonproductive, NVA time. A 1985 Harvard Business School report defined the implications of processes that produce waiting. In the paper, *The Psychology of Waiting Lines*, the author states (Maister, 1985):

$$\text{Satisfaction} = \text{Perception} - \text{Expectation}$$

Waiting was subsequently broken down into core principles. For service delivery organizations, those principles help identify opportunities to manage customer expectations in order to influence their satisfaction with waiting. Using patients as the customer, four of the article's eight principles follow:

1. *Unoccupied time feels longer than occupied time.* Time passes more slowly when there is nothing for a person to do while waiting. This void in activity makes the perception of waiting longer.

   – Example: a patient sits in a waiting room that does not have reading material, music, or a television.

- Strategies to address this principle: provide resources or distractions for patients while they wait. By providing magazines or even informational television shows, the time spent waiting could be seen as productive, especially if the patient is learning something related to his or her visit.

2. *Pre-process waits feel longer than in-process waits.* The time it takes before the process actually starts is unproductive. From the patient's viewpoint, nothing is happening or moving forward in the pre-process phase. The lack of forward-moving progress can create anxiety and dissatisfaction with service delivery.

    - Example: consider two scenarios: (1) a patient signs in at the physician's office front desk and then sits down and waits, and (2) a patient waits in the exam room to see the physician. The first scenario describes a pre-process wait. The patient has not entered the clinical space and therefore the process, from the patient's perspective, has not yet begun. In the second scenario the patient is in-process. By then, the patient has had his vitals taken, was interviewed by the medical assistant or nurse, and now awaits the physician. If the waiting time for each scenario was 10 minutes, the perception would be that the pre-process wait felt longer since nothing had started yet.

    - Strategies to address this principle: apply various process changes to expedite patients getting into the process. For example, immediately take patients back to the exam room (rather than sign in and wait) and complete registration in the room.

3. *Anxiety makes the wait seem longer.* When a person is anxious, time can appear to slow down. Anxiety can arise from many sources, including fear of the unknown.

    - Example: a patient is going to the hospital for a major operation. She has to wake up early, drive to the hospital, navigate the building to find registration, and then go through the presurgical preparation. She is unsure of the procedure duration, the subsequent length of stay, and the expected clinical outcome.

    - Strategies to address this principle: identify potential sources or reasons for patient (and family) anxiety. For components within your control (e.g., communicating expectations regarding the process, procedure, and expected outcomes), develop mechanisms/processes to anticipate and ease patient worrying.

4. *Unexplained waits seem longer than explained waits.* Waiting can seem infinite if the person does not know when to expect something to happen.

    - Example: after being triaged, a patient sits in the ER and waits to be called back by a clinician. The patient is not told how long that will take. To make matters worse, the patient is not updated as to when to expect service. Think about when you call a customer service representative and are put on hold. How do you feel when the representative clicks hold and all you get is an endless loop of songs without any idea how long that will go on? What if you were told the wait would be 10 minutes? Remember, Satisfaction = Perception – Expectation. If the representative returned in six minutes, you would be delighted with how quick it was. Alternatively, if you were not given a time and waited six minutes, it would seem much longer and you would not be happy.

– Strategies to address this principle: develop a communication approach (consider visual management) to notify patients of expected waits. In the example, when the customer service representative notifies you of the 10-minute wait, you are able to adjust your expectation. During the defined waiting time period you might even multitask by performing a brief activity while waiting.

Achieving flow and addressing the principles of waiting are critical in delivering VA services to customers. There are three core components to meet this end:

1. *Determine customer demand.* Know the pace or rate of demand. Serve customers more readily and nimbly by understanding the rhythm of a process.

2. *Balance the process.* Balance the workload and sync process timing with demand. Process balance is essential in optimizing resource utilization.

3. *Standardize the work.* Follow the same steps and practices to ensure a consistent outcome every time.

DETERMINE CUSTOMER DEMAND

Demand will vary depending on the process (Figure 5.2). Understanding the process rhythm enables workload balancing to maximize flow and reduce waiting. To meet this goal and create smooth flow, we need to define the demand. The term used to calculate this is *Takt time* (Figure 5.3). The objective is to match the pace of

$$\text{Takt time} = \frac{\text{Available time (minutes per working day/shift)}}{\text{Volume (daily customer demand)}}$$

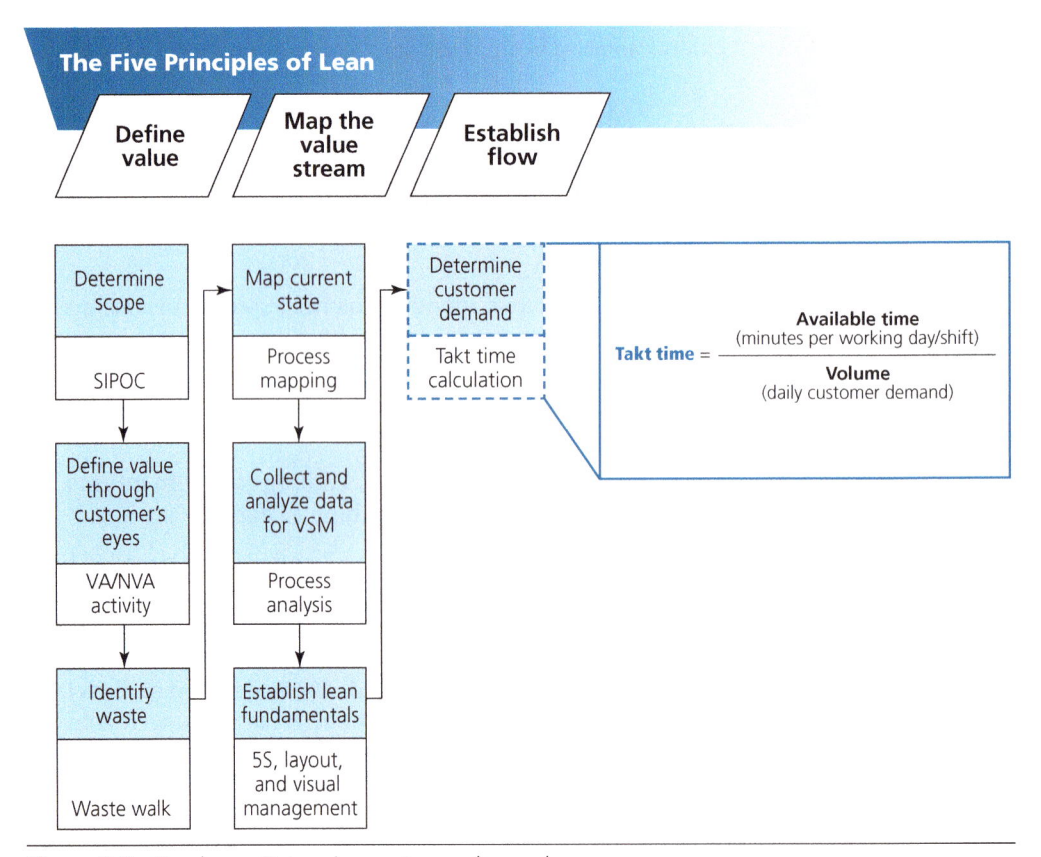

Figure 5.2 Roadmap: Determine customer demand.

$$\text{Takt time} = \frac{\text{Available time (minutes per working day/shift)}}{\text{Volume (daily customer demand)}}$$

Figure 5.3 Takt time equation.

the process to the pace of customer demand. Takt time is the rhythm of the process based on customer demand (Liker & Meier, 2006).

> Takt *is German for the beat that an orchestra conductor uses to regulate the speed at which the musicians play (Lean Enterprise Institute).*

Example of Takt Time Calculation

- Physician's office operates from 7 a.m. to 5 p.m. (with an hour for lunch).
  - Available time = Total time excluding breaks and lunch
  - Total time = 10 hours
  - Breaks and lunch = 1 hour
  - Available time = 9 hours
- Patients go through an eight-step process (from arrival to checkout)
- Average patient volume = 30 per day

What is the Takt time?

- Takt time = (9 hrs. * 60 mins.)/30 = 540/30 = 18 mins./patient

Interpretation of results: In order to keep pace with demand, complete each process step within 18 minutes.

> Note: Unevenness in demand occurs naturally. However, most imbalances result from our own scheduling approach, policies, and other decisions that drive variability. Patient arrival is challenging because it is an important component out of our control. The best way to address demand variation is to appropriately inform and prepare patients prior to arrival as well as design a process capable of managing variation.

BALANCE THE PROCESS

Once customer demand is determined, process balancing follows (Figure 5.4). The goal is to balance and equalize the amount of time required to complete each process step. The duration should be in sync with the Takt time. A balanced process ensures the ability to meet customer demand based on the Takt time rate (Liker & Meier, 2006).

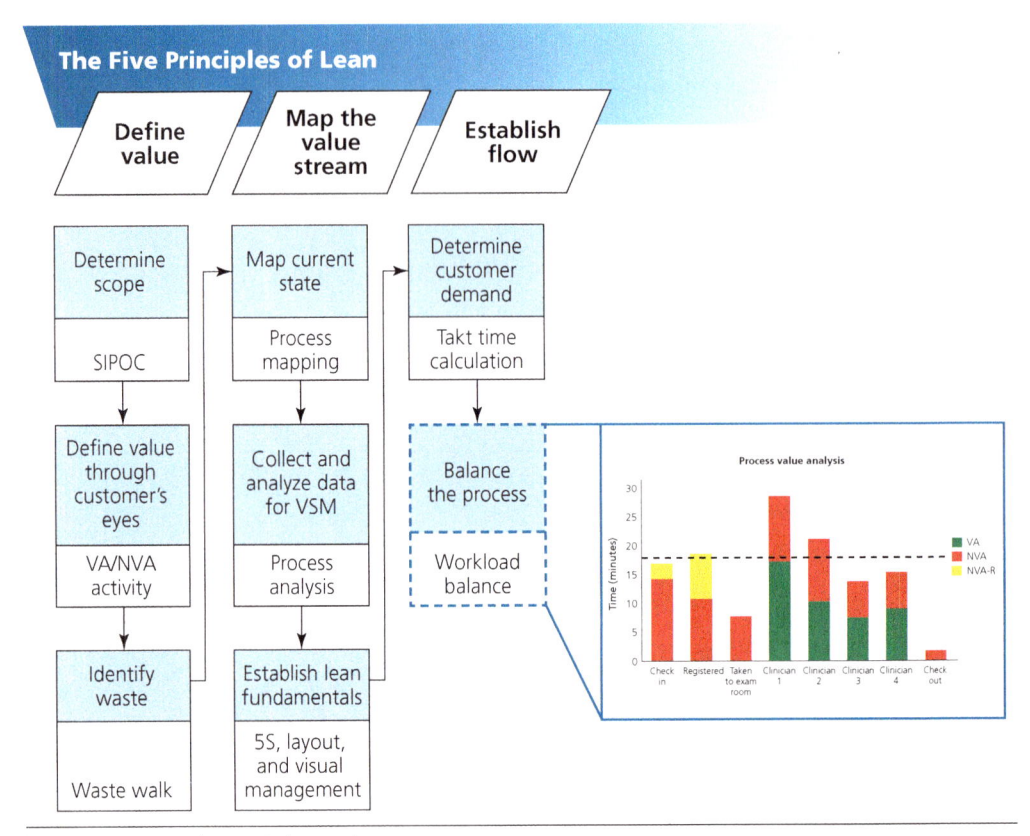

Figure 5.4 Roadmap: Balance the process.

Case Study: Evaluating Gastroenterology Physician's Office Visit

The best way to describe the importance and effectiveness of balancing a process is using a real-world example. Physicians' offices offer a good example of understanding demand and matching the process to meet customer needs. In the gastroenterology (GI) physician's office, patient flow was not smooth. Visits by new patients often took longer than scheduled, which had a compounding effect on subsequent delays. To improve the process, a team of lean leaders observed the physician and medical assistant workflow and matched the process times to demand.

One of the key tools used was the workload balance.

How to Determine Whether the Process Is Balanced

1. Conduct process observations and complete the process value analysis (Figure 5.5).

Process value analysis

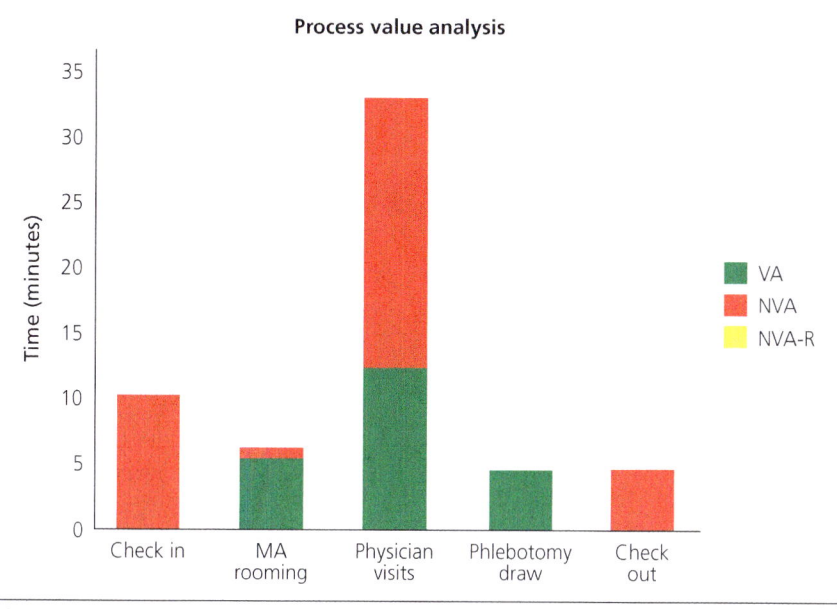

Figure 5.5 Process value analysis example.

2. Calculate Takt time.
   - The physician's office operates from 8 a.m. to 5 p.m. (with an hour for lunch).
     - Available time = Total time excluding breaks and lunch
     - Total time = 9 hours
     - Breaks and lunch = 1 hour
     - Available time = 8 hours
   - Patients go through a five-step process (from check-in to checkout)
     - Average patient volume = 30 per day
   - Takt time = (8 hrs. * 60 mins.)/30 = 480/30 = 16 mins./patient
3. Compare Takt and cycle times to create the workload balance chart (Figure 5.6).
4. Identify sources of unevenness.
   - Once the Takt time line is overlaid on the process value analysis graph, it's easy to see where the internal resources do not match up with customer demand and where the bottlenecks occur.
5. Develop countermeasures to reduce NVA activity and redistribute work in an even manner.
   - In the GI physician's office visit example, the primary issue was the third high-level step, "Physician visits." This step was associated with a large portion of waiting. To remediate, two countermeasures were implemented. First, patients change into a gown before the physician enters. This reduces the amount of time a physician waits for the patient to be ready for the exam. Previously, the physician would do a brief interview and then ask the patient to put on a gown. The physician would leave and come back after a period of time to do the full evaluation. The second countermeasure

(continued)

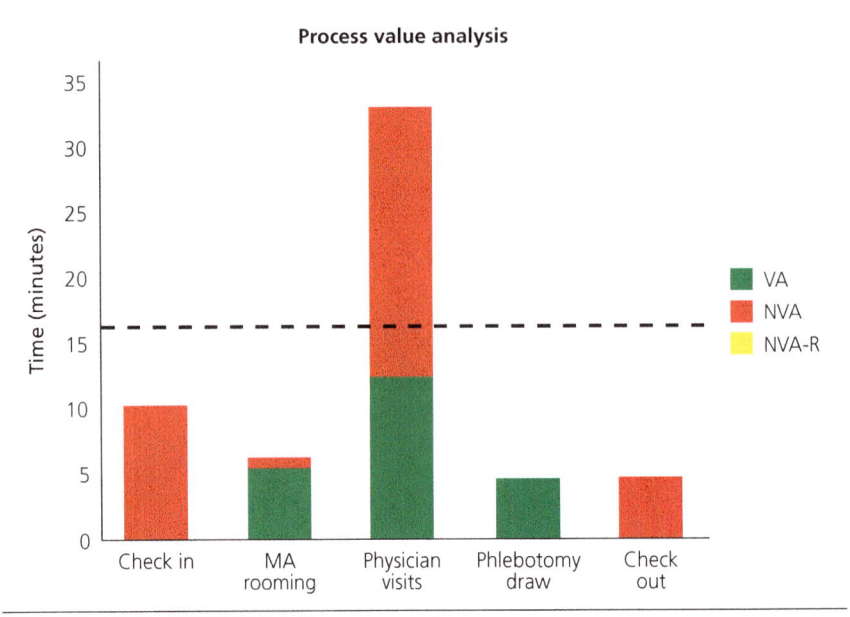

Figure 5.6 Workload balance example: Before intervention.

uses visual cues to alert the medical assistant and physician when the patient has changed into the gown. Exam room flags indicate when the patient is ready (similar to Figure 4.20).

6. Repeat step 3 post-intervention and assess opportunities for improvement.
   – The post-intervention workload balance chart shows a level process that better aligns with the Takt time line (Figure 5.7). Two of the high-level steps still exceed the Takt time line; however, the impact diminishes compared with the pre-intervention process.

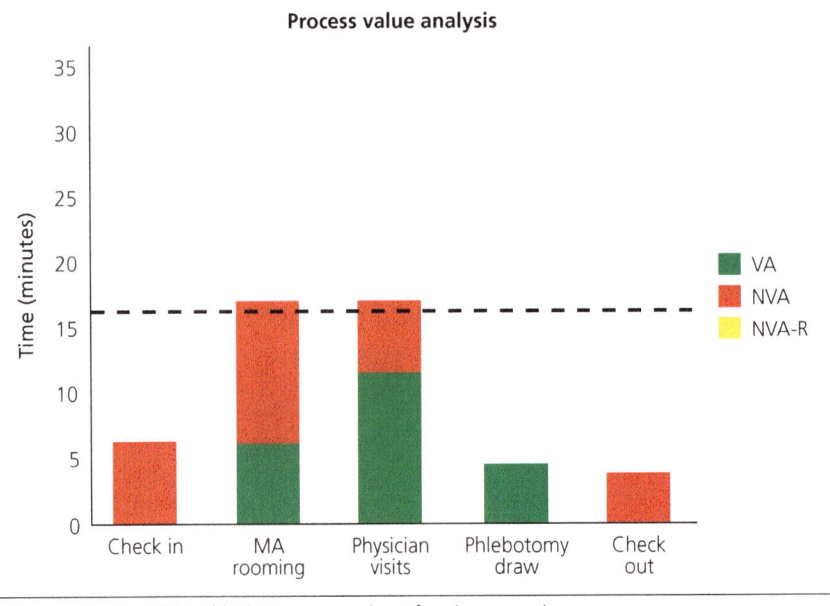

Figure 5.7 Workload balance example: After intervention.

Side-by-side comparison demonstrates the effectiveness of simple solutions leveraged by workload balancing (Figure 5.8). The end result of this effort reduced the length of new patient visits by 26.7% (from 62.5 minutes to 45.8 minutes). The physician visit portion of the process was reduced by 18.3 minutes (51%), with the proportion of VA time increasing from 34% to 69%.

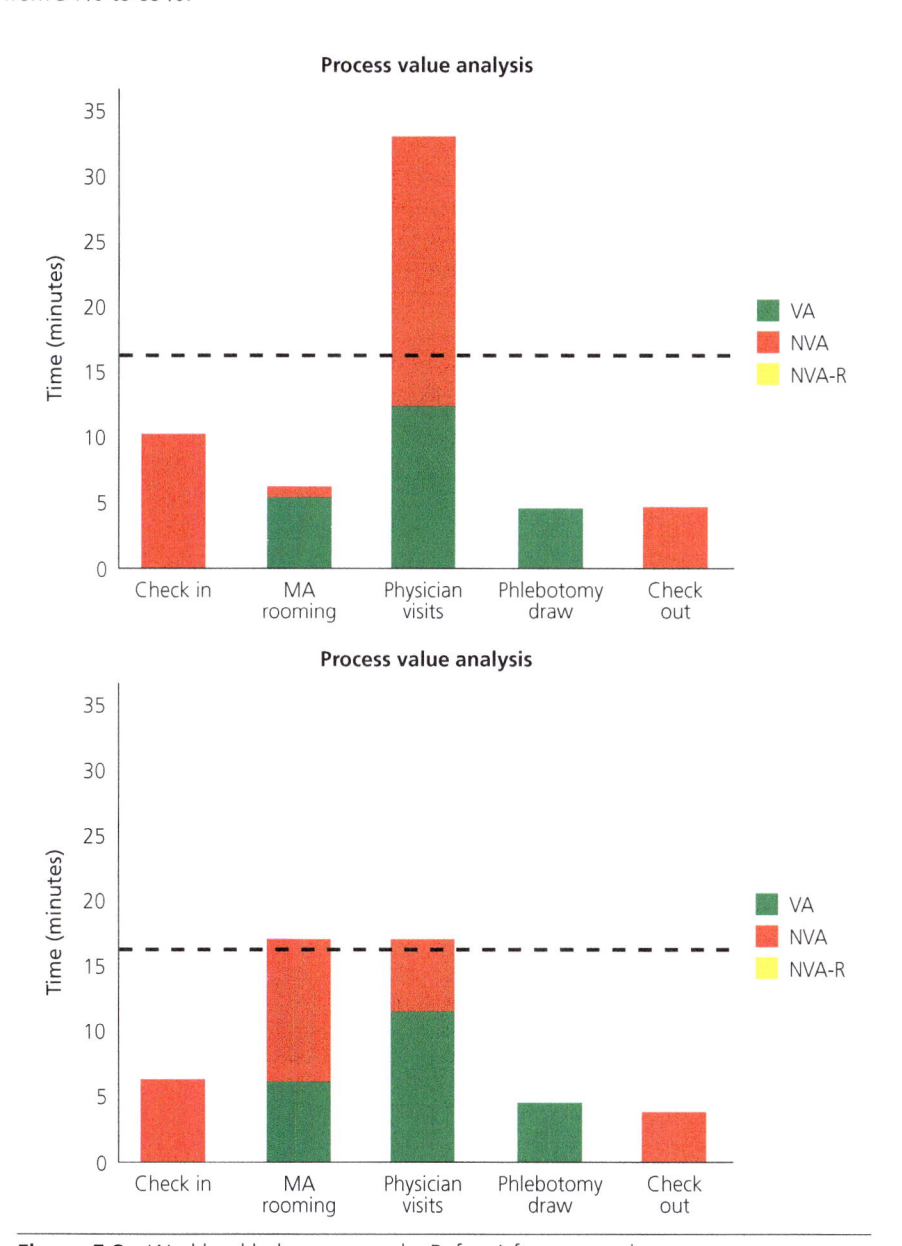

Figure 5.8 Workload balance example: Before/after comparison.

92 *Chapter Five*

Figure 5.9 describes how to analyze the workload balance chart. The Takt time depicts the expected process rhythm compared with the cycle times. When there is a mismatch between them, there are three outcomes: idle time, work-in-process (WIP), and overtime. For cycle times that are short (e.g., step 3), the person working that particular step completes his or her work at a faster rate than the subsequent step. As a result, there is an excess of WIP. In other words, the work will pile up for the person working step 4 because he or she cannot keep up with the pace of production. The person working step 3 will also have a lot of idle time because the task is quick and he or she will not have any incoming WIP.

Employees working down the line will subsequently experience a high volume of WIP and incur overtime to complete the required work. This example demonstrates the significant negative consequence of an uneven process. The goal is to create a process where the cycle times are slightly below the Takt time, creating a cushion. This results in decreased waiting, inventory, and nonutilized skill.

Redistribution or reallocation of work is an effective strategy to balance workflow (Jacobs & Chase, 2008). Ways to reallocate include combining tasks, shifting the sequence of steps, and redistributing work assignments based on quantity, duration, and complexity. It is important to note that workload balancing is not about workforce reduction but rather appropriate utilization of available human

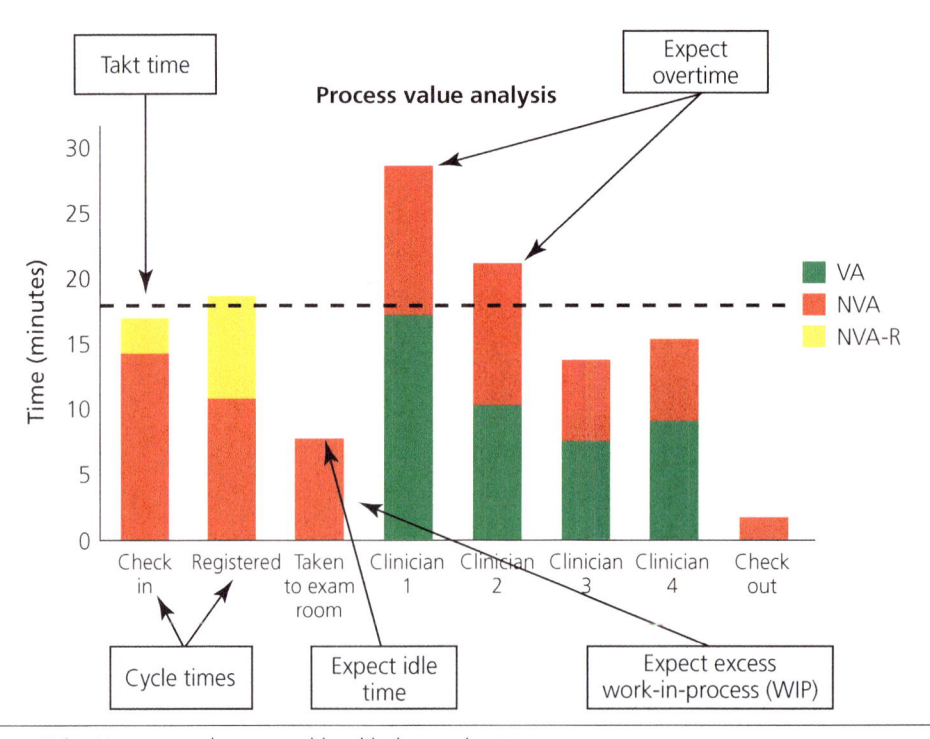

Figure 5.9 How to analyze a workload balance chart.

resources. Other methods that are effective include cross-training and standard operating procedures.

Rapid Changeover

Rapid changeover is an effective method for creating continuous flow and directly reducing the interruptions between steps (Chalice, 2007). The main emphasis is on reducing the amount of time between process steps. The best analogy for rapid changeover is a professional racing pit crew. The pit crew has one goal: service the race car effectively in as short a time as possible. Essential to this effort are preparation and a well-orchestrated plan.

> *Rapid changeover is a common tactic for ORs, inpatient beds, and exam rooms. The organization is not creating any value when these rooms are not in use. Therefore, it is essential to get the room ready for the next patient as quickly as possible.*

Efficient changeovers reduce bottlenecks, decrease overall lead time, and improve process reliability. Changeovers, going from one process step to the next, are NVA activities because they interrupt VA steps. Implementing rapid changeover involves four steps:

1. Document all process steps. List all of the tasks start to finish.

2. Segment external and internal steps. External steps are those steps that can be completed before the current process starts or after it begins. Internal steps are required to be completed between the transition. For example, you must transport the patient out of the OR before you can clean the operating table and the floor (internal). However, you can pack up the surgical equipment and begin throwing out used supplies before the patient leaves the room (external).

3. Reorganize tasks. What NVA activity can be eliminated? What internal steps can be done externally? Move everything to external steps unless it is absolutely necessary to keep them as internal steps. Through proper preparation and timing, most of the changeover can occur before the process step ends. This reduces the amount of work that needs to be completed between steps (time between steps is NVA—waiting). For example, airline flight attendants begin cleaning the cabin before the plane lands. The crew has a limited cleanup job once the plane has landed and the passengers exit. This gives them the ability to quickly prepare the plane for the next wave of passengers.

4. Improve processes by reducing NVA activity. Continuous improvement demands that all processes be consistently evaluated and refined to meet customer needs.

Case Study: Rapid Changeover in the OR

Delays in the OR cause bottlenecks and workflow inefficiencies, and negatively impact both patient and staff satisfaction. A lean team was assigned to help facilitate the reduction of OR turnover time. Streamlining the room changeover process would enable the department to effectively manage the daily schedule while delivering efficient, customer-focused service. The time interval selected was "close to cut." This means the first process step begins when the physician starts closing the surgical site of patient 1 and ends upon initiation of the subsequent case (patient 2) by way of incision.

The lean team evaluated the process through gemba walks and time study observations (Figure 5.10). The team completed the first two steps of rapid changeover with the process experts (i.e., OR nurses, technicians, nursing assistants, and managers).

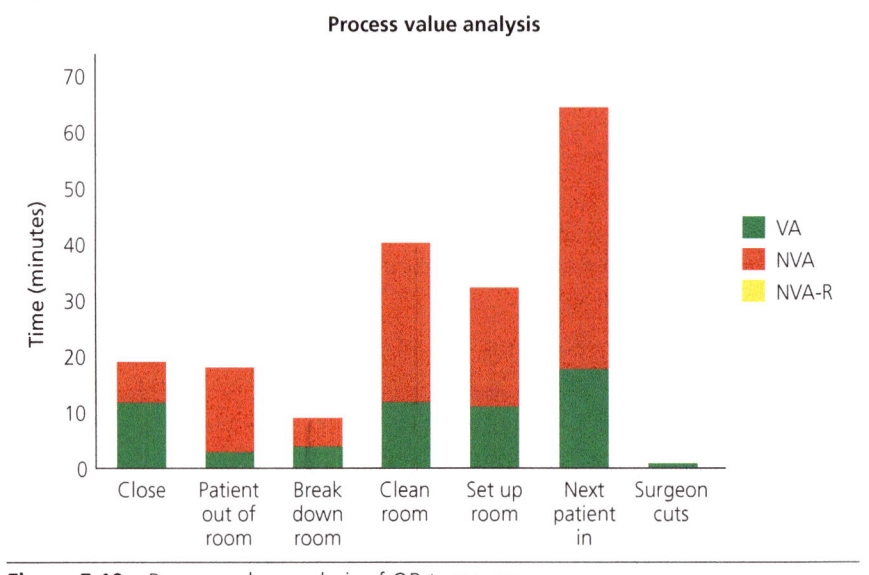

Figure 5.10 Process value analysis of OR turnover.

The process value analysis illustrates the distribution of VA and NVA activities throughout. The process was 60% NVA. The team used a swimlane map to break the process into manageable chunks (Figure 5.11).

The team identified primary issues that led to inefficient room turnovers. These issues included lack of clarity and structure (who is supposed to do what by when), limited staff availability due to scheduled breaks and staffing model, and lack of a standard process. To address these challenges the team defined specific responsibilities for each role using the swimlane map as a method to communicate. The team also developed a "Next Case Checklist" to appropriately prepare for the upcoming patient (Figure 5.12).

The countermeasures implemented led to a statistically significant improvement in turnaround time (from 48 minutes to 44 minutes, $p = .003$). The post-implementation process also demonstrated less variation, as evidenced by the standard deviation (pre-improvement 6.7, post-improvement 3.7). By stabilizing and standardizing the process, future improvement efforts will have a higher impact.

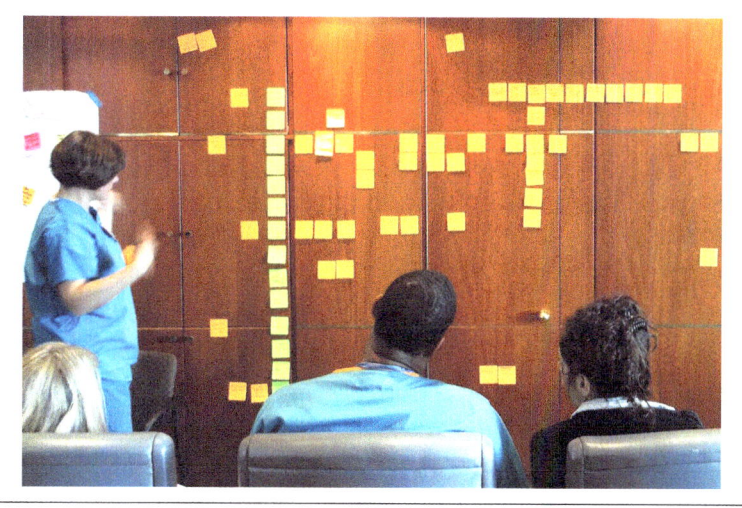

Figure 5.11 Improvement team creating a swimlane map of OR turnover.

Next Case Checklist

Bed position
____ Gel arm rolls
____ Head at bottom
____ Lateral/arm board and vac pack
____ Lateral/arm board without vac pack
____ Lithotomy/stirrups—head at bottom
____ Prone/check rolls with 3 pillows
____ Sleds
____ Supine/head at top

Equipment needed
____ Argon
____ Bair hugger
____ C arm and monitor
____ CO_2 tank
____ D&E machine
____ Doctor's specialty cart
____ Double bovie
____ EGD tower
____ Fluid warmer
____ Harmonic generator
____ Headlight and box
____ Ligasure machine
____ Nitrogen tank
____ Pediatric warmer
____ Pediatric cart
____ Sharps/recyclables exchange
____ Slave monitor
____ Universal arm board
____ Video tower
____ X-ray shield

Other:
_____
_____

Equipment to remove from room:
_____
_____

Figure 5.12 Next case checklist.

STANDARDIZE THE WORK

The last component of principle 3, establishing flow, is to standardize work (Figure 5.13). Standardized work is an approach that creates consistent processes that reduce variability (Lean Enterprise Institute). Standardized work (or standard work) is the current best way to do a process/step. It is the foundation for improvement. Lack of standard work leads to waste (primarily defects), which inhibits process capability and employee effectiveness. Without a standard in place, there is no base from which to improve (Jones & Mitchell, 2006). Improvement advice usually follows as (Mann, 2010):

1. *Stabilize:* Get the process in control. Call a time-out if necessary so you can wrap your head/arms around what is currently happening.

2. *Standardize:* Develop the current best approach and train everyone to do the same thing, everywhere, every time.

3. *Improve:* Using the standard as a baseline for improvement, refine and improve.

The process experts define standard work. To start, identify the process steps and determine the best method to perform each of them. These steps should define who does what, when. Everyone performs steps in the same way, every time

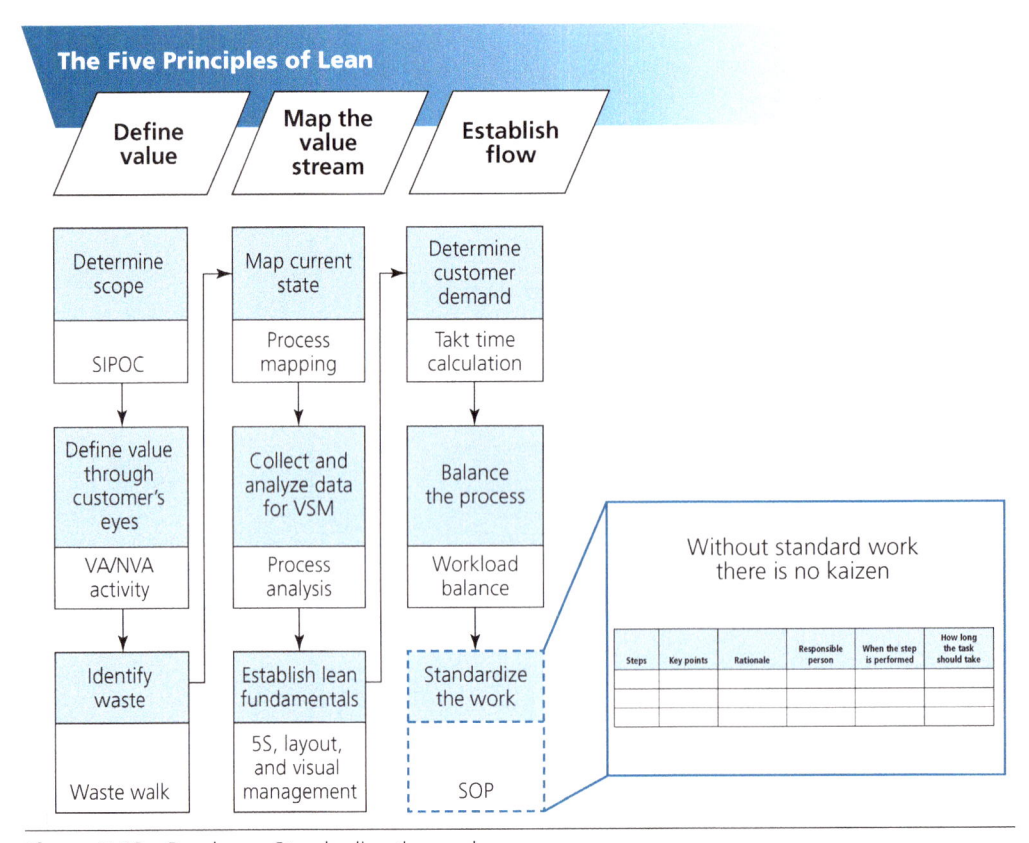

Figure 5.13 Roadmap: Standardize the work.

(Toussaint & Gerard, 2010). Standard work frees your mind of the simple tasks and processes because they are hardwired and consistent. Therefore, you have more time and energy to address anything else that comes your way.

Processes should be mostly standard (80%–95%) and only a small portion customizable (5%–20%). There are tacit activities, or those things that require a more artful approach or interpretation, that cannot be written as instructions. Standardizing care through vehicles like clinical pathways has met significant resistance over the years (Martens et al., 2014; Shortell et al., 2007). The cooking analogy works best to explain the importance and impact of standardizing tasks.

Recipes serve as the basis for creating a consistent meal. The recipe describes the ingredients and method of cooking in detail. However, there are built-in components that require an "art" or sense that cannot be articulated in a list or directions. For example, every grill or oven cooks slightly different. It is therefore important to have an understanding of the performance of the grill or oven in order to interpret instructions that say "cook for 8–12 minutes." The message is powerful. When the kitchen concept is applied to clinical pathways, it does not promote cookie-cutter medicine but rather a standard and consistent way (as demonstrated by the best clinical evidence) to do the majority of work and make the majority of the decisions while still leaving room for interpretation and latitude to diverge if indicated (Rycroft-Malone et al., 2002; Shortell, 1998).

There is some degree of stability and known variation throughout a normal workday. For the most part (perhaps 80% of the time), you get what you expect. You might encounter unique or challenging scenarios (maybe 20% of the time) in which you have to do something different. How you prepare and standardize the 80% greatly affects your capacity to effectively and efficiently address the 20%. If you do not have control around the "typical" tasks and processes (what we are calling the 80%), then everything will appear and feel chaotic.

> *There is a reason for recipes when you cook. You want to have limited variation in the outcome. You want your mother's chicken soup to taste like her chicken soup every time you make it. If you do not follow a recipe, it will taste different every time. It also is impossible to improve the dish if there is no baseline from which to refine. You can draw the same correlation to care delivery. For 65%–75% of patients, there is a standard of care that does not need to be individualized patient to patient. These steps should be standardized based on best practice and refined as appropriate. The remaining 25%–35% of the care delivery process relies on the clinical team's experience, knowledge, and so forth (the art and science of medicine). The overall goal is to reduce the unnecessary variation in outcomes by doing the same thing every time (as appropriate).*

Creating standard work requires the input of process experts. Developing standard work is straightforward.

1. *Identify problems or sources of variation.* Determine what you are trying to improve.

2. *Document the process steps in the current state.* The content experts are likely to develop the best method of completing tasks given their experience and technical expertise. Remember to look for external best practices as well.

3. *Evaluate the current state and determine which steps to eliminate.* Then, identify the steps to be standardized.

    a. For standardizing steps, use the standard work template in Table 5.1. Document the step and key points for performing it correctly. Provide a rationale for the defined best method. Identify who is doing the task, when they are doing it, and how long it should take to complete.

    b. Questions to consider when evaluating the process and building the standard include the following: What is the purpose? Where should the step be completed? How should the step be performed? Who should do it?

4. *Train and cross-train staff.*

5. *Implement.*

6. *Monitor, refine, and continuously improve.*

Standard operating procedures (SOPs), a manual, training presentations, or other methods can document standard work. The method of documentation is not as important as the fact that the documentation serves as the standard. Developing standard work should coincide with the lean fundamentals. Workspace layout and organization have a major impact on process efficiency and the ability of staff to consistently perform tasks.

Standard work is a dynamic approach to streamline processes and reduce variation. The operative word is "current best" approach. Continuous improvement aims to make things better on an iterative basis. Standard work should live through the staff and be refined periodically to ensure compliance with the current best methods. Figure 5.14 shows how standard work acts as a wedge to reduce performance regression while the next iteration of improvements drives toward the future state.

> *Without standard work there is no basis from which to improve.*

Table 5.1 Standard work template.

Steps	Key points	Rationale	Responsible person	When the step is performed	How long the task should take

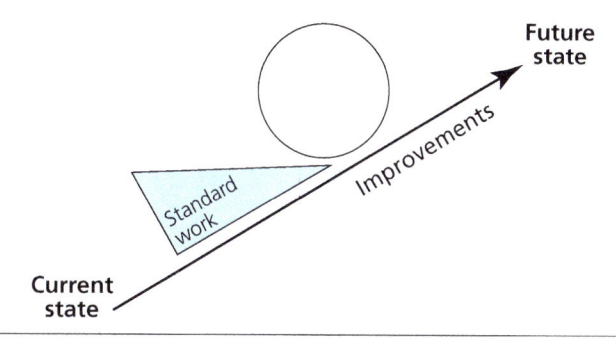

Figure 5.14 Standard work and continuous improvement.
Source: Adapted from Rother 2010.

Checklists

The "single-person" process is something encountered frequently. One could argue that a "single-person" process means there is no process. Relying on one person to do something is not systematic or sustainable. If that person wins the lottery tomorrow, does the process look entirely different for whoever takes over? If yes, no process exists. Processes that are people-dependent make sustainability essentially impossible. This also applies to employees who customize their approach to work in a way that reduces standardization and challenges sustainability. Leaders often fall victim to relying on individuals instead of designing and improving processes that maximize everyone's capabilities.

Aviation has driven the use of checklists in healthcare given the high reliability and safety within the industry (Gawande, 2009). Though at times fatiguing, a checklist provides the required reminders that could be overlooked due to the nature of human beings and their tendency to make mistakes unknowingly or unintentionally (Gawande, 2009). Checklists remove the need to remember everything that needs to be done. This frees up an individual's mind to think about the other things requiring attention.

At some point, checklists become hardwired into the tasks and are no longer necessary or are used as a reminder rather than a core checkpoint. There is a balance between the quantity of checklists and the frequency of their use, which is why reviewing their use and effectiveness periodically is critical. There is a significant difference between "checking the box" and actually doing the work. A useless checklist is a terrible waste of time.

CHAPTER CHALLENGE

Identify a process that needs to be standardized. Develop a standard operating procedure with staff in the area. What are the challenges in implementing standard work? Why do these issues/barriers exist? How can you overcome them?

QUESTIONS

1. What flows within your area (e.g., patient, specimens, paperwork)?
2. How does waiting affect the processes in your area? How are waiting expectations managed?
3. Why is it important to understand customer demand?
4. What types of waste can an uneven process produce?
5. What is the impact of an uneven process on employee productivity and morale?
6. Is there a process in your area where rapid changeover can be applied? If so, what internal tasks can be moved externally or eliminated?
7. Why do standards need to be in place before improvements can occur?
8. Are standards static or dynamic?
9. How does standard work promote creativity?
10. What are the benefits of checklists?
11. How can checklists be utilized in your area?

Chapter 6
Principle #4: Implement Pull

Simplicity is the ultimate sophistication.

—Leonardo da Vinci

Establishing flow creates smooth processes. Interruptions of VA activity are reduced or eliminated. Once flow is established, the goal becomes just-in-time production. The two principles of flow and pull are closely related (Figure 6.1). Each emphasizes the balance of resources to improve

The Five Principles of Lean

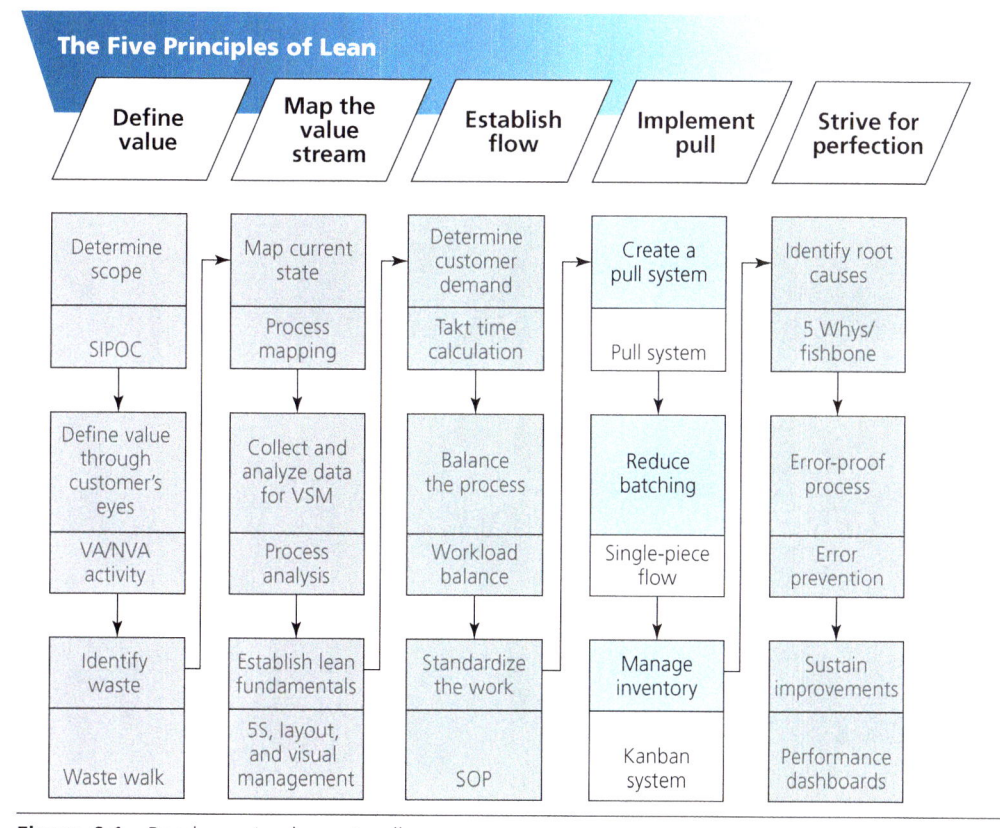

Define value	Map the value stream	Establish flow	Implement pull	Strive for perfection
Determine scope	Map current state	Determine customer demand	Create a pull system	Identify root causes
SIPOC	Process mapping	Takt time calculation	Pull system	5 Whys/ fishbone
Define value through customer's eyes	Collect and analyze data for VSM	Balance the process	Reduce batching	Error-proof process
VA/NVA activity	Process analysis	Workload balance	Single-piece flow	Error prevention
Identify waste	Establish lean fundamentals	Standardize the work	Manage inventory	Sustain improvements
Waste walk	5S, layout, and visual management	SOP	Kanban system	Performance dashboards

Figure 6.1 Roadmap: Implement pull.

throughput. Without flow, it is difficult to implement a pull system. Without a pull system, it is difficult to ensure flow and just-in-time production.

Implementing pull, especially in the healthcare environment, is challenging. From batching to inventory management, the requirement for process reliability and responsiveness is mandatory. The fourth principle of lean comprises three components: (1) create a pull system, (2) reduce batching, and (3) manage inventory. Pull highlights the right product/service in the right amount at the right time.

Sometimes it is surprising to learn what you need versus what you have. We live and work in a world of excess. In the current healthcare environment, it is becoming clear that this mentality is not sustainable. Organizations cannot afford (literally) to manage supplies haphazardly as reimbursement rates continue to decline. Unfortunately, many organizations will need to employ drastic cost-saving measures in order to reduce the impact of operational expenses.

CREATE A PULL SYSTEM

A pull system is a method of controlling and balancing the flow of resources (Liker, 2004; Tapping et al., 2009). Processes are designed to eliminate waste and unevenness while producing only what has been requested. This concept is just-in-time production (Liker & Meier, 2006). Just-in-time production emphasizes a pull approach to demand rather than the traditional push mentality (Figure 6.2).

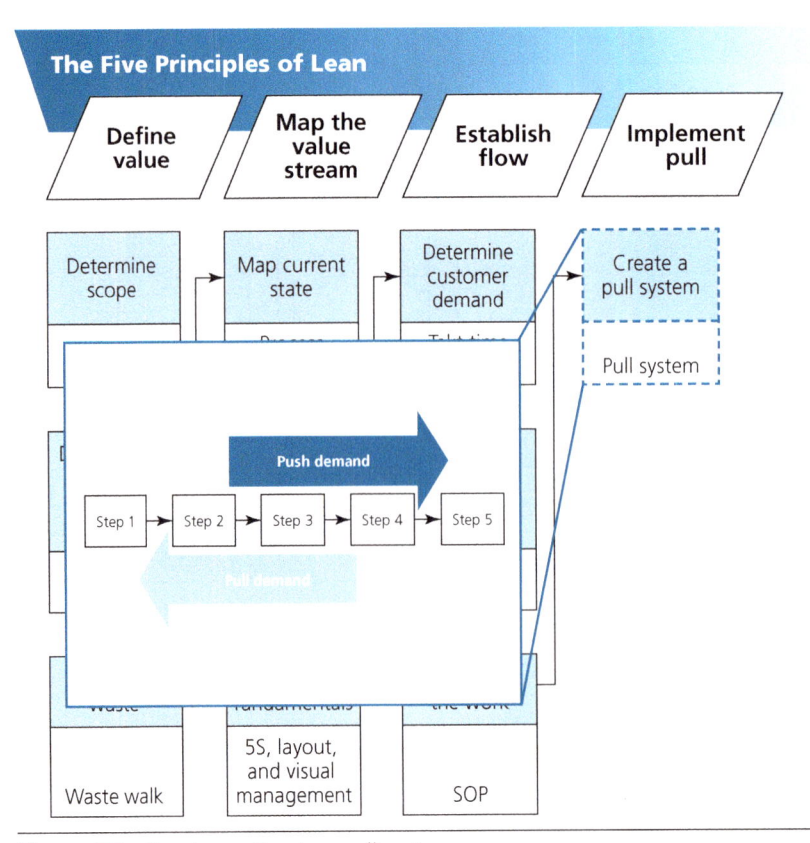

Figure 6.2 Roadmap: Create a pull system.

Push Systems

The push approach produces products/service regardless of demand (Figure 6.3) (Womack & Jones, 1996). Processes are contingent on demand forecasting. If the predicted demand is not accurate, it will lead to excess inventory and wasted resources (i.e., time, equipment, materials). These types of systems push work to employees whether or not they are ready. As a result, a significant backlog of WIP accumulates.

Take the following scenario as an example. A department is predicting its customer demand tomorrow to be 10. Based on the forecast, the employees prepare 10 boxes of supplies (represented by the blue boxes in Figure 6.4). The "day before" diagram shows the 10 boxes ready for processing. If the customer demand

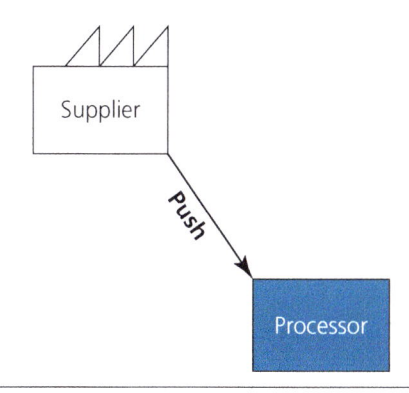

Figure 6.3 Push process.

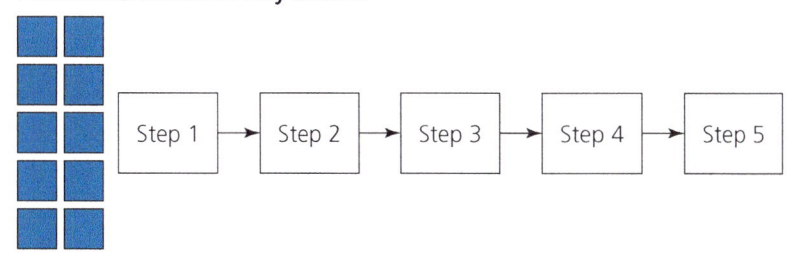

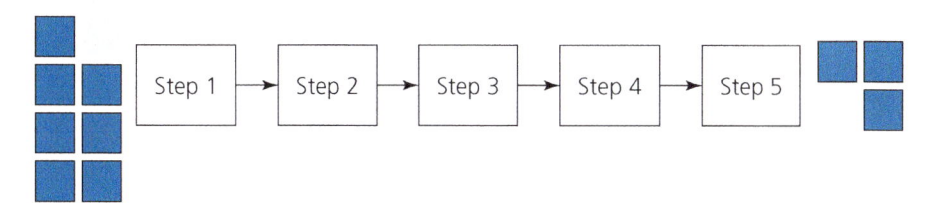

Figure 6.4 Push process example.

for the "day of" service is only 3, there is an inventory of 7 excess boxes. These supplies can be reserved for the next day's operation; however, if the supplies are perishable, they will be waste.

Similarly, evaluating push systems at the process level demonstrates the impact of WIP on productivity. Using the same example, if the system pushes all 10 boxes through regardless of demand and the employees' ability to process them, an excess of WIP will build. Figure 6.5 demonstrates what happens when all 10 boxes are pushed to step 1. If step 2 takes a longer time for processing, the WIP will pile up here, thus creating a bottleneck. In this push system, the uneven workload interrupts flow.

Pull Systems

In contrast to the push system, a pull system balances resources and workflow (Lean Enterprise Institute). Demand or a request initiates the process. Demand is upstream rather than the downstream push effect (Figure 6.6). A pull system aims to improve flow through limiting interruptions caused by overloading and uneven distribution of work.

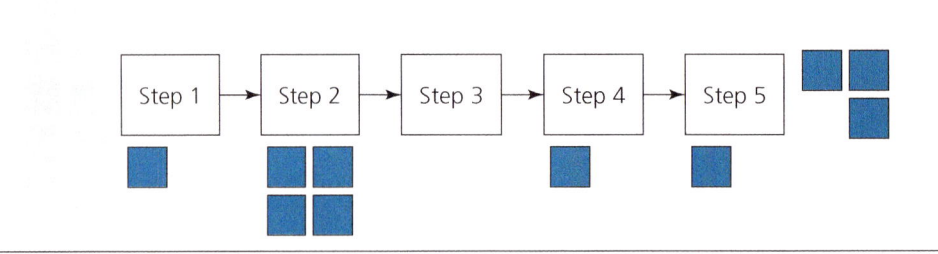

Figure 6.5 Push process example: WIP.

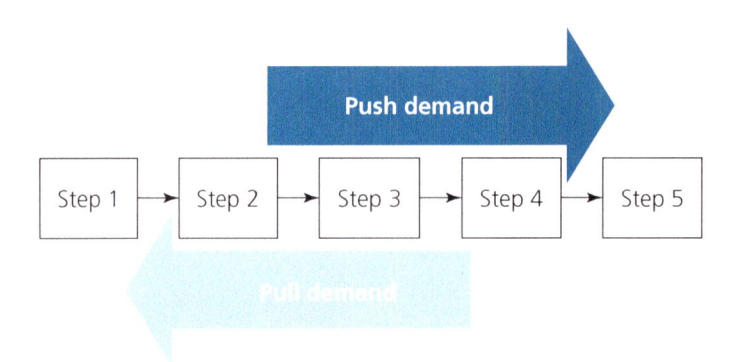

Figure 6.6 Push versus pull.

Pull system examples include inpatient nursing units pulling patients from the ED or departments utilizing par levels to manage supplies (Figure 6.7). Vending machines are another example of common pull systems.

Figure 6.8 illustrates how pull systems work. Diagram A shows an inventory of 10 boxes ready for processing. In the pull system, the inventory level is determined by historical demand, the time from order to replenishment, and a buffer to ensure required resource availability. Once the first product is requested (Diagram B), one box is processed through all five steps. Additionally, one box remains at each step, ready to be pulled through the process upon the second request.

Diagrams C and D show what happens once the second box is requested. At step 5, the box is finished and delivered to the customer. There is an empty slot now at step 5. In order to replenish, the employee in step 5 pulls the resource from step 4. The cascading effect continues as step 4 pulls the box from step 3, and so on. Step 1 will then pull a new, unprocessed box of supplies from the inventory. By each step having a box ready to pull from the subsequent step, the process is highly responsive to demand and reduces the throughput time. In this scenario, customer demand pulls the product through the process.

The example shows WIP throughout the process. For inventory management within a lean system, the goal is not zero inventory but rather a process that reduces disruption of flow caused by lack of available resources when needed. It is important to control WIP based on the signaling cue to pull as well as the initial supply for step 1. Flow will be smooth and consistent if inventory and processing are managed effectively. Processes that push demand through steps produce bottlenecks and delays. Similarly, processes that do not have steps ready for just-in-time production are not reaching their potential. Pull enables maximal throughput by positioning every step to perform what is requested, at that time, in the specified amount necessary. In other words, work entering a process step initiates once work exits that step. The approach is simple in explanation but difficult to implement. The next two sections discuss strategies and tools to enable flow and efficient use of resources.

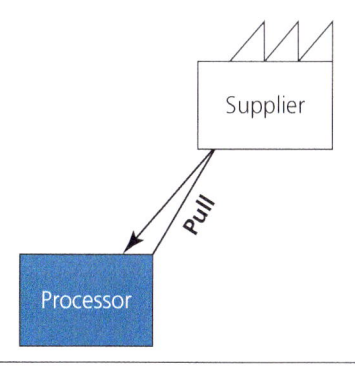

Figure 6.7 Pull process.

106 *Chapter Six*

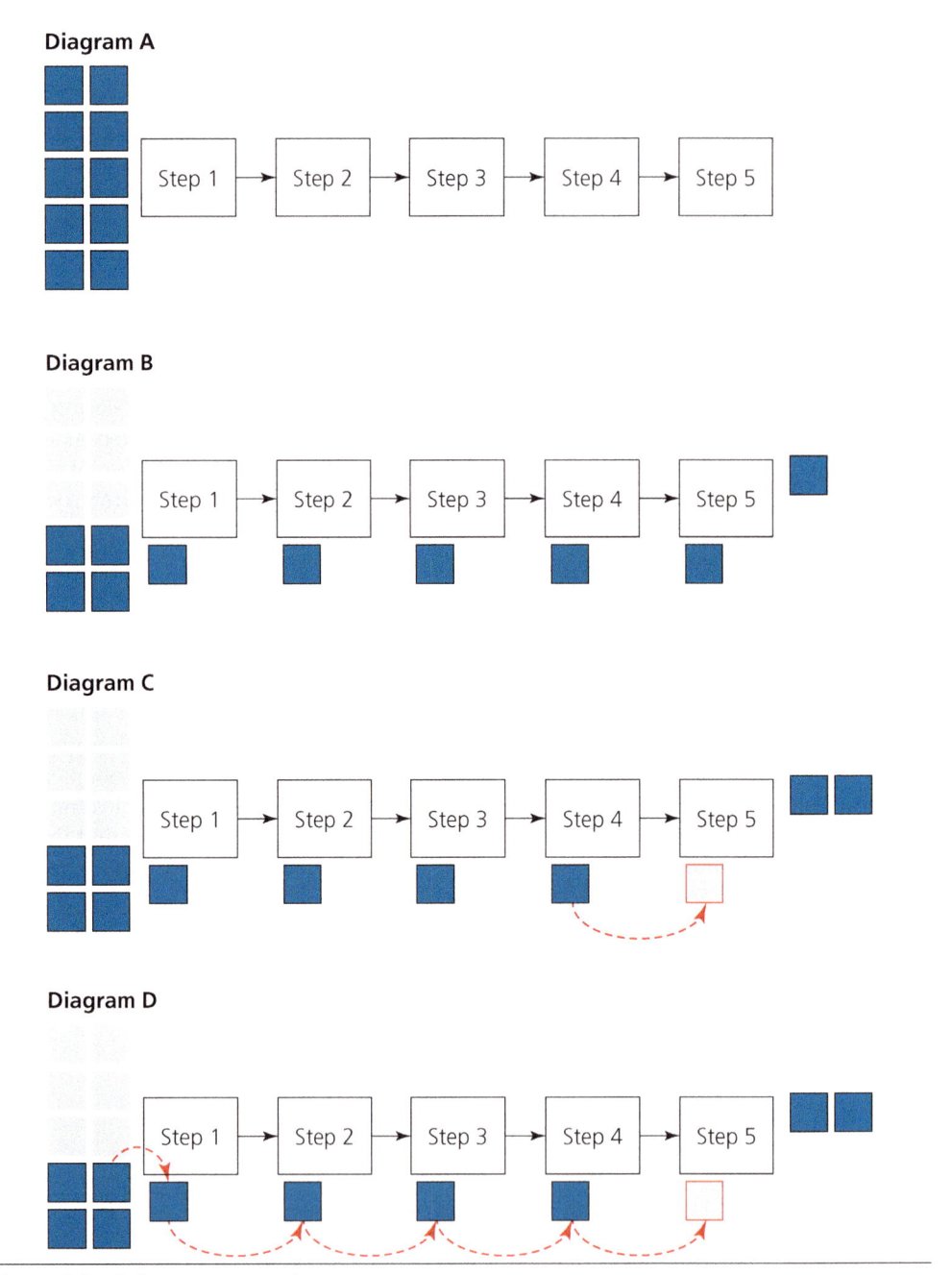

Diagram A

Diagram B

Diagram C

Diagram D

Figure 6.8 Pull process example.

Case Study: Patient Transportation

A team of lean leaders utilized the pull system approach to improve the patient transportation process. Transport request delays, cancellations, and rescheduling have a negative systemic effect on patient flow. The project focused on inpatient nursing unit transportation requests. Due to the high volume of transportation requests, the need for an efficient process is critical in ensuring high-quality and timely care, as well as promoting patient and employee satisfaction through reliable service. The overall project objective was to reduce the number of pickup delays, cancellations, and transportation rescheduling requests.

The team worked with key stakeholders (i.e., nurses, unit clerks, transportation aides, and management) to identify the root causes and develop targeted solutions. The main issue was a push approach to transportation. A unit would request a transportation aide (e.g., send patient to radiology for MRI). The transport aide was dispatched to the unit without any notification to the unit (a push). As a result, the patient and/or clinical staff were not ready for transportation, causing delays and cancellations. The team devised a pilot to test a transportation aide pull system in order to address these issues.

Upon transportation request confirmation, the requesting nursing unit would receive a call notifying when the transport aide would arrive on the floor. This provided unit staff time to prepare the patient or cancel the request prior to the transport aide arriving. If the patient or staff were not ready, the dispatcher notified the transport aide prior to his or her arrival on the unit, reducing the possibility of delaying subsequent assignments.

The pull system created improved communication between departments and ensured services provision when ready. As a result, the overall percentage of successful transfers increased from pre-pilot 54.8% to post-pilot 89.6% (Table 6.1). The two pilot units experienced a large uptick in successful transportation requests. The pilot debrief revealed lessons learned:

- Coordination and communication can significantly reduce waste, delays, cancellations, and reschedules.
- Inbound information provided to the nursing unit allows more timely service to patients and internal customers.

Table 6.1 Transportation pilot results.

	Successful request before	Successful request after
Pilot Unit 1	51.1%	95.1%
Pilot Unit 2	60.3%	83.3%
Combined	54.8%	89.6%

REDUCE BATCHING

Establishing flow is a challenge. The just-in-time mentality is not always embraced in healthcare, so shifting from batching to single-piece flow is difficult, but doable. There are two ways in which products or services are processed: batching or single-piece flow (Figure 6.9). Batching emphasizes processing large amounts/quantities of the same item at a time (e.g., elevators batch individuals, fill up before moving to next floor) (Liker, 2004). Alternatively, single-piece flow focuses on processing items based on customer demand. Single-piece flow provides the customer what they want, when they want it, and in the right amount (Womack & Jones, 2005). Escalators, unlike elevators, operate in a single-piece flow transporting individuals up and down floors continually rather than doing batch runs.

Batching interrupts VA steps. The result is elongated throughput times and delays. Batching processes also make it difficult to detect issues at the time of occurrence. In a batching process, a defect is not easily or quickly identifiable since there can be long times between the start and completion of the batch. Single-piece flow enables rapid identification of issues and problem solving, creating a more nimble and responsive system. Batching is not always a bad thing, though.

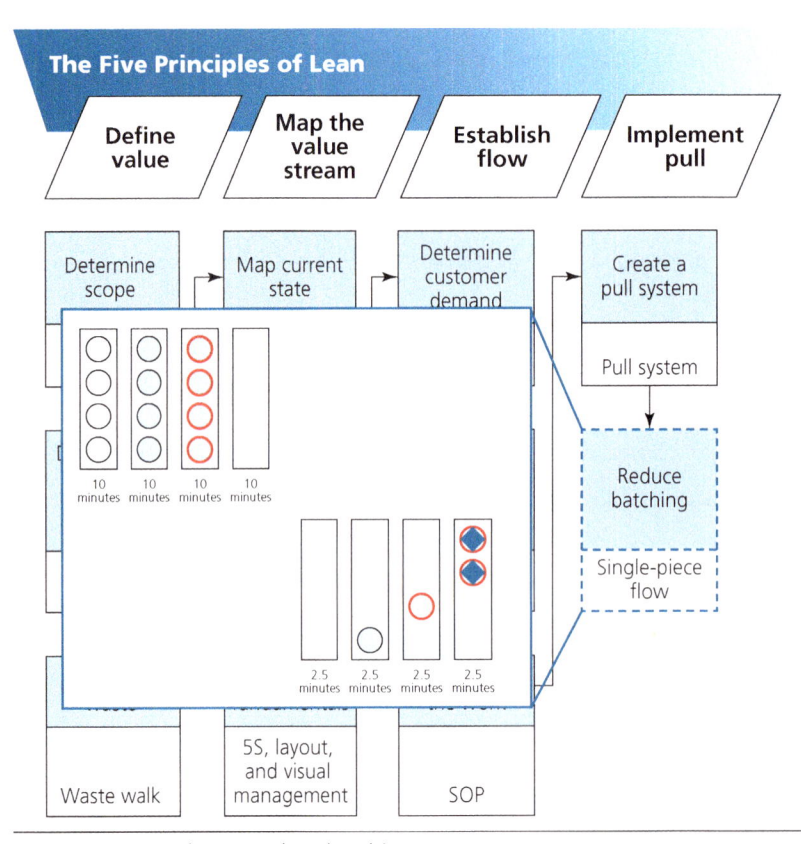

Figure 6.9 Roadmap: Reduce batching.

Batching is advantageous in the following scenarios (Breakthrough Management Group International):

- Time-consuming setups
- Steps that cannot be synchronized due to specific restraints/requirements
- Geography/physical distance between processing steps

Figure 6.10 demonstrates the impact of batching versus single-piece flow. There are four processing steps in the example. Each item (indicated by a circle) requires 2.5 minutes of processing per step. In the Batching A example, each step takes 10 minutes to complete (2.5 minutes per four items). The cycle continues through completion. The overall lead time for one individual item is the same as the entire batch, 40 minutes.

The single-piece flow process can move the item through independently (remember the escalator analogy). Each item must spend 2.5 minutes at processing steps before advancing. The lead time is 10 minutes. Batching B (Figure 6.10) shows the process through three steps. The batch cannot be completed until every item has been processed. In comparison, Single-piece flow B shows how items can move along the process independent of one another. This approach enables continuous flow and reduces the delays and bottlenecks batching produces.

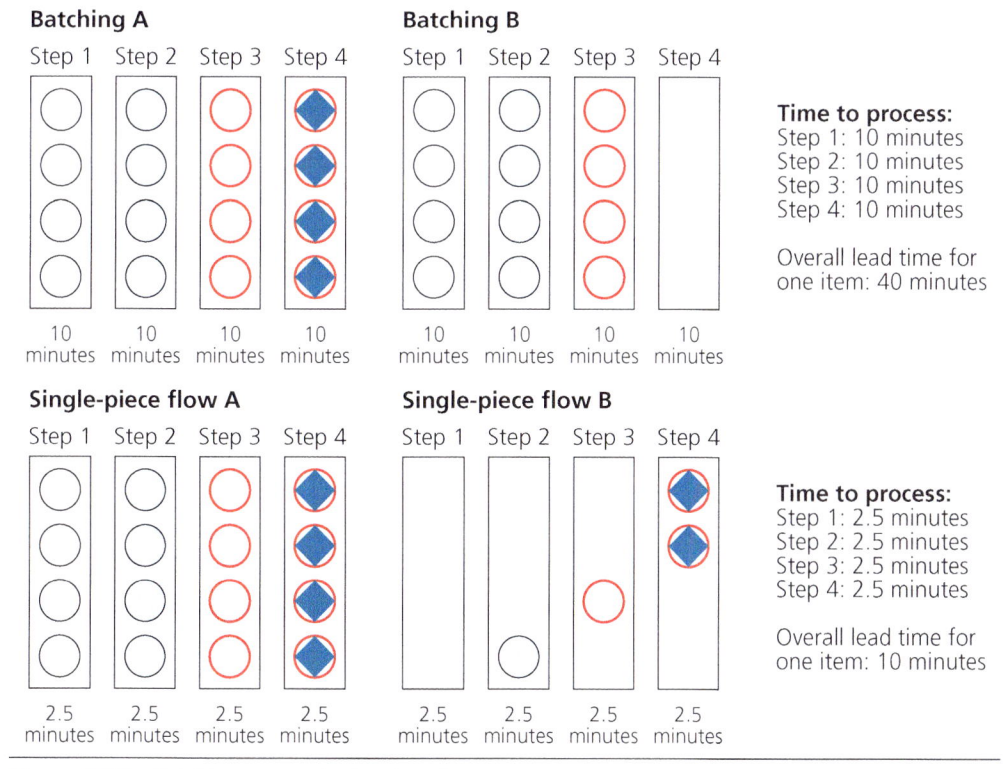

Figure 6.10 Batching versus single-piece flow.

Case Study: Pharmacy Batching

The pharmacy department was evaluating opportunities to improve workflow processes, reduce waste, and manage inventory. One of the areas of opportunity was the process for preparing and distributing small volume parenterals (SVPs). SVPs are solutions used to deliver medications in small quantities. Before the lean project, the SVP process was batched (one time per day). Pharmacy technicians would complete all SVP orders for the upcoming 24 hours.

The batch process led to excess waste. Patient needs could change between order submission and batch production. As a result, the pharmacy technician could end up preparing an unneeded SVP. To meet customer demands (patients and ordering clinicians), the process needed to be redesigned and responsive to changes in needs.

A team of lean leaders, all of whom served as clinical pharmacists in their full-time responsibilities, evaluated the process. There were several issues that contributed to wasted supplies and suboptimization of resources, including staff and physical space. The team facilitated a 5S rapid improvement event to redesign the workspace and develop a new workflow.

The SVP batch process was broken down to three times per day, rather than once. Though still batching, the more frequent time intervals yield production closer to just-in-time. Given the other responsibilities of the pharmacy technicians and staff, true single-piece flow was not an option. A checklist accompanied the new process to ensure consistency and sustainability, along with a log for documenting production.

The SVP process redesign led to a decrease in wasted supplies. Pharmacy staff indicated a noticeable drop in calls from nursing units regarding missing SVP doses. The team targeted medication usage of those most likely to be affected by the project based on volume/utilization. Based on four of the top five high-cost drugs monitored, annual cost savings are over $140,000.

MANAGE INVENTORY

Inventory management aims to provide customers and staff what they need, when they need it, and in the right amount (Figure 6.11). To accomplish this, use the lowest level of required resources and inventory as needed. Inventory management is difficult to apply in the healthcare setting. Supplies tend to be overstocked since the risk or consequence of not having something can be catastrophic for patient outcomes. There are, however, ample opportunities to streamline and standardize supply management in order to optimize resources. Small changes make a huge impact due to the large volume of patients a hospital will see. The one-off supplies in rare cases make systematic storage/inventory management nearly impossible. Planning for such instances is not always practical and often it makes more sense to keep excess supply since the risk of not having it when needed is much greater than the cost and burden of storing it. This section focuses on the more common inventory-related issues.

Why is excess inventory a bad thing? As described in earlier chapters, excess inventory is NVA. Excess inventory is a symptom of underlying distribution and utilization issues. Take, for example, supplies on a nursing unit. If the nursing unit does not trust the replenishment system, employees are likely to hoard supplies. Issues include supplies replenished at a variable rate (e.g., order to replenish ranges from 1 to 10 days) and incomplete or inaccurate order fulfillment. Excessive inventory takes up valuable storage space, ties up available cash, and creates the

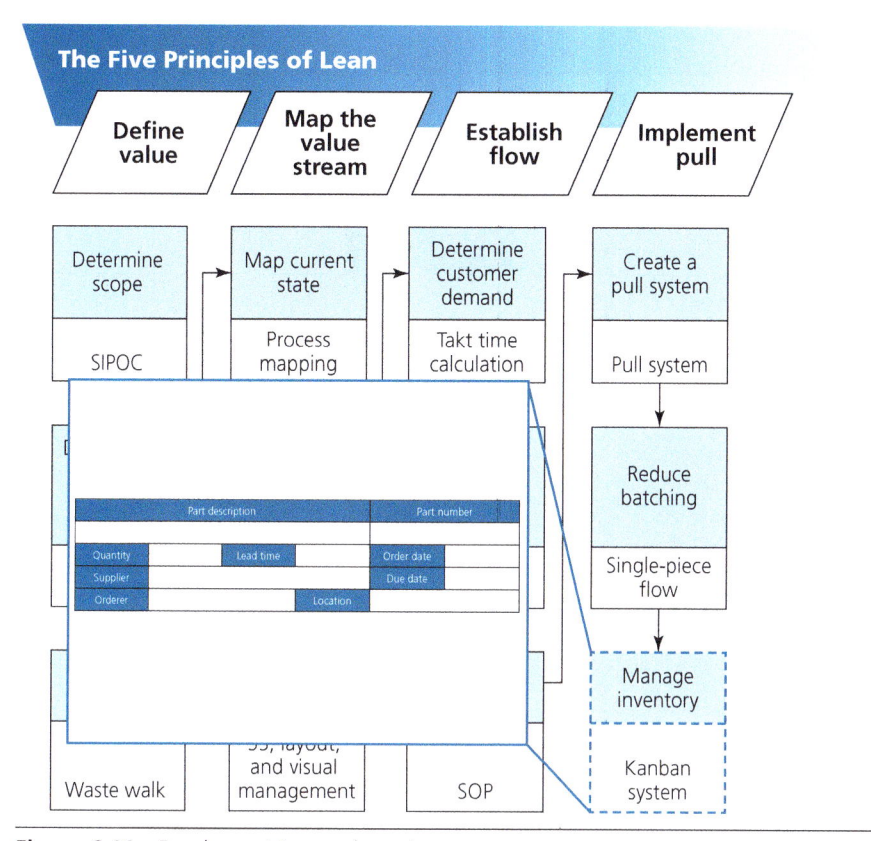

Figure 6.11 Roadmap: Manage inventory.

risk of expiration (especially with medications). However, excessive inventory is appropriate in some scenarios. Unknown or uneven demand, long lead times from order to replenishment, and the consequence of stock-outs all justify higher inventory levels (Womack & Jones, 2005).

Par Levels

Inventory management systems attempt to create a pull process from the user of the supplies to the supplier. The goal is to replenish items in the quantities in which they are used. Par levels offer a simple approach to identify the time and quantity needed to reorder. Par levels are based on average use of supplies as well as the delivery frequency and lead time. A buffer is included to remediate the risk of a stock-out. Inventory management requires oversight and control of supplies. If you cannot keep track of it, you cannot control and manage it.

The kanban card is the implementation tool of pull systems and par levels. *Kanban* is a Japanese word that means "sign" or "card" (Graban, 2012). The tool provides a visual cue that indicates supply replenishment (e.g., red strip on receipt roll indicates paper is running low and a new roll will be needed soon). Kanbans reduce inventory by creating a reliable replenishment system. The kanban card identifies the part (description and number), quantity to order, and replenishment lead time, along with order and due dates (Figure 6.12).

Part description			Part number	
Quantity		Lead time	Order date	
Supplier			Due date	
Orderer		Location		

Figure 6.12 Kanban template.

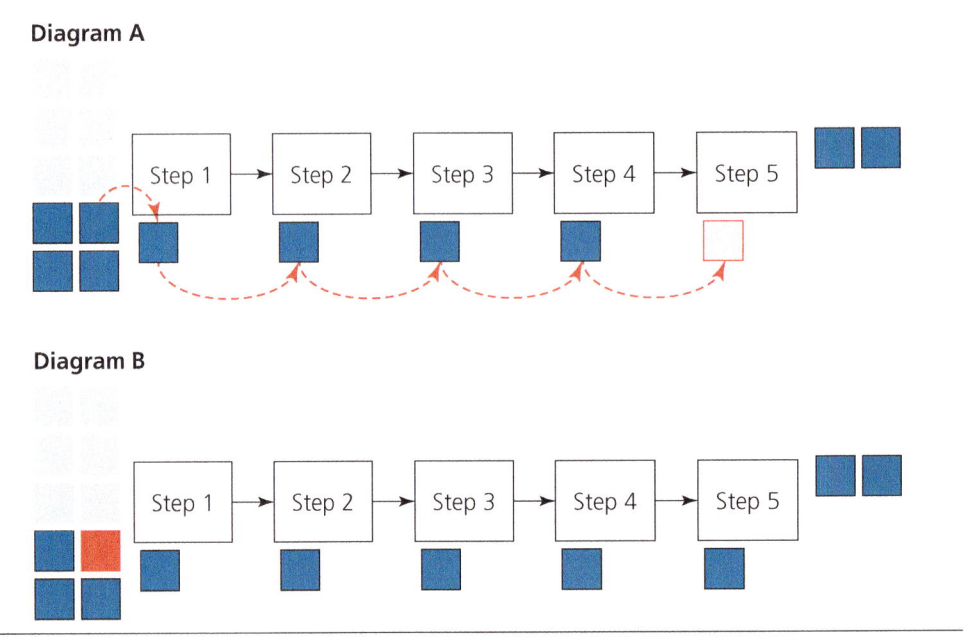

Diagram A

Diagram B

Figure 6.13 Kanban example.

Figure 6.13 explains kanbans using the prior example for creating a pull system. Diagram A shows the pull system taking a box from step 4 and transitioning it to step 5. Subsequently, the boxes are pulled until step 1 pulls from the inventory. Diagram B indicates use of a kanban card. The red box signals the employee at step 1 to order seven boxes to replenish the stock. The three remaining blue boxes are a buffer to reduce the likelihood of running out.

Case Study: Pharmacy Inventory

Due to shortages and stock-outs, the pharmacy is in a different arena when it comes to supplies. There are known and unanticipated shortages that promote the hoarding behavior as an organizational defense mechanism. Uninterrupted patient care is paramount, and at times hoarding-like behavior is acceptable due to the dynamic nature of pharmaceutical supply availability. The pharmacy storerooms provide inventory/stock to central and satellite locations. The pharmacy department wanted to improve workflow and inventory management by consolidating storerooms on the second, fourth, and fifth floors into a singular storeroom on the second floor.

The pharmacy storeroom was decentralized and did not have a systematic process for inventory management. It was difficult for staff to find requested supplies and led to wasted motion and nonutilized skill. Also, due to the inefficient practices, several non-storage locations held supplies. These practices affected ordering accuracy and appropriateness as well as distribution (Figure 6.14).

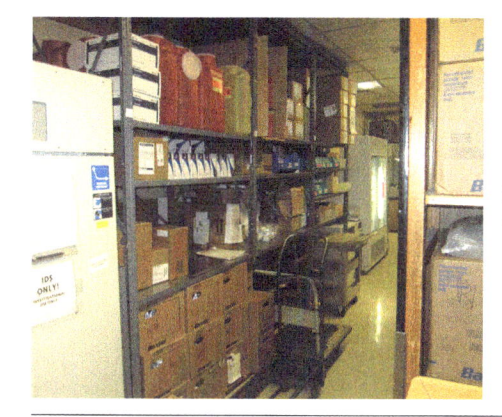

Storeroom shelves were overstocked with unneeded supplies and not organized.

Figure 6.14 Pharmacy storeroom before improvements.

A team of lean leaders led the pharmacy storeroom project. The goal was to create a systematic inventory management process that enabled staff to readily retrieve and distribute supplies on demand. The team also aimed to reduce inventory levels and put processes into place to control ordering, distribution, and use of supplies (Figures 6.15–6.17).

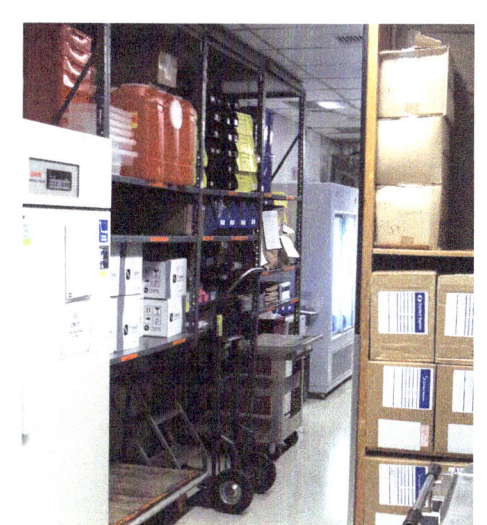

All supplies were sorted and stored based on frequency of use.

Figure 6.15 Pharmacy storeroom after improvements.

(continued)

114 Chapter Six

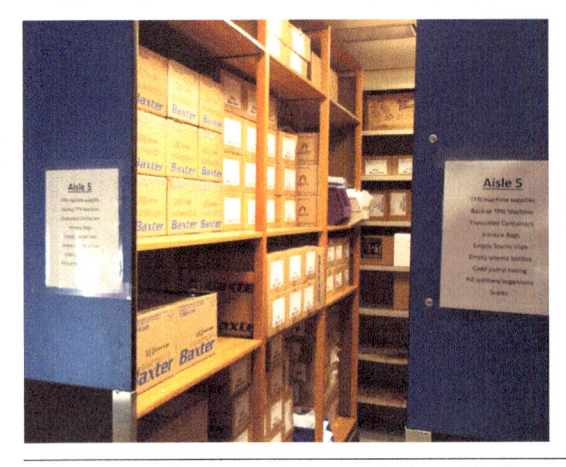

Shelves were organized and properly labeled to help guide staff to appropriate locations.

Figure 6.16 Pharmacy storeroom shelves after improvements.

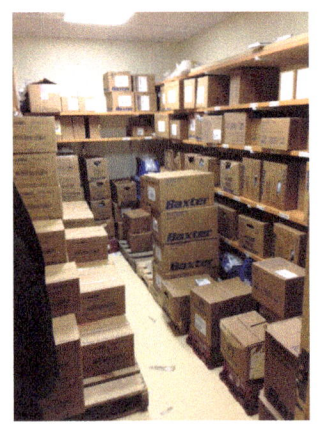

Before: Decentralized storage areas were unorganized. It was nearly impossible to manage inventory because no one knew what exactly was on hand.

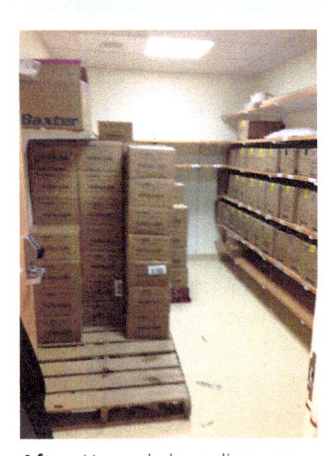

After: Unneeded supplies were appropriately discarded or returned. Supplies that belonged in the main storeroom were relocated and the decentralized storerooms were organized.

Figure 6.17 Pharmacy decentralized storerooms before and after improvements.

The improvement effort served as a transition prior to a complete physical redesign of the pharmacy storeroom (pending one year from project date). The countermeasures developed modeled the future layout and processes. The team used the 5S approach to remove and restock all medications from the satellite storerooms to the main storeroom. As a result, storage space was reclaimed in the main storeroom, unused items were removed, and excess stock of medications was returned to the wholesaler.

CHAPTER CHALLENGE

Streamline your inventory, either in the office or at home or both. How hard is this to do? Are there certain things/items in which the inventory can be more easily managed? What visual cues are in place to determine the appropriate amount as well as the reorder points?

QUESTIONS

1. How do flow and pull relate to each other?
2. Why is a pull system more favorable than the traditional push approach?
3. What processes in your area can apply the pull methodology? How difficult is it to do?
4. How does excess inventory hide system and process issues?
5. Why is single-piece flow ideal?
6. What are batching examples in your workflow? Can they be converted to single-piece flow? Why or why not?
7. Why are kanbans useful in managing inventory? How can they be applied to supplies in your area?

Chapter 7
Principle #5: Strive for Perfection

The experience taught me that when you see a problem, run toward it or it will only get worse.

—Mitt Romney

Continuous improvement demands focusing on reducing errors and rework. Perfection underlies the previous four principles. As you have seen and read throughout the book, the philosophy of lean thinking is to identify and eliminate NVA activity, much of which derives from errors not eliminated or dealt with directly, in a timely manner. The fifth principle of lean, strive for perfection, consists of three core components: (1) identify root causes, (2) error-proof processes, and (3) sustain improvements (Figure 7.1).

IDENTIFY ROOT CAUSES

Seek first to understand, then to be understood.

—Stephen Covey

The quality of a Lean Thinker is not in the answers they provide but rather the questions that they ask.

—Breakthrough Management Group International

Lean improvements emphasize a focus on improving systems and processes rather than working harder or faster (Graban, 2012). Lean thinking is not about having solutions to all problems. Effective problem solvers focus time and observation on the current state process. Before any meaningful change can be developed and implemented, you must first truly understand the underlying root causes (Figure 7.2). Covey's quote eloquently makes this point. A lean thinker leverages the knowledge and experience of process experts to help uncover problems and develop effective solutions. The measure of an effective lean thinker lies in his or her ability to discover such root causes through interviews, observations, and analysis.

118 Chapter Seven

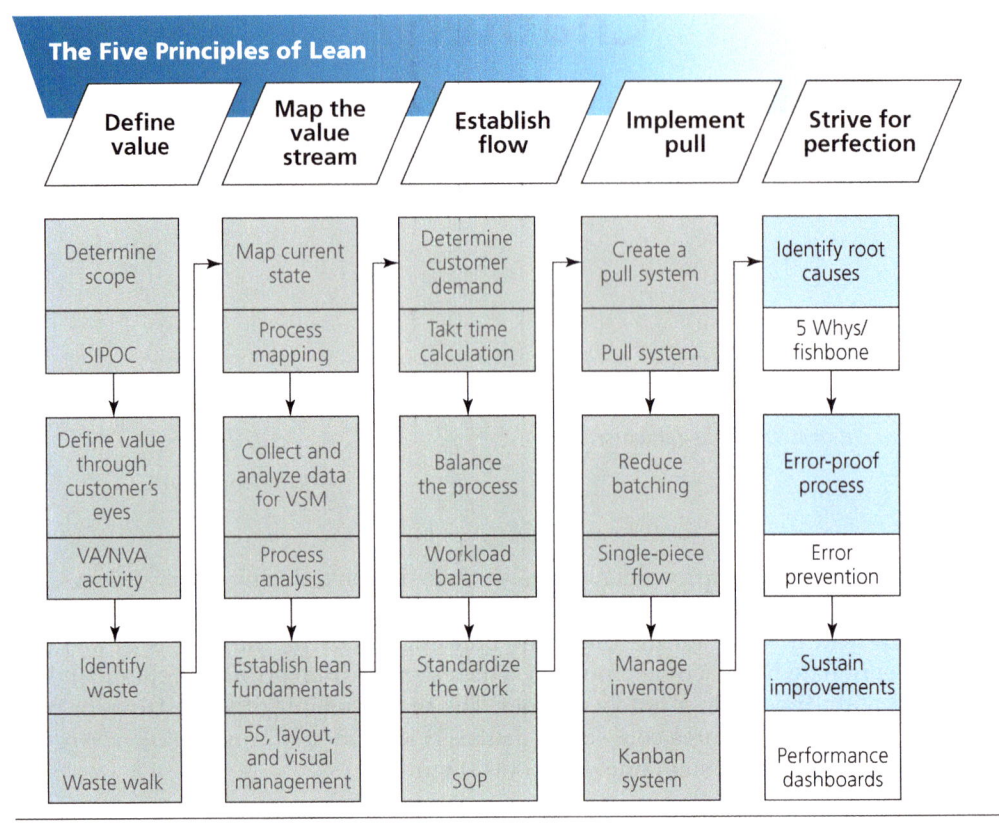

The Five Principles of Lean				
Define value	**Map the value stream**	**Establish flow**	**Implement pull**	**Strive for perfection**
Determine scope	Map current state	Determine customer demand	Create a pull system	Identify root causes
SIPOC	Process mapping	Takt time calculation	Pull system	5 Whys/ fishbone
Define value through customer's eyes	Collect and analyze data for VSM	Balance the process	Reduce batching	Error-proof process
VA/NVA activity	Process analysis	Workload balance	Single-piece flow	Error prevention
Identify waste	Establish lean fundamentals	Standardize the work	Manage inventory	Sustain improvements
Waste walk	5S, layout, and visual management	SOP	Kanban system	Performance dashboards

Figure 7.1 Roadmap: Strive for perfection.

Root causes are at the heart of problem solving. Addressing symptoms rather than the root cause of the problem can lead to ineffective solutions and build customer and employee frustration. For the clinicians out there, if a patient presents in the Emergency Department with a fever, do you just simply say, "Take an Advil, and if it persists, come back in a few days"? Or do you explore the issue by doing a physical exam, diagnostic tests, and so on, to find out what is causing the fever? If there is an underlying bloodstream infection, you need to address it. Dealing with symptoms does not solve the problem. The same applies to processes. Operational problems might show themselves as poor patient/customer satisfaction or slow turnaround times. However, the root cause might be limited visual management, poor communication, or lack of coordination of tasks. The key is to ask why!

The root cause is the underlying issue that leads to the observed symptoms. Identifying root causes starts with going to the gemba. Go to the work area, talk with the staff, and use the tools and concepts you have learned throughout the book to ask probing questions. When errors are identified, the system/process issues are isolated and remediated with an end goal of eliminating the likelihood or chance for it to occur again in the same or a similar place. That is the mark of an effective root cause analysis and remediation. If it happened once, it is highly likely that it will happen again (Mann, 2010).

PRINCIPLE #5: STRIVE FOR PERFECTION   119

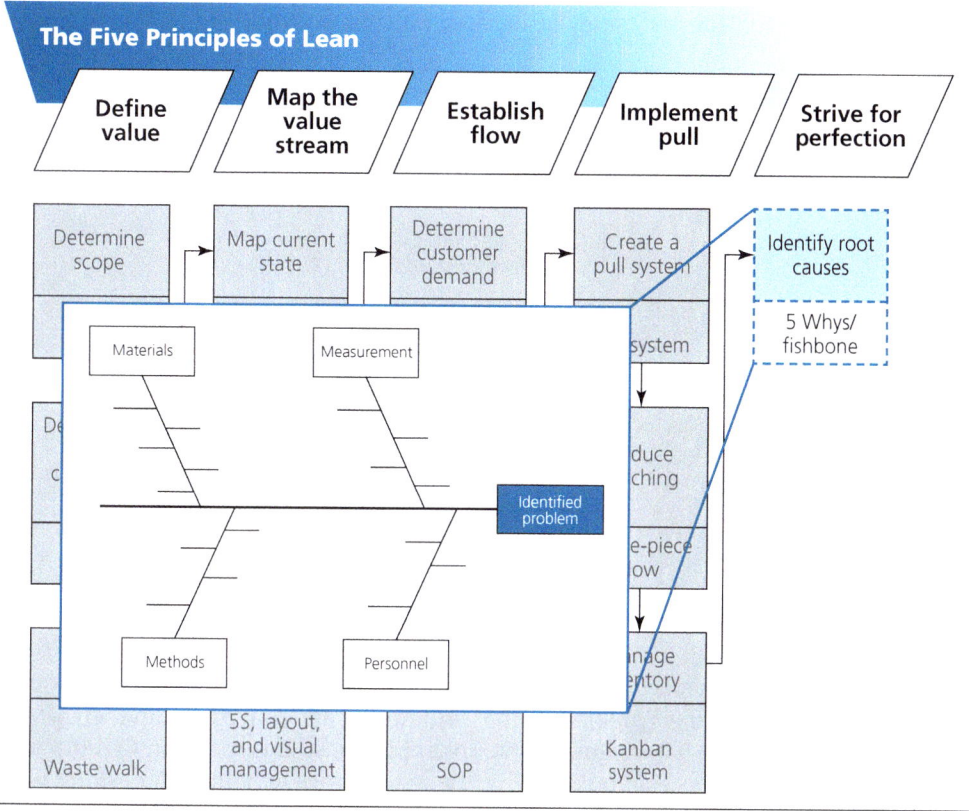

Figure 7.2 Roadmap: Identify root causes.

Tools to Help Identify Root Causes

Two tools that are highly effective in identifying root causes are the 5 Whys and the fishbone diagram.

5 Whys

The 5 Whys method explores potential root causes by diving below the surface of a presenting symptom. Upon discovering the underlying root cause, applied countermeasures reduce or eliminate the likelihood of future occurrences.

> *Root cause analysis for process improvement mirrors that of clinical diagnostics.*
>
> **Symptoms versus Root Causes**
> - Illness
>   - **Symptoms:** headache, fever
>   - **Ask 5 Whys:** diagnostic tests, physical exam
>   - **Root cause:** bloodstream infection
> - Process
>   - **Symptoms:** slow turnaround times, long throughput, dissatisfied customers/patients
>   - **Ask 5 Whys:** observations, staff rounding, data analysis
>   - **Root cause:** lack of visual management and coordination of workflow

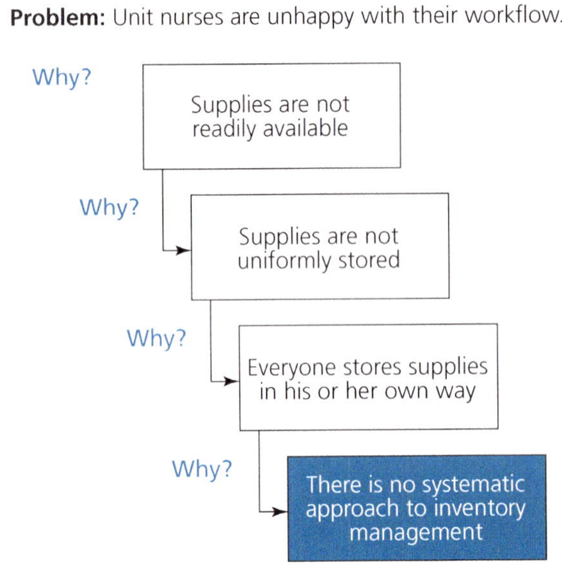

Problem: Unit nurses are unhappy with their workflow.

Why? → Supplies are not readily available

Why? → Supplies are not uniformly stored

Why? → Everyone stores supplies in his or her own way

Why? → There is no systematic approach to inventory management

Figure 7.3 Example of 5 Whys.

The 5 Whys approach is straightforward. Figure 7.3 is an example of how to employ it. The identified problem is that unit nurses are unhappy with their workflow. It is not clear what is causing the unhappiness, so it is too soon to jump to a conclusion or solution. As you ask why, the issue comes to light. After asking why four times, the root cause is unmasked: there is no systematic approach to inventory management. This root cause is the reason nurses are unhappy with the workflow. In this example, you had to ask why only four times. You may need to ask it 10 or more times, or sometimes, as in this example, there is a direct path to the root cause.

Another way to look at this flow diagram is to take it in reverse. Start with the root cause and work your way back up to the identified problem. The reverse, using *therefore*, tells the story of the consequences a root cause produces:

- There is no systematic approach to inventory management, *therefore*
- Everyone stores supplies in his or her own way, *therefore*
- Supplies are not uniformly stored, *therefore*
- Supplies are not readily available, *therefore*
- Unit nurses are unhappy with their workflow

Fishbone Diagram

Dr. Kaoru Ishikawa developed the fishbone diagram. Other names for the tool include the Ishikawa diagram or cause-and-effect diagram. The tool guides systematic identification of issues and causes of the problem under review (Lighter, 2013). This type of analysis is qualitative and effective in group brainstorming sessions.

Building a Fishbone

1. Select the problem (effect) (Figure 7.4)

2. Create the body (structure) (Figure 7.5)
3. Label categories (Figure 7.6)
4. Brainstorm potential causes (Figure 7.7)

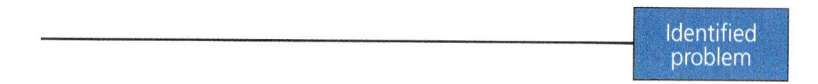

Figure 7.4 Fishbone problem.

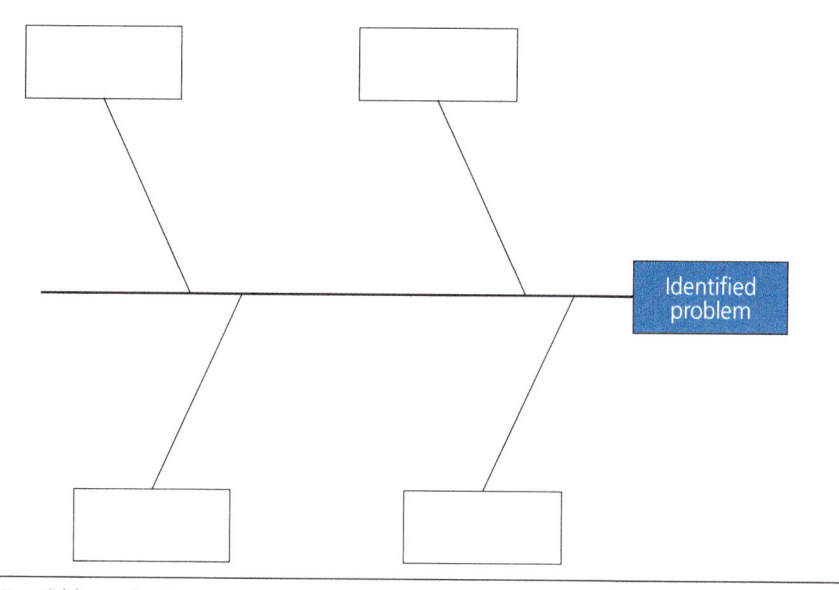

Figure 7.5 Fishbone body structure.

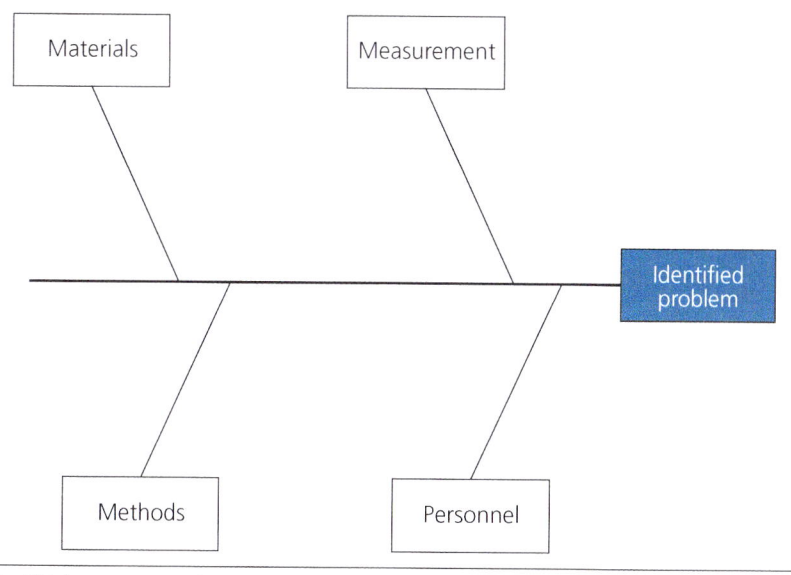

Figure 7.6 Fishbone categories.

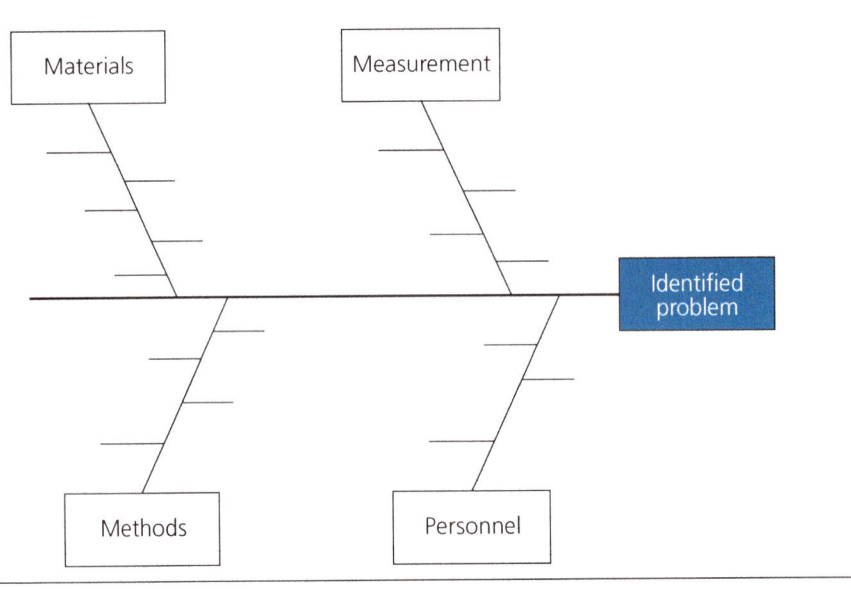

Figure 7.7 Fishbone with potential causes.

Typical Fishbone Categories
- Personnel
- Materials/supplies
- Measurement
- Method/processes
- Machine/equipment

A completed fishbone analysis enables the team to narrow the focus toward the probable causes of the problem. This type of analysis leads to the issues that are directly within your control as opposed to those barriers and issues you cannot impact. Data can accompany the analysis to verify potential sources of the problem.

Case Study: Inpatient Admission from the Emergency Department

The patient flow management center (PFMC) is a comprehensive, best-practice center overseeing patient flow within and across units/organizations at Jefferson. The PFMC integrates seven departments: Bed Management, Transfer Center, Environmental Services, External Transportation (air and ground transport), Nursing, Patient Transportation, and Case Management. The multidisciplinary PFMC utilizes a robust information system to assign inpatient beds, among other functions.

For patients awaiting admission from the Emergency Department (ED) to an inpatient floor, employees use the information system to submit the request. ED nursing staff enter the attribute data (i.e., patient demographics, isolation precautions) into the system. While the PFMC has dramatically improved patient flow, inaccurate and omitted attribute

PRINCIPLE #5: STRIVE FOR PERFECTION   123

selections continue to delay bed assignments. Delays in inpatient bed assignments result in longer ED boarding hours and wait times for new ED patient arrivals. Accordingly, these delays manifest in reduced patient satisfaction levels. Bed assignment delays may also indirectly contribute to a greater number of patients leaving the ED before having a physician evaluation.

In order to drill down to the main issues, the lean team utilized the fishbone diagram (Figure 7.8). The team compiled the fishbone through voice-of-customer interviews, data analysis, and gemba walk observations. The tool was vetted with process experts and refined to reflect the current state. The fishbone depicts the issues leading to "delays in ED admission process." The two root causes are "attributes not entered in timely fashion" and "incomplete or inaccurate attributes."

To address these root causes, the improvement team developed a standard checklist of required patient attributes along with a process for who completes the checklist, by when. The mandatory attributes require ED staff to supply the PFMC with the information it needs to assign the appropriate bed as quickly as possible. The improved process reduces rework by way of reassigning beds, phone calls between departments for status updates or troubleshooting, and delays in subsequent process steps.

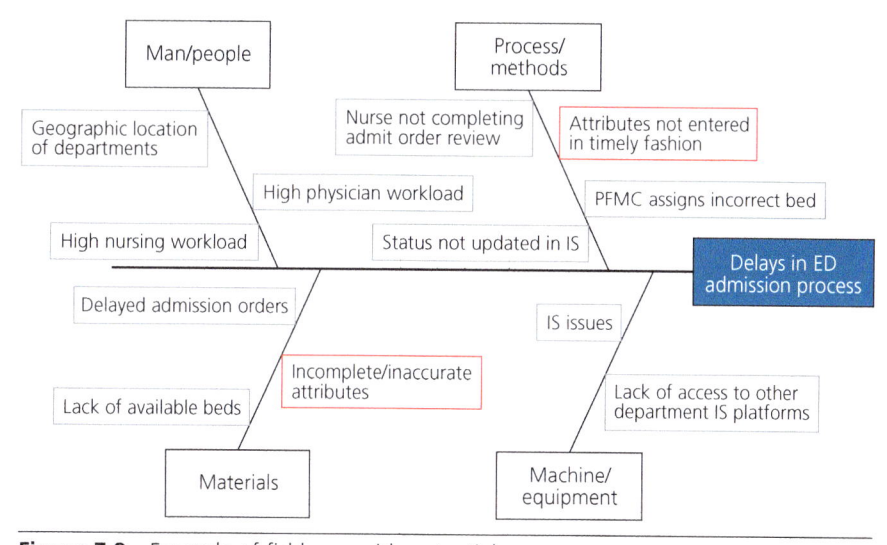

Figure 7.8 Example of fishbone with potential causes.

ERROR-PROOF PROCESSES

> *Human error is inevitable. We can never eliminate it. We can eliminate problems in the system that make it more likely to happen.*
> — Sir Liam Donaldson, World Health Organization

Errors are learning opportunities. The goal is to prevent the error from occurring again. Error-proofing is one lean strategy to achieve this (Figure 7.9). Using the error-proofing approach, the likelihood of an error occurring is designed out

The Five Principles of Lean

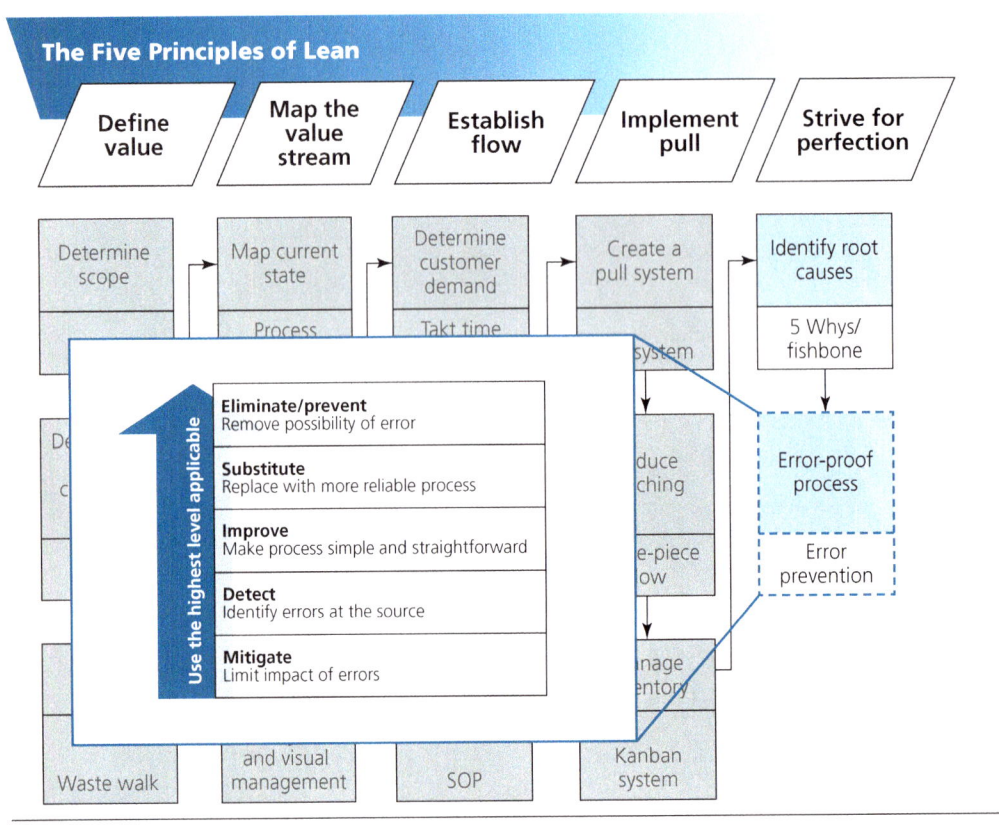

Define value → Map the value stream → Establish flow → Implement pull → Strive for perfection

Use the highest level applicable:
- **Eliminate/prevent** — Remove possibility of error
- **Substitute** — Replace with more reliable process
- **Improve** — Make process simple and straightforward
- **Detect** — Identify errors at the source
- **Mitigate** — Limit impact of errors

Figure 7.9 Roadmap: Error-proof process.

of the process (Grout, 2007; Lean Enterprise Institute). The focus is prevention and avoidance of errors by building quality directly into the system/process. This approach derives from the Toyota Production System (*jidoka*—preventing errors at the source) (Liker, 2004). Lean thinking emphasizes doing things correctly the first time, every time (Toussaint & Gerard, 2010). The term *error-proofing* may seem foreign but its application is not. Many everyday items use error-proofing strategies. Examples include the following:

- New cars have keys that detect when they are inside or outside the vehicle, thereby making it impossible to lock your keys inside the car
- Microwaves stop when you open the door
- An alert pops up if you try to send an e-mail without a subject line
- Three-pronged plugs cannot fit into an ungrounded two-prong electrical outlet

These are just a few examples that you might encounter throughout the day. In the healthcare setting, there are simple and sophisticated error-proofing mechanisms:

- Medical gas connection safeguards
- Medication labeling/identification

- Bed alarms
- Radio-frequency identification surgical sponges

> Mistake-proofing the Design of Health Care Processes, *a publication of the Agency for Healthcare Research and Quality (AHRQ), provides a comprehensive overview with examples of error-proofing applied in the healthcare setting (Grout, 2007). The literature uses "mistake-proofing" and "error-proofing" interchangeably. "Mistake" has a negative connotation, which is why in this book I use the term "error-proofing."*

Error-proofing is an effective intervention when there are consistent defects within the process. The lean thinking philosophy supports this approach toward defects:

1. Do not accept a defect
2. Do not produce a defect
3. Do not pass along a defect

The price of prevention is insignificant compared with the cost of intervention once an error has occurred. Error-proofing leads to lower costs as a result of improved quality and decreased rework (Martin et al., 2009).

Error-proofing occurs in a few simple steps (Silverstein, Samuel, & DeCarlo, 2009):

1. Identify the defect/error and its location
2. Determine the root cause
3. Review the current process and standard work
4. Identify any deviation from the standard work
5. Develop intervention/countermeasure to correct for future occurrences
6. Implement improvement and evaluate for effectiveness

Identifying the source of the defect is paramount. Root causes are system and process based. Remember to ask why, not who. Employees will devise creative workarounds to deal with poor process design, but remember that creativity and rework can sometimes be the same thing (Womack, 2011). Error-proofing targets the design of processes that lead to errors. Learning from mistakes is the fastest way to improve (Bicheno & Holweg, 2004). There are a variety of methods to apply to drive defects out of the system. These include flags, inspection, alerts/warnings, and standard operating procedures.

Error-proofing should progress from mitigation to elimination/prevention (Figure 7.10). Over time, a more sophisticated approach detects issues as they arise. Subsequently, an improvement approach is taken to clean up the process and reduce variation of outcomes. Where possible, higher-performing and reliable processes replace less efficient ones. The ultimate goal is to design errors out of the system.

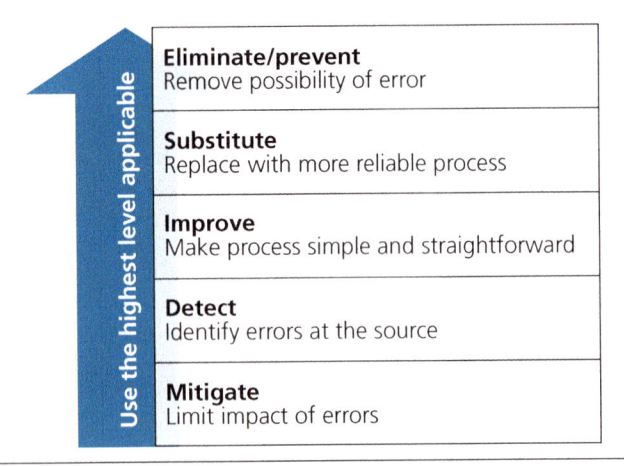

Figure 7.10 Progression of error reduction.
Source: Adapted model based on Lean and Six Sigma International Board, 2011.

Preventing Human Error

Humans are the main processors in the healthcare environment. As described in *To Err Is Human*, people are fallible; thus, process designs should reduce and eliminate the potential for human error (Kohn, Donaldson, & Committee on Quality of Health Care in America, Institute of Medicine, 2000). Shigeo Shingo, a key influence in the Toyota Production System, identified common reasons humans make errors (Breakthrough Management Group International):

- *Lack of experience:* Employees with little experience or knowledge of the process.

- *Misunderstanding:* Not understanding the situation and subsequently choosing an inappropriate course of action.

- *Forgetfulness:* Despite repetition and familiarity, an employee might still forget to do a particular step or task.

- *Lack of standards or supervision:* Employees are more likely to create errors if they do not know what is expected or do not receive training on how to properly perform tasks.

- *Willful errors:* Intentional mistakes made without bad intentions. An example is someone doing a process "her own way" because she believes it is more efficient.

- *Inadvertent errors:* Caused by lack of attentiveness, discipline, or a standard operating procedure.

- *Intentional errors*: Malicious errors made to the process without the goal of providing a better result (unlike willful errors).

Understanding these sources of deviation enables proper identification of error-proofing tactics. Lean thinking encourages empowering individuals to solve problems and own their work. From a leadership perspective, it is essential to position employees to be successful by designing processes that promote high-quality, consistent outcomes and prevent errors from occurring. Errors will occur. How you learn from them is what makes the difference.

SUSTAIN IMPROVEMENTS

Sustaining gains is the biggest challenge in an improvement effort (Figure 7.11). A multifaceted approach supports sustainability. The main goal for sustainability is to monitor performance against expected outcomes and course-correct as indicated. There are many ways to monitor progress (e.g., dashboards, run charts, balanced scorecards). What you employ is largely dependent on your environment and available tools and data.

As mentioned earlier, errors will occur. The response to these errors makes the difference in quality outcomes and sustainable progress. Early identification of problems will enable rapid remediation and elimination. Employees should be positioned to produce high-quality outputs. To that end, evaluate several factors:

1. *Priority of tasks:* Employees understand the priority and nature of urgency for tasks

2. *Distractions:* Distractions should be removed or reduced in order to encourage focus

3. *Workload balance:* Workloads should be appropriate and evenly balanced to support flow

4. *Direction/guidance:* Instructions and expectations should be clear

Many factors threaten sustainability. Table 7.1 describes the various factors and potential countermeasures to address each.

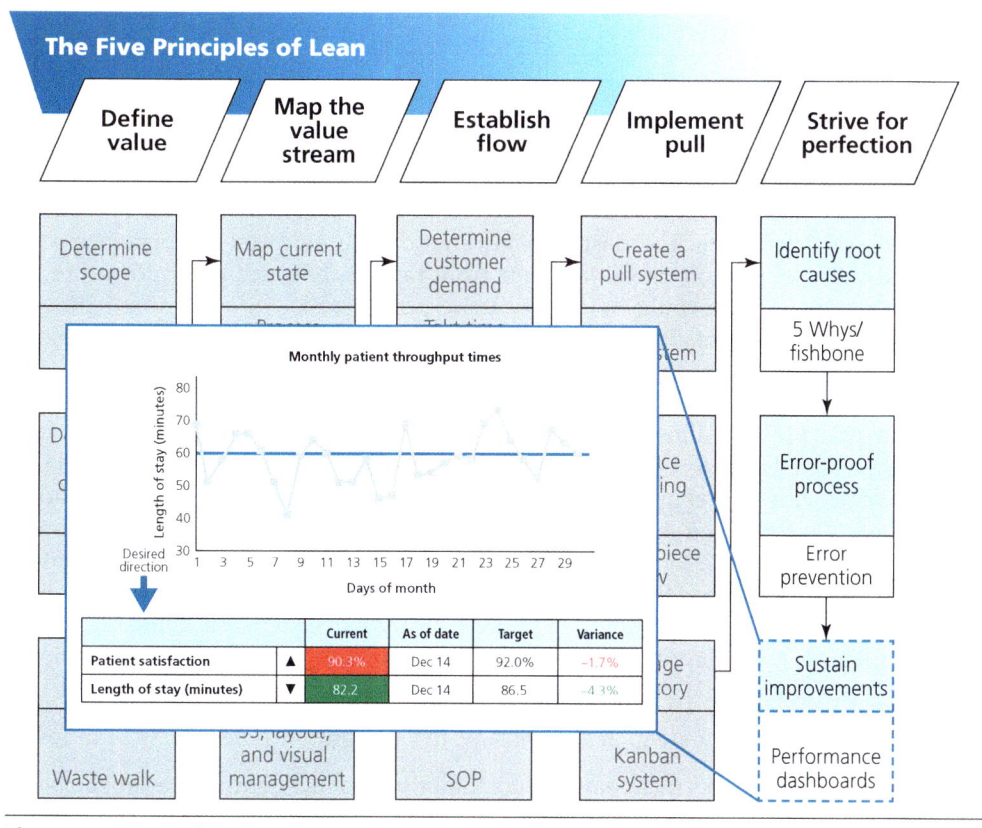

Figure 7.11 Roadmap: Sustain improvements.

Table 7.1 Threats to sustainability.

Issue	Description	Potential countermeasure
Process variation	Uneven flow (too much, too little)	• Standard work • Pull system • Performance dashboards
Unanticipated events	Equipment malfunction/failure, accidents, external events (e.g., weather)	• Error-proofing • Visual management (alerts)
Cultural resistance	Individuals stuck in the "old way" of doing things	• Standard work • Training
Lack of standards	No consistent approach to perform work	• Standard work • Visual management
Poor training	Employees not trained on how to do the job correctly	• Standard work • Training
No visual management	No readily accessible information to support work	• Visual management
No performance dashboards	No feedback mechanism to depict progress versus goals	• Visual management • Performance dashboards
Poor quality	Lack of understanding of customer needs, lack of standard process, variation in outcomes	• Voice of customer • Standard work • Error-proofing

Performance Dashboards

Performance dashboards are visual management tools that monitor and communicate actual versus expected outcomes. Dashboards can be created by using a variety of chart types. The dashboard design displays current performance compared with set goals/targets. Variance from targets indicates an opportunity for improvement. There could be quality issues, bottlenecks, or system and process problems that are creating underperforming outcomes. Consistent visual assessment of performance is critical to sustainability.

In Chapter 4 we discussed visual management, one of the lean fundamentals. Visual management aims to create an immediate snapshot of the current state and communicate key information to appropriate stakeholders. Visual cues like dashboards provide status updates and make performance gaps or problems readily obvious. Performance dashboards can provide feedback on process adherence, productivity, and customer satisfaction. Feedback is an essential component to foster employee buy-in in both the short term and the long term.

Dashboards can be created through information systems (if available) or by using simple charts in tools like Microsoft Excel (Bass, 2007). There are two common types of metrics:

- Operational metrics (e.g., length of stay, throughput, turnaround, wait times)
- Satisfaction metrics (e.g., patient/customer satisfaction, employee satisfaction)

Table 7.2 Performance update table.

As of date	Metric	Target	Actual	Variance	Reason for variance	Action plan

Table 7.2 is a simple tool that can serve as a performance dashboard. The table compares a metric's target with the actual performance as of the date indicated. Variance is either favorable or unfavorable (positive or negative depending on the desired direction for change). If there is an unfavorable variance, a reason should accompany it, followed by a corresponding corrective action plan. Continuous monitoring and course correction limit regression.

There are many chart options for performance dashboards. Important things to consider when creating charts include the following:

- *Frequency of data reporting.* Present data in appropriate intervals based on the nature of the process (e.g., daily, weekly, monthly). Where possible, use the lowest possible interval for more rapid identification of issues, for example, tracking daily patient throughput in the Emergency Department. Metrics like 30-day readmissions should be reported monthly.

- *Targets.* Use performance goals/targets as a comparison. Base targets on known best practices (i.e., top decile, top quartile, mean, median, or internal benchmark). Without an appropriate comparison, it is not possible to assess whether the current performance is acceptable or requires intervention.

- *Display.* Keep charts clean and simple. Adjust the scale (y-axis) to reflect the appropriate range of performance. Additionally, include an arrow to indicate the desired direction of change. This arrow enables quick assessment of progress compared with expected directional movement along the x-axis.

- *Lagging and leading metrics.* As discussed in Chapter 1, the lag measure represents the desired result, whereas the leading metrics are variables that the team can directly affect.

Run charts are an effective way to show performance of operational and satisfaction metrics over time. The charts in Figure 7.12 display the daily length of stay (in minutes) and patient satisfaction over the course of a month.

Bar graphs provide a similar visual and might be more effective in certain instances because of their ease of interpretation or display (Figure 7.13).

Pie charts are simple displays for compliance or other data that emphasize a segmentation or proportion of results (e.g., yes, no). These graphs provide a straightforward assessment of the current state and make opportunities obvious (Figure 7.14).

Summary tables, like Table 7.3, provide a consolidated view of metric performance. If charts are too cumbersome or space is an issue, tables are an easy solution. These tables are referred to as scorecards or dashboards and may contain

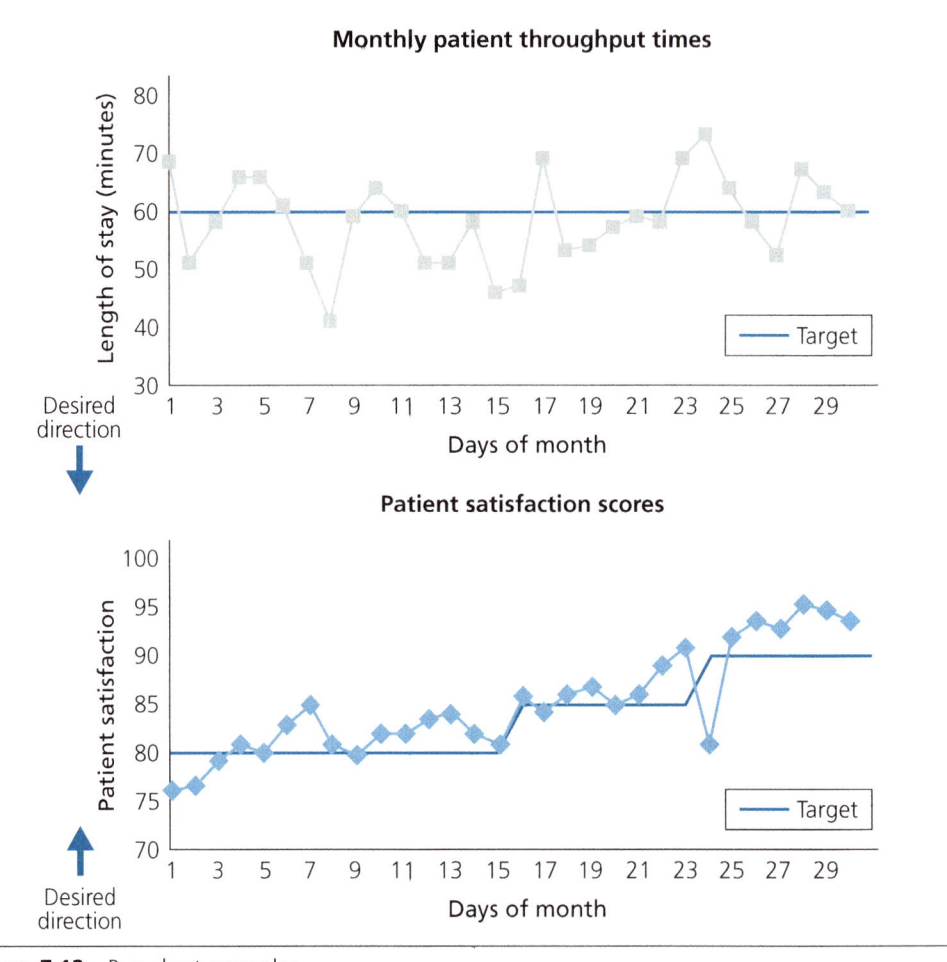

Figure 7.12 Run chart examples.

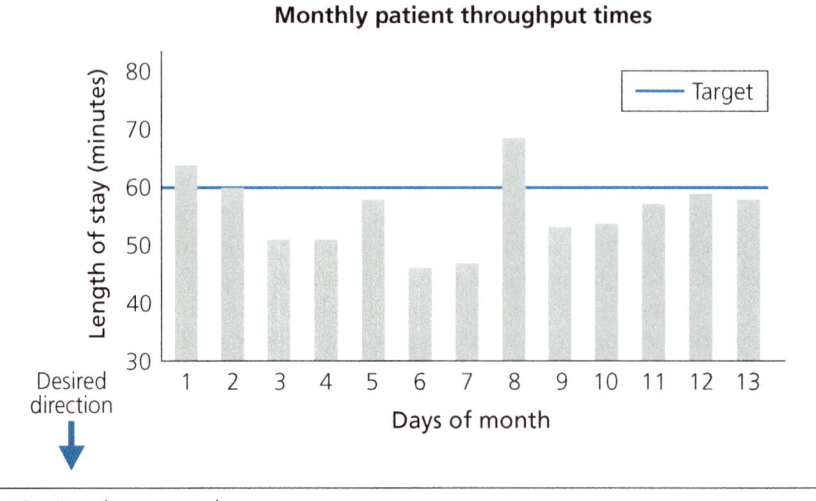

Figure 7.13 Bar chart example.

Quality control dashboard

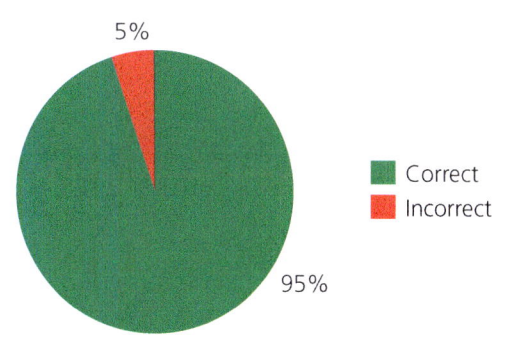

Figure 7.14 Pie graph example.

Table 7.3 Performance dashboard example.

		Current	As of date	Target	Variance
Patient satisfaction	▲	90.3%	Dec 14	92.0%	−1.7%
Length of stay (minutes)	▼	82.2	Dec 14	86.5	−4.3%

over 10 performance metrics depending on the area. The considerations outlined earlier apply to these tables as well. The direction of desired performance and current state should be obvious. Using colors provides an added visual cue for quick assessment of favorable or unfavorable performance.

Case Study: Operating Room Performance Dashboards

The perioperative department applied lean improvement strategies across the entire value stream. As part of the evolution of the department, leadership employed a performance dashboard to evaluate the daily progress of OR operational metrics to ensure streamlined patient flow. A comprehensive review of previous Jefferson OR projects was published by the American Society for Quality (*Systematically Improving Operating Room Patient Flow through Value Stream Mapping and Kaizen Events*, October 2013). Using the OR information system, leadership developed a tracking dashboard that monitors four performance indicators: (1) cases completed and in progress, (2) OR turnover by floor, (3) on time to holding area (HA) for first-case starts, and (4) on-time first-case starts. Figure 7.15 is an example of the OR performance dashboard.

These data represent indicators for efficiency within the daily OR patient flow. As you can see, there is a focus on first-case starts. If the day starts off slow and behind schedule, there is a compounding effect on the remainder of the day. For the OR, it is critical to start on time and efficiently turn operating rooms over to enable continuous flow.

(continued)

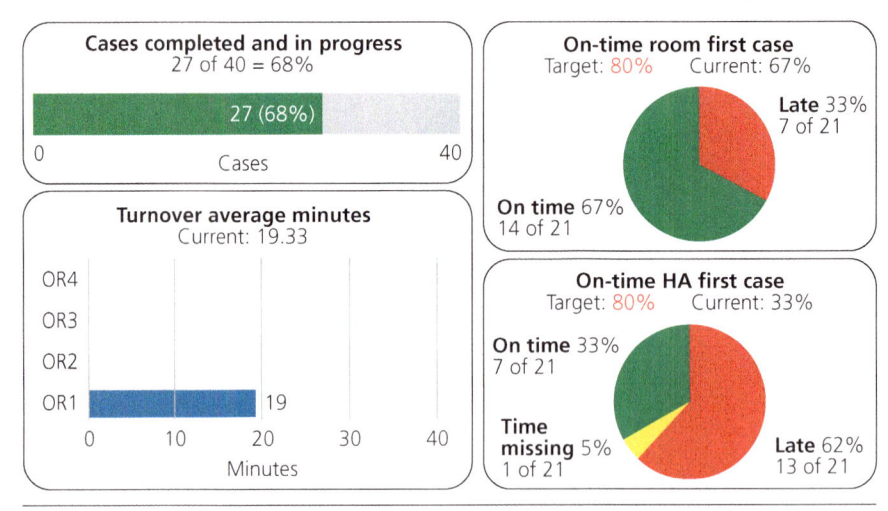

Figure 7.15 Performance dashboard example in the OR.

CHAPTER CHALLENGE

Go on a gemba walk through a department (can be your department) and look for signs that remind or tell employees to be careful. Signs can be an indicator of a process problem and that root cause has not been properly addressed. Are there any root causes not being addressed? Are there any opportunities to apply error-proofing?

QUESTIONS

1. Why do you need to identify root causes before developing a solution?
2. How is a tool like the fishbone diagram used to diagnose key issues?
3. How can you learn from errors?
4. What processes in your area can apply error-proofing? Are error-proofing tactics already in place? Are they effective? Can they be replicated or adapted for other processes?
5. What is the progression of problem solving? Why is prevention at the top?
6. What are ways in which humans can make errors? How do you address or anticipate these concerns?
7. Why is performance feedback an important part of sustainability?
8. What types of information (data, charts, etc.) are provided in your area with regard to performance versus target? If there are not any, why not? What should they be?
9. What are the different ways in which sustainability can be threatened? How can you counter these scenarios?
10. Why do you need to include targets with performance dashboards?

Chapter 8
Executing a Project through Lean DMAIC

Failure to prepare is preparing to fail.

—Ben Franklin

The first seven chapters provide the conceptual model for executing lean improvements. The five principles of lean are critical in systematically identifying opportunities for improvement and developing effective countermeasures. This chapter covers the project management framework for executing lean improvement projects. Similar to Six Sigma, creating a lean process follows the DMAIC structure (Define, Measure, Analyze, Improve, Control) (Bicheno & Holweg, 2008). We will review the key deliverables within each phase and discuss the importance of a systematic approach to performance improvement. The structured checklist-driven approach to improvement enables consistent outcomes.

Lean improvement projects emphasize the collaboration of content and process experts. Individuals who do the work where the problem lives are responsible for helping develop solutions and fixes (Graban, 2012). Lean practitioners are responsible for facilitating the problem-solving process, leveraging the expertise and experience of the employees who work the process (Aij, Simons, Widdershoven, & Visse, 2013). Chapter 9 details the facilitation approach. The lean DMAIC checklist allows individuals to execute projects in a systematic, structured way.

KAIZEN

Kaizen is a Japanese term that means "change for good" (Imai, 1997). A rapid improvement event (RIE) is a type of facilitated kaizen focused on changing a process for the better. The focus is incremental process improvement. RIEs can range from two hours up to three days depending on the problem complexity and project scope. However, kaizen and rapid improvements occur more commonly on the front lines, where the work happens (Graban & Swartz, 2012). Kaizen represents any opportunity to change for the better—not just formal improvement projects.

The kaizen mentality and approach follow the format of the Plan-Do-Check-Act (PDCA) cycle. Walter A. Shewhart developed the PDCA model. The model emphasizes piloting improvements, reviewing the impact, refining, and then repeating (Figure 8.1) (Langley et al., 2009). A future state defines what direction to go in based on the current state. An implementation plan outlines key tasks for moving

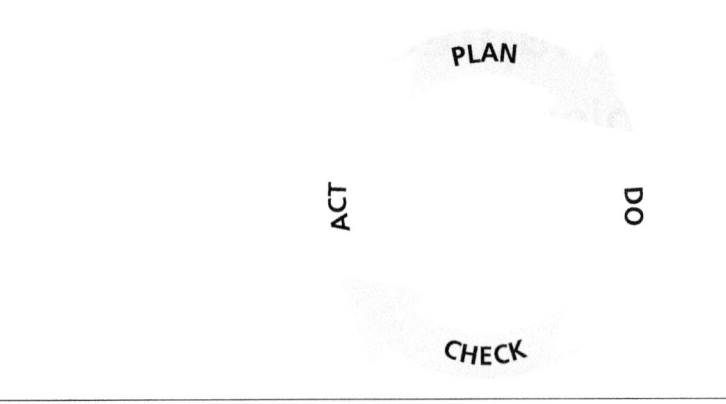

Figure 8.1 PDCA cycle.

toward the future state. Progress and impact are evaluated during and after implementation. The iterative cycle consists of the following:

- *Plan:* Define the objective. Prepare for the improvement changes/actions to be implemented. Identify who will do what, how, and when. Define the expected outcomes of the changes.
- *Do:* Implement the planned changes.
- *Check:* Evaluate the impact of the implemented changes against the expected outcomes. Did the changes have the desired effect? Does the process need to be further refined?
- *Act:* Make refinements to the changes, plan the next iteration of experimentation, and then implement the revised changes and assess their impact compared with expectations.

Of the four phases of the PDCA cycle, Check is probably the most important. In the Check phase, the effectiveness of the plan and execution are evaluated, asking:

- What are we trying to accomplish? Why?
- What is the expected outcome?
- How will we know it is an improvement?
- What worked or did not work? Why?
- What do we need to refine to achieve our goals?

The PDCA model aligns with a lean concept called improvement kata. *Kata* is a Japanese word that means the description and practice of detailed choreography of patterns and movements (Lean Enterprise Institute). Traditionally from martial arts, practicing kata provides the systematic framework for people to tackle problems. Popularized by the book *Toyota Kata* (Rother, 2010), the four-step model (Figure 8.2) defines the structured approach from problem/goal identification to intervention implementation. The improvement kata approach

```
Understand          Grasp the           Establish the next      PDCA toward the
the direction  -->  current direction   target condition   -->  target condition

What problem are    What is the current  What is your objective    PLAN
you trying to address?  state?           (future state)?
                    Are there patterns?                         ACT         DO

                                                                    CHECK
```

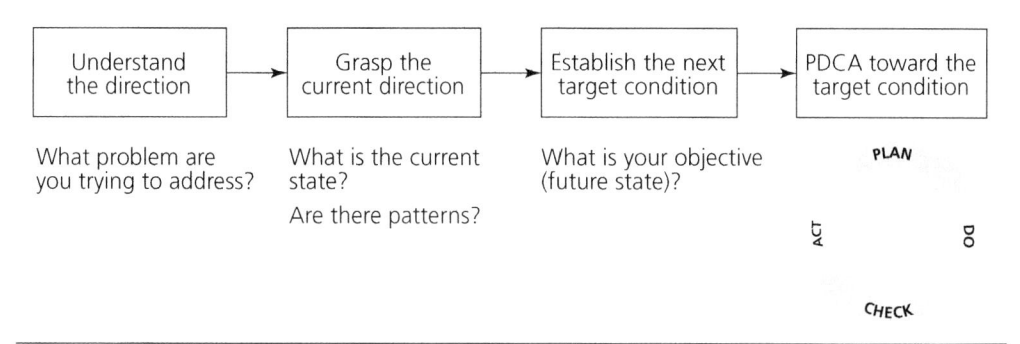

Figure 8.2 Improvement kata model.

isolates the next target condition as the incremental improvement step. The next target condition represents an advancement from the current state that begins to resemble the desired future state. Incremental improvement strategies make transformation efforts manageable and less overwhelming. Remember, don't boil the ocean.

The questions to ask when implementing the improvement kata model are as follows (Rother, 2010):

1. What problem are you trying to address?
2. What obstacles or barriers are preventing you from reaching your goal?
3. Which obstacle or barrier (choose only one) are you going to address?
4. What is your next step (PDCA cycle) and what do you expect to happen?
5. When are you going to the gemba to see what you have learned and what you need to do next?

The PDCA model is powerful. Implement something (pilots and trials work best), evaluate the impact, and refine as needed. Review results and ensure process compliance. Reassess and redesign after changes are hardwired, seeking a new level of performance... "rinse and repeat." Sometimes you pilot new ideas only to find that what you were doing previously worked best. Each effort is a learning opportunity to identify the strengths and limitations of the intervention and use that knowledge to improve the next experiment (Langley et al., 2009).

Figure 8.3 depicts the scope and frequency of problems an organization likely experiences. System- and organization-level improvements are lower in frequency. These processes and problems are complex in nature and involve various value streams and functional areas. The scope is broad and comprehensive. Department- and team-level opportunities are multifaceted. Opportunities involve only a few (or one) functional departments or teams. The most abundant opportunities are at the frontline level (Graban & Swartz, 2012). Processes and problems at the front line tend to be straightforward and less complex. The power of lean is leveraging this section of the pyramid. By empowering staff to solve problems at the source, these small improvements (kaizen) have a compounding effect across the organization.

System/organizational level
Complex processes and problems crossing various value streams and functional areas

Department/team level
Multifaceted processes and problems involving core departments or teams. Narrower in scope than system/organization level efforts.

Frontline level
Straightforward and often less complex processes and problems

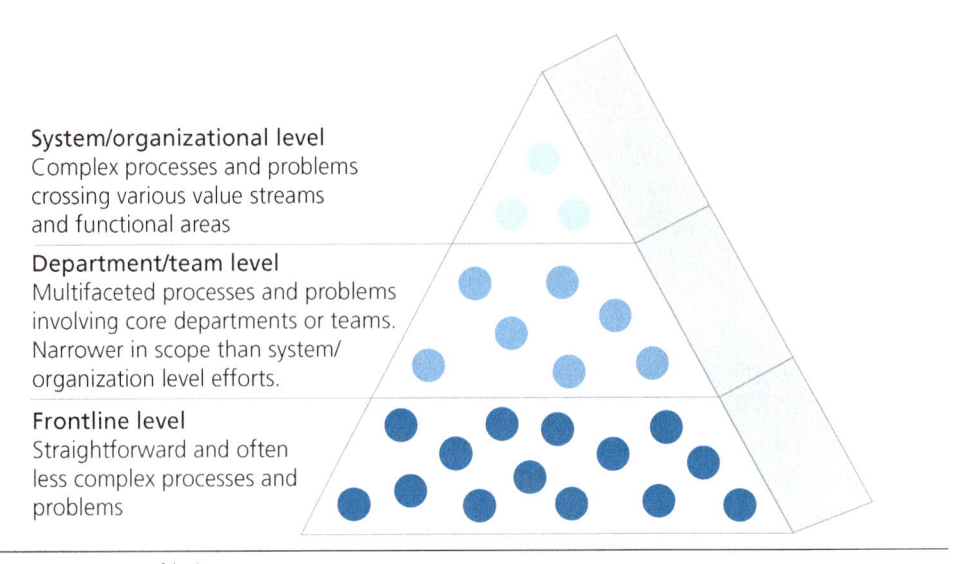

Figure 8.3 Types of kaizen.
Source: Adapted from Liker 2004.

LEAN DMAIC MODEL

The lean DMAIC model is a checklist-driven, systematic approach used to deploy the roadmap. The overlay of DMAIC on the roadmap depicts how the checklist applies the lean principles to a project (Figure 8.4).

- *Define:* Establish the scope and clearly define the problem to be addressed
- *Measure:* Document and validate the current state using process maps, data, and analysis to quantify current capability
- *Analyze:* Analyze data and identify opportunities
- *Improve:* Utilize the lean fundamentals, flow, and pull to implement countermeasures for the identified opportunities
- *Control:* Emphasize sustainability and process and outcome quality

Remember, kaizen (change for good) is an ongoing process. Lean is the relentless pursuit of waste reduction. Checklists, like other processes and systems, should be continually evaluated and improved to ensure they drive quality and efficiency. You do not want these types of documents to be static. For example, when the lean DMAIC checklist was first developed at Jefferson, it was six pages long. There was a lot of detail for everything that needed to take place. After each RIE, the teams would evaluate the checklist and discuss what was missed and unused. Over the course of six years, the list narrowed to a single page, which continues to be refined. Keep notes as you apply the tool. Document tasks you might have missed or details that were overlooked. Include your own revisions on details and steps to consider in advance based on prior or new experiences. The DMAIC checklist helps provide project management structure (Hina-Syeda, Kimbrough,

EXECUTING A PROJECT THROUGH LEAN DMAIC   137

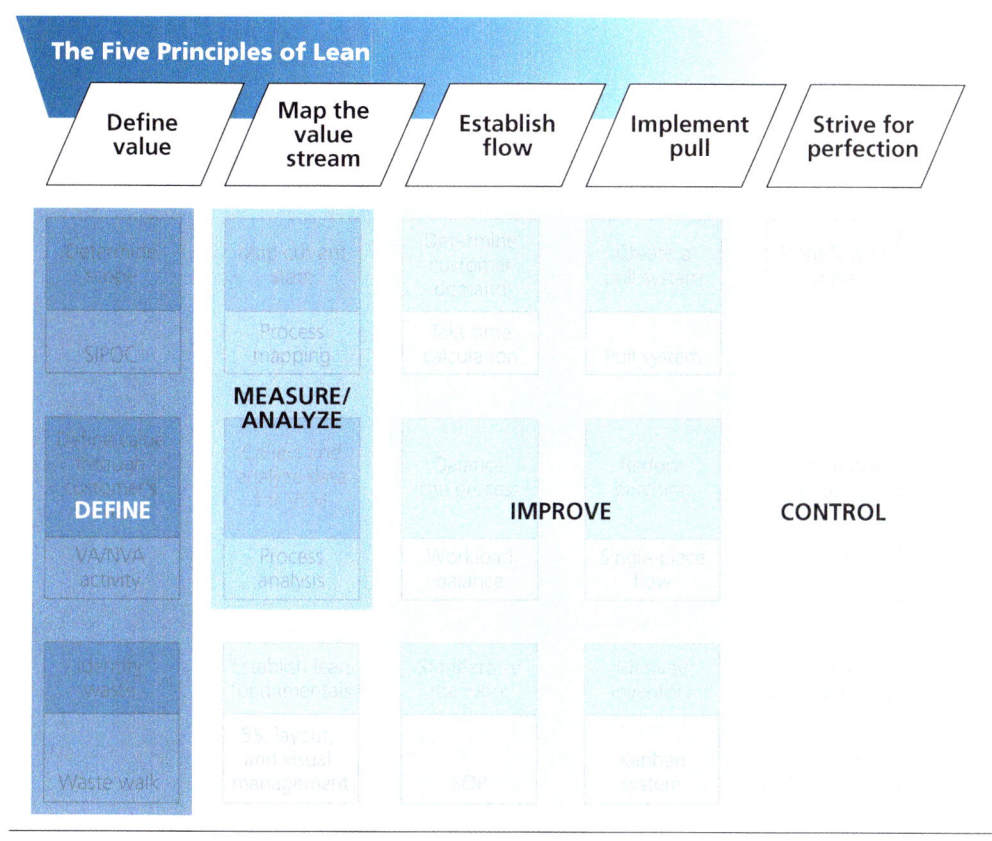

Figure 8.4   Roadmap with DMAIC overlay.

Murdoch, & Markova, 2013). You can apply the checklist to non-lean projects, bypassing tools or activities that do not apply; however, the framework is the same.

The lean DMAIC checklist includes deliverables and logistics for initiating, planning, executing, and closing lean improvement projects (Figure 8.5). The appendixes contain a detailed review of all tools and templates provided on the CD. The time frame for each phase is an approximate guideline for how long the planning, execution, and control/close processes take. Depending on the scope and resource availability, the project might vary significantly. Use your organizational knowledge and experience to determine what works best for you.

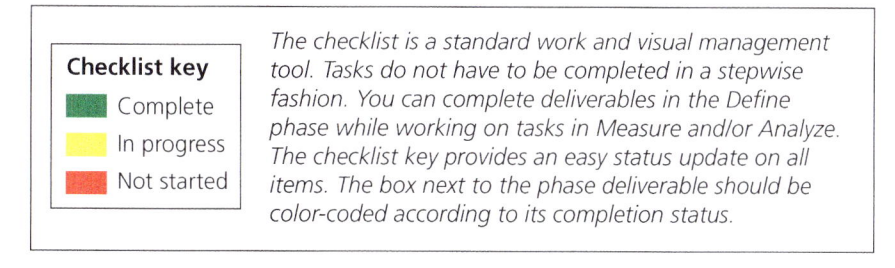

Checklist key
- Complete
- In progress
- Not started

The checklist is a standard work and visual management tool. Tasks do not have to be completed in a stepwise fashion. You can complete deliverables in the Define phase while working on tasks in Measure and/or Analyze. The checklist key provides an easy status update on all items. The box next to the phase deliverable should be color-coded according to its completion status.

Lean DMAIC Checklist Project name: _____ Date last revised: _____

Date of event: _____ Facilitators: _____

DEFINE Phase Checklist
5–6 weeks before event

- [ ] Assign facilitator team roles
  - Leader, communications, logistics
- [ ] Kickoff meeting with sponsor(s)
  - Define problem/goal
  - Identify individuals to interview/draft communication plan
- [ ] Review current IS or other projects in area
  - Review potential/upcoming IS changes
- [ ] Conduct voice of customer (VOC) interviews
- [ ] Conduct a waste walk
- [ ] Develop high-level process map
- [ ] Begin project charter
- [ ] Assess change readiness using profile tool
- [ ] Use systems and process profile tool
- [ ] Schedule event (location/date/times)
- [ ] **Close DEFINE phase**

MEASURE Phase Checklist
4 weeks before event

- [ ] Review previous rapid improvement events, kaizens, or other projects
- [ ] Formulate data collection plan (if needed)
- [ ] Conduct process value analysis
- [ ] Conduct workflow value analysis
- [ ] Create current state value stream map (VSM)
- [ ] Determine event improvement metrics (2–3)
  - Identify data sources
  - Collect and graph baseline data
  - Calculate potential financial impact
- [ ] Consolidate VOC interviews into key themes
- [ ] Select team of process experts/stakeholders (ideal size is 6–8)
- [ ] Complete project charter
- [ ] Assess equipment, IS, and facilities support requirements
- [ ] **Close MEASURE phase**

ANALYZE Phase Checklist
3 weeks before event

- [ ] Perform data analysis
- [ ] Determine key stakeholders
  - Conduct stakeholder analysis
- [ ] Develop vision statement and elevator speech

1–2 weeks before event

- [ ] Confirm event location, time, and attendance
  - Confirm sponsor attendance at kick-off
- [ ] Prepare team information packet
  - Charter, VOC summaries, other relevant documentation
- [ ] Complete rapid improvement event agenda
- [ ] Prepare needed supplies (flip charts, markers, tape, sticky notes, PowerPoint, handouts, etc.)
- [ ] **Close ANALYZE phase**

IMPROVE Phase Checklist
Event duration 2 hours to 3 days

The Rapid Improvement Event

- [ ] Prepare event room (1hr before start)
  - Post all flip charts, prepare supplies
- [ ] Kickoff (sponsor welcome)
- [ ] Current state validation—where we are today and what we need to do to get to future state

Problem-solving process:

- [ ] 1. Brainstorm issue/barriers
- [ ] 2. Filter and prioritize
- [ ] 3. Brainstorm potential solutions
- [ ] 4. Filter and prioritize
- [ ] 5. Develop action plan
- [ ] Develop recommendations
- [ ] Develop communication plan
- [ ] Finalize Control phase action plan
  - Determine Control phase meeting schedule, time, and location
- [ ] Create sponsor/process owner report-out
  - Review Control phase action plan
  - Present recommendations
  - Discuss next steps
- [ ] Report out to sponsor(s) and process owner(s)
- [ ] **Close IMPROVE phase**

CONTROL Phase Checklist
4–8 weeks after event

1 week after
- [ ] Review communication plan/deliverables
- [ ] Monitor event metrics
- [ ] Control phase team meeting

2 weeks after
- [ ] Monitor event metrics
- [ ] Control phase team meeting

3–4 weeks after
- [ ] Monitor event metrics
- [ ] Control phase team meeting
- [ ] Develop control plan with sponsor(s) and process owner(s) to monitor sustainability
- [ ] Calculate any financial impact
  - Cost savings/avoidance, etc.
- [ ] Conduct process analysis (before/after)
- [ ] Conduct change readiness profile (before/after)
- [ ] Begin kaizen A3 report

5 weeks after
- [ ] Project handoff
- [ ] Finalize kaizen A3 report
- [ ] Send thank-yous to participants
- [ ] **Close project and CONTROL phase**

6–8 weeks after
- [ ] Formal results presentation/sharing

NOTES:

Checklist key:
- Complete
- In progress
- Not started

Figure 8.5 DMAIC checklist.

Define Phase

Appendixes A and B describe tools presented here in further detail. The Define phase initiates the project (Figure 8.6). Once the scope is defined, the Define phase checklist is employed. The work put into the first three phases (Define, Measure, and Analyze) will pay big dividends downstream, reducing rework and other issues (Toussaint & Gerard, 2010). The focus is on processes, not outcomes. If the focus is on improving the correct process, outcomes will follow. It is like the analogy of losing weight: if you focus on the process (burning more calories than you consume), the weight reduction will follow. An additional note, before engaging in

DEFINE Phase Checklist
5–6 weeks before event
- ☐ Assign facilitator team roles
    - –Leader, communications, logistics
- ☐ Kickoff meeting with sponsor(s)
    - –Define problem/goal
    - –Identify individuals to interview/draft communication plan
- ☐ Review current IS or other projects in area
    - –Review potential/upcoming IS changes
- ☐ Conduct voice of customer (VOC) interviews
- ☐ Conduct a waste walk
- ☐ Develop high-level process map
- ☐ Begin project charter
- ☐ Assess change readiness using profile tool
- ☐ Use systems and process profile tool
- ☐ Schedule event (location/date/times)
- ☐ **Close DEFINE phase**

Figure 8.6 Define phase checklist.

an improvement project, make sure the area under evaluation is within your circle of control. If you do not have the ability to change it (e.g., another department's process), you will have to assess your effectiveness in influencing the desired change; otherwise you could be fighting a losing battle.

Assign Facilitator Team Roles (Leader, Communications, Logistics)

An improvement team, especially one led by lean practitioners, needs defined roles. These individuals serve as the core team driving the project. Ideally at least three individuals are assigned to the team in order to distribute the workload. The leader is responsible for delegating project tasks to the team. The communications person manages the communication plan. The logistics person oversees the coordination of tasks required to schedule and host an improvement event.

Kickoff Meeting with Sponsor(s)

The project sponsor is typically the person with decision-making authority (e.g., vice president or director). The kickoff meeting is between the improvement team and the sponsor. The problem and objective of the project are reviewed and agreed upon. The sponsor provides a list of individuals for the team to interview and include in the improvement event. The sponsor identifies the process owner, the individual with direct day-to-day oversight of the functional areas affected by the project. Lean projects typically have several process owners since the project flows horizontally across functional departments. The team also drafts the communication plan.

Communication Plan

The communication plan defines the groups of stakeholders that need to be kept informed throughout the DMAIC project phases (Snee & Hoerl, 2003). For each specified group there is a key message about the project or impending change that needs to be articulated. Depending on the group, the delivery mechanism and frequency of providing communication will vary. For example, clinicians typically prefer communication through huddles rather than e-mail. The person responsible for delivering the message is from the improvement team or the sponsor.

Review Current Information Systems or Other Projects in Area

It is important to do an environmental scan of previous, current, or upcoming projects related to the effort. Are there projects that you can leverage? Are there individuals or teams of importance that you can include? This will help reduce the likelihood of rework, redundant projects, or counterproductive efforts.

Conduct Voice of Customer Interviews

VOC interviews are critical for understanding the context of the problem. Since a variety of stakeholders are usually involved, shadowing is a great way to learn the process (Pande & Holpp, 2002). Remember to "go and see, ask why, and show respect" (Womack, 2011). If you do not understand the issues that staff are dealing with, how can you help support and empower them to resolve them? Talk with employees and look beyond surface issues. Drill down to the root causes (5 Whys), and look across the value stream (Graban, 2012). Ask the following questions during VOC interviews: (1) What is working? (2) What is not working? (3) What frustrates you at work? and (4) If you could change one or two things, what would you change and why?

Conduct a Waste Walk

The waste walk is an observational assessment of process inefficiencies at the gemba. The improvement team allocates time to observe the process and employee flow and documents all DOWNTIME wastes observed.

> **Waste Walk Questions**
> - How does the process work?
> - How do you know if it is being performed correctly?
> - How do you know when an error occurs?
> - What do you do when a problem arises?
> - What cues are there to indicate you need to do something?
> - Do you do tasks the same way as others?

Develop a High-Level Process Map

Draft a high-level process map using the project scope.

Begin Project Charter

The project charter is the contract between the improvement team and the sponsor. The charter includes the scope, problem, and objective. Additional information includes what data are used, individuals of value, and anticipated issues or barriers to address. To begin, complete page 1 of the two-page charter.

Assess Change Readiness Using Profile Tool

The change readiness profile tool assesses the current environment of the targeted improvement area (Figure 8.7) (Palmer, 2004). The six domains (detailed in Chapter 10) evaluate the current, transition, and future state components to leading change. Through VOC interviews or a survey, the improvement team can estimate the area's level of change readiness.

Use Systems and Process Profile Tool

Another tool used to determine the impact on change is the systems and process profile (Figure 8.8). This assessment tool evaluates the potential effect a change could have on various elements like staffing, information systems, and resources. This tool, along with the change readiness profile, provides a better understanding of the environmental current state and enables the improvement team to identify vulnerable areas and leverage strengths.

Schedule Event (Location, Date, Times)

The logistics leader works with the sponsor to determine the date and duration of the improvement event. As described earlier, the event could be two hours or up to three days depending on the project scope and problem complexity.

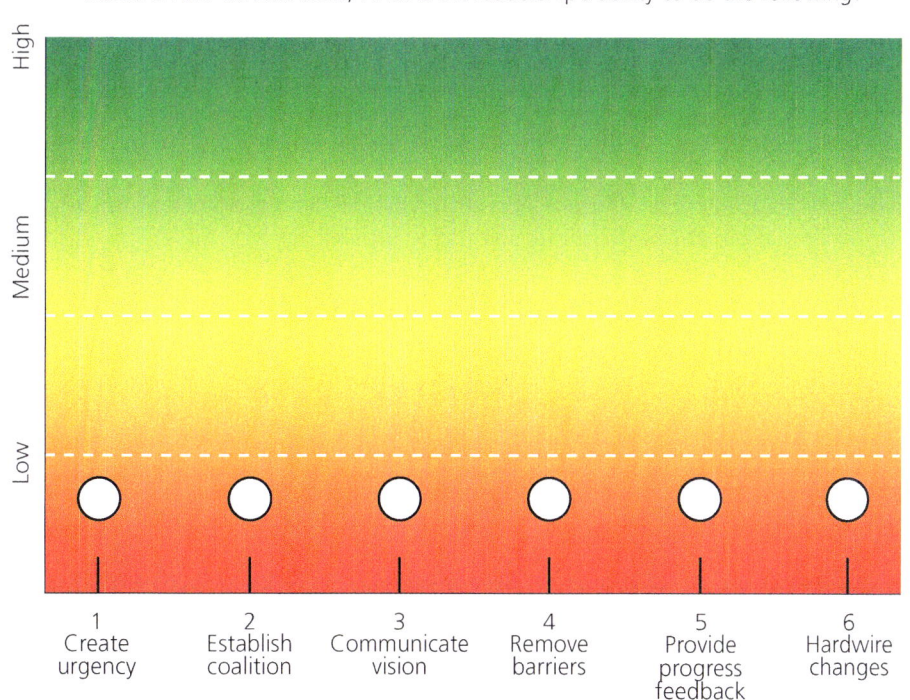

Figure 8.7 Change readiness profile tool.

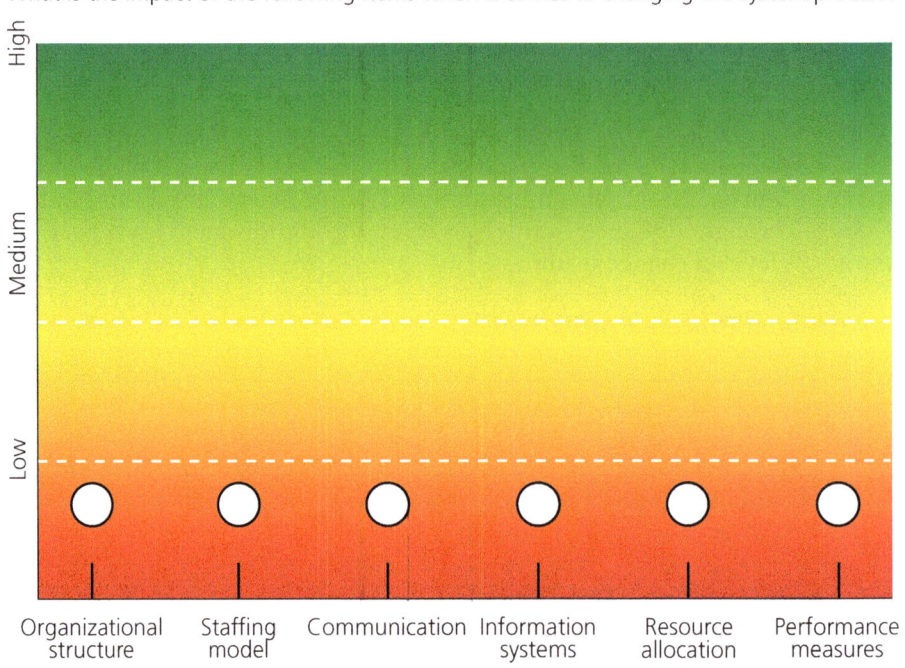

What is the impact of the following items when it comes to changing the system/process?

Figure 8.8 Systems and process profile tool.

Close Define Phase

The Define phase closes once all applicable deliverables have been completed.

Measure Phase

Tools presented here are further described in Appendixes A and C. The Measure phase introduces data collection (Figure 8.9). The following deliverables help paint a picture of where opportunities for improvement exist within the process. Improvement event participants are also identified.

Review Previous Rapid Improvement Events, Kaizens, or Other Projects

If the problem was previously addressed, review what that team did. Lessons learned and strategies applied will provide insight as to how you can move your team forward. If there were similar projects in other areas, you might be able to adopt and adapt their improvement approach. Also, remember that kaizen happens everywhere. Talk with staff and see if they have previously tried to solve the problem. Solutions and lessons learned are generated by more ways than just projects. Where possible, do not reinvent the wheel.

Formulate Data Collection Plan (if Needed)

Providing data in order to drive improvements is critical. How can you get better if you do not even know how you are doing in the first place? How will you know where your vulnerabilities and strengths are? We have to arm people with actionable information and then hold them accountable for the outcomes. Develop a data collection

MEASURE Phase Checklist

4 weeks before event

☐ Review previous rapid improvement events, kaizens, or other projects
☐ Formulate data collection plan (if needed)
☐ Conduct process value analysis
☐ Conduct workflow value analysis
☐ Create current state value stream map (VSM)
☐ Determine event improvement metrics (2–3)
  –Identify data sources
  –Collect and graph baseline data
  –Calculate potential financial impact
☐ Consolidate VOC interviews into key themes
☐ Select team of process experts/stakeholders (ideal size is 6–8)
☐ Complete project charter
☐ Assess equipment, IS, and facilities support requirements
☐ **Close MEASURE phase**

Figure 8.9 Measure phase checklist.

plan if there are no information systems or automated data collection tools in place. This can be an interim log to calculate baseline performance. A post-improvement audit will occur in the Control phase to assess the impact of change.

Conduct Process and Workflow Value Analyses

Using the Microsoft Excel–based tools, conduct time study observations following the process and employee flow. As described in Chapter 3, process value analysis is one of the most powerful lean diagnostic tools.

Create Current State Value Stream Map

Using the high-level SIPOC and process value analysis observations, complete the current state VSM. Remember to include waiting in between steps.

Determine Event Improvement Metrics (Two or Three)

Improvement metrics should reflect the operational performance of the area (Lawal et al., 2014). The metrics should align directly with the problem and objective. Using the appropriate chart (see "Performance Dashboards" in Chapter 7), collect and graph baseline data. The baseline is the foundation from which to assess the impact of planned changes. If applicable, calculate the financial impact of any change (e.g., overtime or rework reductions).

Consolidate VOC Interviews into Key Themes

Sort key themes that were consistent throughout the VOC interviews conducted by the improvement team. Themes usually include lack of communication; unavailable information, tools, and equipment; poor coordination between or within teams; issues with information systems; and no accountability. The themes might indicate potential root causes.

Select Team of Process Experts/Stakeholders

Involving stakeholders is critical to the success of any improvement or change effort. You have likely experienced a project stall or fail because the right people were not included. Lean thinking comes from a horizontal perspective. Who is involved upstream and downstream? Include all parties across the continuum of a process. For example, when improving patient flow in the operating room, include the departments that see the patient first (i.e., admissions/registration, pre-procedure nursing), the operating room itself, and the areas that may see the patient after surgery (i.e., nursing unit, recovery unit). Horizontal thinking breaks the vertical "silo" approach. The ideal number of improvement event participants is six to eight individuals, not including the improvement team facilitators.

Complete Project Charter

Finalize the charter by completing page 2.

Assess Equipment, Information Systems, and Facilities Support Requirements

Depending on the scope, area, and problem, assess whether ad hoc support services will be needed during the scheduled improvement event.

Close Measure Phase

The Measure phase closes once all applicable deliverables have been completed.

Analyze Phase

Tools presented here are further described in Appendixes A and D. The Analyze phase includes analysis of collected data as well as final logistic planning for the improvement event (Figure 8.10).

ANALYZE Phase Checklist

3 weeks before event

- [ ] Perform data analysis
- [ ] Determine key stakeholders
    – Conduct stakeholder analysis
- [ ] Develop vision statement and elevator speech

1–2 weeks before event

- [ ] Confirm event location, time, and attendance
    – Confirm sponsor attendance at kickoff
- [ ] Prepare team information packet
    – Charter, VOC summaries, other relevant documentation
- [ ] Complete rapid improvement event agenda
- [ ] Prepare needed supplies (flip charts, markers, tape, sticky notes, PowerPoint, handouts, etc.)
- [ ] **Close ANALYZE phase**

Figure 8.10 Analyze phase checklist.

Perform Data Analysis

Using data, determine opportunities for improvement. What are the key drivers of the problem? If you are not comfortable with data analysis, seek help from individuals with this skill set. Data analysis will help verify and target root causes.

Determine Key Stakeholders

Use VOC and process observations to conduct a stakeholder analysis with the improvement team. Identify individuals or groups that support the project and those who oppose it. If there is resistance to the effort, develop a strategy to win their support or, at the very least, address their concerns and limit the negative impact they might cause. Project success is contingent on leveraging the leaders and influencers within the improvement area. Build a guiding coalition to help communicate and disseminate changes rapidly.

Develop the Vision Statement and Elevator Speech

The elevator speech provides a concise summary that defines the project, objective, and what staff can do to help. This becomes a consistent message delivered between the improvement team and the sponsor throughout the life cycle of the project. When combined, the vision statement provides the destination and direction of the improvement strategy, while the elevator speech outlines the script to communicate important aspects of the change (i.e., what, when, how, what you can do to help, how it affects you).

Confirm Event Location, Time, and Attendance

The logistics person confirms all required resources are available (e.g., audio/visual equipment, food/snacks, and supplies such as sticky notes, markers, and flipcharts). The sponsor undertakes the improvement event kickoff to set expectations.

Prepare Team Information Packet

The improvement team shares information gathered and analyzed through the first three project phases. The charter, VOC summary, and other relevant analyses are distributed to the improvement event participants. This information provides context for where identified opportunities exist and the current state baseline.

Complete Rapid Improvement Event Agenda

The agenda details are in Appendix A.

Close the Analyze Phase

The Analyze phase closes once all applicable deliverables have been completed.

Improve Phase

Appendixes A and E further define tools presented here. The rapid improvement event (or improvement event) is the problem-solving portion of the project (Figure 8.11). The first three phases provided a detailed understanding of the current

IMPROVE Phase Checklist
Event duration 2 hours to 3 days
The Rapid Improvement Event

- [ ] Prepare event room (1hr before start)
    - Post all flip charts, prepare supplies
- [ ] Kickoff (sponsor welcome)
- [ ] Current state validation—where we are today and what we need to do to get to future state

Problem-solving process:
- [ ] 1. Brainstorm issue/barriers
- [ ] 2. Filter and prioritize
- [ ] 3. Brainstorm potential solutions
- [ ] 4. Filter and prioritize
- [ ] 5. Develop action plan
- [ ] Develop recommendations
- [ ] Develop communication plan
- [ ] Finalize Control phase action plan
    - Determine Control phase meeting schedule, time, and location
- [ ] Create sponsor/process owner report-out
    - Review Control phase action plan
    - Present recommendations
    - Discuss next steps
- [ ] Report out to sponsor(s) and process owner(s)
- [ ] **Close IMPROVE phase**

Figure 8.11 Improve phase checklist.

state through VOC interviews, observations, and process analysis. Now with an assigned team of process experts, the improvement team is ready to facilitate the problem-solving process. Chapter 9, "Facilitating Rapid Improvements," provides a systematic approach to develop a high-impact action plan.

Prepare Event Room (One Hour before Start)

Verify that all needed supplies are ready in advance of the participants arriving.

Kickoff

Led by the sponsor, participants get an overview of why the project was selected, what the objective is for the improvement event, and the expectations for their participation and commitment into the Control phase.

Current State Validation

The team reviews the informational packet with the participants. Remember that some participants may not understand process maps or other basic lean concepts like VA versus NVA activity. Depending on the level of knowledge, you might need to provide a simple introduction or tutorial on concepts and terms. This can also be done in advance of the improvement event.

Problem-Solving Process

The five-step problem-solving process is explained in Chapter 9. The steps are (1) brainstorm issues and barriers, (2) filter and prioritize, (3) brainstorm solutions, (4) filter and prioritize, and (5) develop and implement an action plan.

Develop a Communication Plan

Once the action plan is developed, create or revise the vision statement and elevator speech. Briefly explain what is changing, why, and how it will happen. Remember that the improvement event participants are representing their area or discipline. Implementing improvements requires the commitment of all employees within the affected area. Therefore, it is essential to communicate (and over-communicate) with everyone not directly included in the development of the action plan.

Finalize Control Phase Action Plan

Before completing the Improve phase, determine how the action plan will be implemented and monitored. Determine when and where to hold the weekly Control phase meetings. Standing meetings (where you literally stand in a circle) are most effective. The meeting should occur as close to the affected area as possible and should be brief and direct, focusing on status updates and next steps.

Report Out to Sponsor(s) and Process Owner(s)

Upon completion of the action plan and Control phase planning, the improvement event participants should report out to the sponsor and process owner. If there are recommendations that require approval or feedback, this is the time for the team to make the pitch.

Close Improve Phase

The Improve phase closes once all applicable deliverables have been completed.

Improvement Team Reflective Questions

Day 1 Review:
- What did you observe the team doing today?
- What would you do differently and why?
- What lean concepts (tools/principles) is the team working on, and do they need help?
- What must be done by the end of day tomorrow?

Day 2 Review:
- What obstacles did you observe with the team seeing waste?
- What specifically did you do that worked well? Why?
- What was today's biggest challenge? How did you deal with it?

(continued)

Participant Reflective Questions

Day 1 Review:
- What are your observations of the process?
- What workarounds exist?

Day 2 Review:
- What are the key wastes you observed?
- What are the root causes of these wastes?
- What changes have you tried or will you try?
- How do you plan to communicate these changes?
- Did you communicate to all people affected by the changes?
- How are you going to sustain the new process?

Control Phase

Tools presented here are further described in Appendixes A and F. The final project phase is the Control phase (Figure 8.12). This phase consists of executing the action plan developed in the Improve phase as well as formally closing the project and handing off the outstanding action items and tasks to the sponsor and process owner.

CONTROL Phase Checklist
4–8 weeks after event

1 week after
- ☐ Review communication plan/deliverables
- ☐ Monitor event metrics
- ☐ Control phase team meeting

2 weeks after
- ☐ Monitor event metrics
- ☐ Control phase team meeting

3–4 weeks after
- ☐ Monitor event metrics
- ☐ Control phase team meeting
- ☐ Develop control plan with sponsor(s) and process owner(s) to monitor sustainability
- ☐ Calculate any financial impact
  –Cost savings/avoidance, etc.
- ☐ Conduct process analysis (before/after)
- ☐ Conduct change readiness profile (before/after)
- ☐ Begin kaizen A3 report

5 weeks after
- ☐ Project handoff
- ☐ Finalize kaizen A3 report
- ☐ Send thank-yous to participants
- ☐ **Close project and CONTROL phase**

6–8 weeks after
- ☐ Formal results presentation/sharing

Figure 8.12 Control phase checklist.

Review Communication Plan/Deliverables

The communications leader ensures execution of the communication plan throughout this phase of the project. At this point changes are being made to the process. Communication and feedback are critical.

Monitor Event Metrics

Data updates continue throughout the Control phase. Figure 8.13 shows the baseline data (gray) compared with the post-intervention data (blue) and the target. The team communicates performance updates to the affected area on a regular basis serving as a feedback loop.

Control Phase Team Meeting

The weekly team meetings involve the improvement team, improvement event participants, sponsor, process owner, and any stakeholder that needs be included. The team reviews the Control phase action plan and participants provide updates on assigned items.

Develop Control Plan with Sponsor(s) and Process Owner(s) to Monitor Sustainability

Before concluding the Control phase, the improvement team develops a control plan with the sponsor and process owners. The control plan includes strategies for ongoing verification of process compliance, data collection and dissemination, and longer-term refinement of the changes. This is an important transition plan, focusing on hardwiring effective changes.

Calculate Any Financial Impact

Where applicable, calculate any cost savings, revenue enhancement, or cost avoidance as a result of the project. Utilize internal expertise to evaluate and estimate the

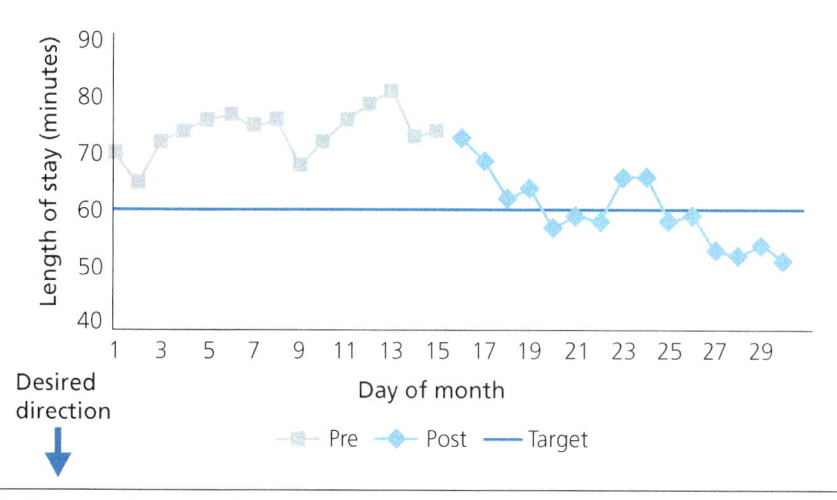

Figure 8.13 Example of run chart, post-improvement.

financial gains. Assessing the impact of improvements can be challenging. Many organizations look for the dollar savings that improvement projects generate, but there are other indicators that show quality output gains (e.g., efficiencies realized, increases in staff/patient satisfaction), all of which are important.

Conduct Process Analysis and Change Readiness Profile (Before/After)

The process analysis (before and after) shows the new distribution of VA to NVA activities. The change readiness profile demonstrates any changes in the work area environment as they relate to change management factors. Results of these analyses support the potential positive impact of the project.

Project Handoff

At the conclusion of the Control phase, the improvement team hands off the project to the sponsor and the process owner. The action plan may not be complete, so it is the responsibility of the sponsor and the process owner to oversee its execution. The improvement team formally closes and hands off the deliverables and assignments so it can move on to the next project.

Finalize Kaizen A3 Report

The A3 report is a standard project documentation template that describes the project's story (Figure 8.14). This becomes the main document for sharing lessons learned and results (Jimmerson et al., 2005). Organizations can accelerate improvements by sharing such information so similar areas and work processes do not encounter the same problem or issue (Sobek & Smalley, 2008). The term *A3* refers to the paper size (11×17). It is a tool that was developed in the late 1960s by Toyota as a standard format for problem solving, proposals, plans, and status reviews (Bicheno & Holweg, 2004; Lean Enterprise Institute).

Send Thank-Yous to Participants

Improvement event participants took time from their workday to help contribute to the project. Be sure to thank them for their time and efforts during both the event and the Control phase. Success and sustainability rely on engaged staff who feel that their contributions are valued.

Close Project and Control Phase

The Control phase closes once all applicable deliverables have been completed.

Formal Results Presentation/Sharing

Several weeks after the close of the Control phase, the sponsor and the process owner provide an update on the project's success and sustainability of results. This is a great opportunity to Check (refine) and Act (from PDCA). Continuous improvement encourages the frequent review of implemented solutions to ensure that they are having the desired, favorable impact. Update the A3 report with final results and distribute to all appropriate stakeholders.

Project title
Participant names

Background
Provide context about the area (organization, department, workspace) under review. What are the core processes/outputs? What is interesting about this project?

Problem statement
What problem is being addressed? How did you validate the problem? What implications/consequences exist if the problem is not resolved?

Project/proposal objective
How do you define success? What specific goals and outcomes define success (e.g., performance metrics)?

Countermeasures (implemented or proposed)
Describe the countermeasures applied or proposed. Explain how the countermeasure addresses the problems identified as well as the expected outcomes.

Pictures/process maps
Provide a current state process map. What are the main issues and gaps in the process? What section are you targeting and why?

Provide a future state map to demonstrate the impact of countermeasures on the process. What is different and why?

Results (metrics to follow/baseline data)
Provide performance dashboard (pre/post if applicable) of metrics described in the problem statement and objectives. Results should link throughout the A3 report.

If an improvement was made, indicate when it occurred so it is easy to see before/after.

Indicate the desired direction of the data (i.e., higher is better).

Next steps
What activities will be required for implementation? Who will be responsible and by when? What other issues/barriers need to be addressed?

Figure 8.14 Example of a kaizen A3 report.

Case Study: Patient Flow through the Short-Procedure Unit (SPU)

The largest volume of surgeries occurs on Jefferson's Center City campus. The OR is a setting abundant in opportunities for improvement. System inefficiencies can lead to suboptimization of OR utilization, thereby decreasing revenue generation. Delays, from patient arrival to entering the preoperative holding area, have an impact on the ability to start scheduled OR procedures on time. Due to high surgical volumes, delays in first cases have a cascading effect on the entire schedule, bottlenecking the pre- and post-procedural areas. These delays have fiscal consequences and are a primary source of patient and employee dissatisfaction.

The project was conducted for 32 of Jefferson's main ORs. On the day of surgery, the patient flow process begins with checking in at admissions and ends after surgery, where the patient is either discharged to home or admitted to an inpatient bed. In order to impact meaningful, incremental improvement, the project scope narrowed to only include patient flow from patient check-in at admissions through arrival at the holding area (HA) (Figure 8.15).

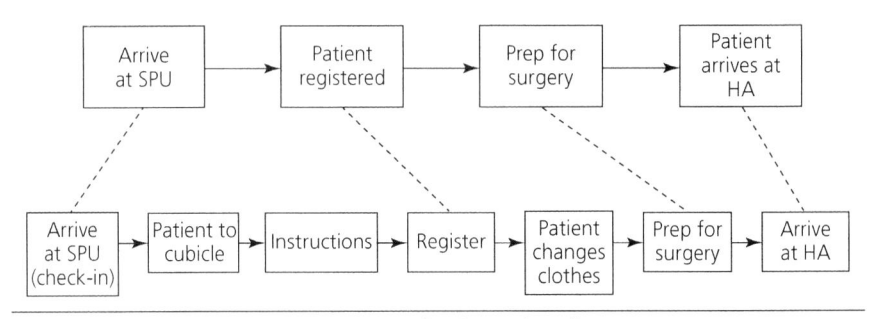

Figure 8.15 Current state process map for OR patient flow.

The study design was a pre/post intervention assessment. The project used the DMAIC framework (Define, Measure, Analyze, Improve, and Control). The primary outcome measure was the time from patient check-in to arrival at the holding area. The patient flow process in the pre-intervention analysis was 54.1 minutes.

Prior to a scheduled RIE, certified lean leaders conducted VOC interviews and process analysis observations. These deliverables established the baseline current state. VOC interviews were conducted with more than 20 staff from all associated areas (registration, SPU, HA, OR, transportation, administration, etc.). The key themes of issues inhibiting process efficiency identified through the VOC interviews and observations were: (1) scheduling; (2) registration delays due to location of department; (3) transportation of patients from SPU to HA; and (4) lack of coordination of activities within the SPU. The inputs from the interviews and process analysis served as the basis for improvement.

Process analysis showed a large proportion (>60%) of NVA activity (Figure 8.16). Within the current state of the process, 43.3% of the process time involved the patient waiting for something to happen (i.e., waiting for a nurse, physician). An additional 8% of the time was committed to patient travel from location to location. In patient flow studies, waiting and transportation are typically the most pervasive forms of waste in the process. These results were expected due to the complexity of the process, geography of work areas, and organizational structure (i.e., admissions, transportation, and OR staff having different reporting structures and managers).

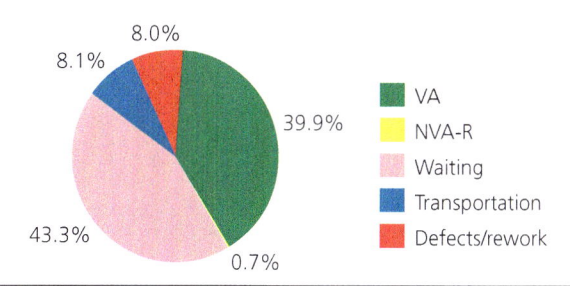

Figure 8.16 Value analysis breakdown for OR patient flow.

After the current state VOC and process analyses were completed, the lean team entered the Improve phase of the project. The lean practitioners facilitated a four-day RIE with a multi-disciplinary group of staff from registration, SPU, HA, and OR (together known as the team). The goal for the team was to develop and pilot countermeasures to address and eliminate identified waste and issues.

During the event, the lean leaders led a structured problem solving process. Participating staff brainstormed barriers and issues that drive inefficiency. The salient issues were prioritized through consensus voting. The priority issues were inefficient patient flow logistics and lack of workflow coordination within the SPU. These issues became targets for improvement. The team developed solutions through structured brainstorming and additional site visits to the work area. There were three core solutions that required detailed action planning:

1. Patient registration moved from the admissions department to SPU at the bedside. This process change removes the need for patients to check in multiple times (previously at admissions then at SPU) (Figures 8.17 and 8.18).

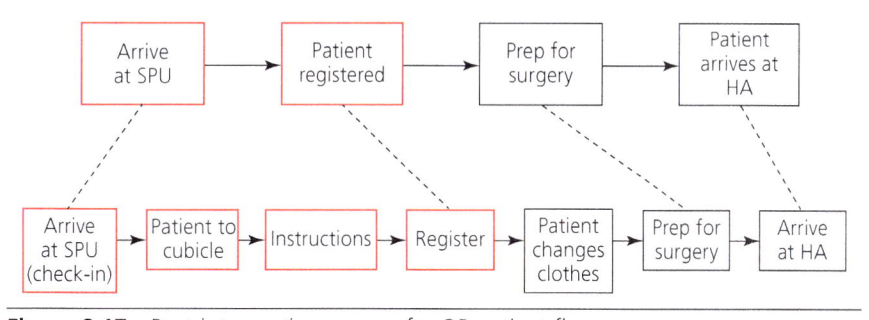

Figure 8.17 Post-intervention process for OR patient flow.

2. SPU charge nurse (responsible for patient flow monitoring) was relocated and tasks were standardized. The charge nurse role is integral in managing flow and assigning nurses to patients based on priority and need. The role rotates between three individuals, which necessitates a standard approach to documentation and responsibilities. The added structure enables staff to work efficiently while the charge nurse monitors the flow of patients, nurses, and registrars.

(continued)

154 Chapter Eight

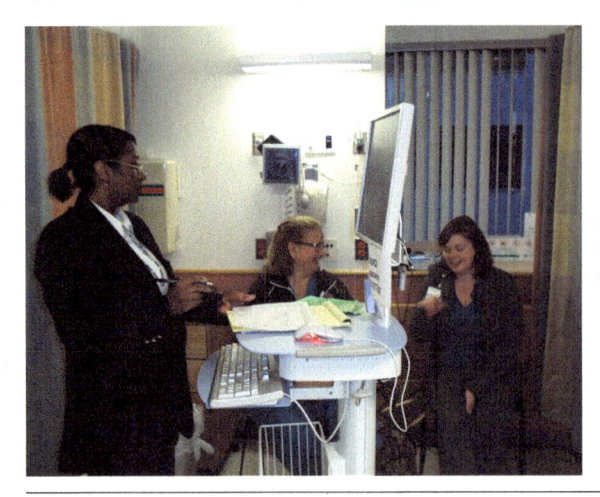

Improvement team piloting registration at the bedside with mock patients

Figure 8.18 Improvement team piloting changes.

3. SPU patient interview processes were streamlined to accommodate the integration of registration staff. The patient interview process performed by the nurse was lengthy. The "need to know" information was identified and re-scripted. This standardized the approach and freed up time for the registrars to complete the admission prior to the patient's surgery preparation.

After the Improve phase, the solutions were hardwired into daily operations. The Control phase included weekly monitoring of action plan progress as well as data updates and reporting. Figure 8.19 provides the pre-/post-intervention monthly processing time trends, including the pre-intervention. Post-intervention data demonstrate a statistically significant improvement in mean processing time from pre-intervention of 54.1 minutes (95% confidence interval 53.3–54.8 minutes) to post-intervention 46.1 minutes (95% confidence interval 45.3–46.9 minutes, $p = 0.000$).

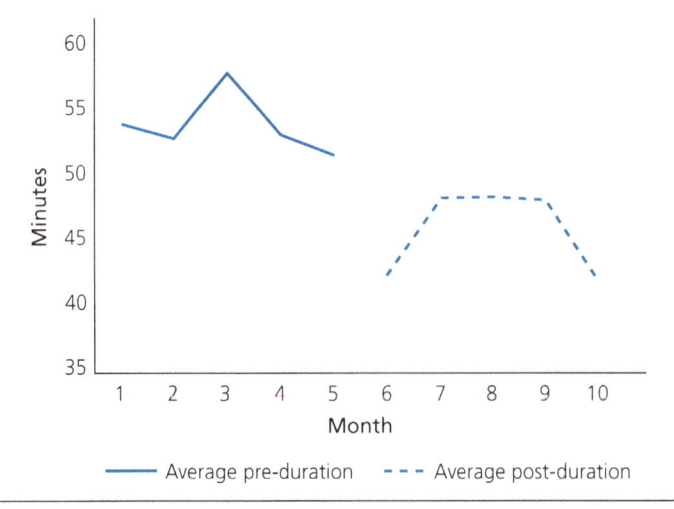

Figure 8.19 Monthly average of SPU processing time.

The process value analysis graph depicts the distribution of VA to NVA activities (Figure 8.20). Post-intervention, the percentage of VA activities increased from 40% to 49%, which was a direct result of reducing and eliminating NVA activities such as transportation and waiting.

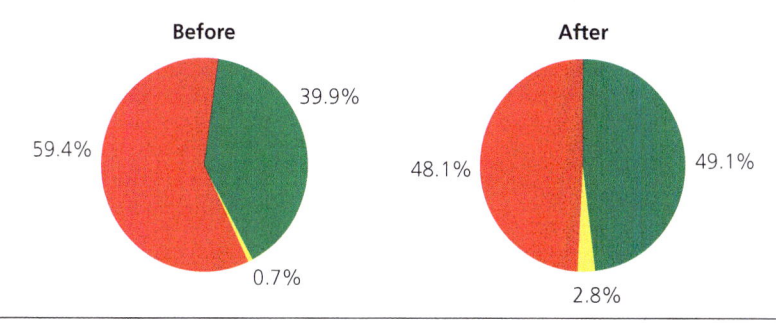

Figure 8.20 Process value analysis before and after intervention.

Source: Modified from Delisle & Jaffe 2015.

CHAPTER CHALLENGE

Develop a project plan using the lean DMAIC checklist. Outline the deliverables with an associated timeline. Execute the plan. What was your experience using the structured approach? Was the checklist helpful? Are there components that need to be added or removed based on your experience?

QUESTIONS

1. What does the kaizen mentality represent?
2. What does everyday kaizen mean?
3. How does the PDCA cycle work? What is the significance of Check and Act?
4. Why do projects require structured phases?
5. What benefit does a project checklist provide? How can you use this in your area of responsibility?
6. Why are VOC interviews important? Who should you talk to when starting a project or process evaluation?
7. What kind of information can a change readiness profile give you? Why is this useful?

8. Why do you need to perform observations and process analyses?
9. Who should be included in a rapid improvement event? Why?
10. What is the importance of weekly Control phase team meetings?
11. Why do projects need to be handed off to sponsors and process owners?
12. How are kaizen A3 reports used to communicate project success and lessons learned?

Chapter 9
Facilitating Rapid Improvements

A plan is an experiment you run to see what you don't understand about the work.

—Steven Spear

Rapid improvement events (RIEs) are an effective management approach that accelerates the pace of change. The RIE ranges in duration from two hours to three days or longer, depending on the scope of the project and complexity of the problem. RIEs involve process experts and stakeholders (usually 6–12 individuals) who are brought together to solve a problem and implement an action plan. The approach expedites the normal business approach of forming committees or working groups that can take months to solve a problem. The rate of change is as important as the scope of it. If you rush something, you will generate strong resistance. If you go too slowly, you will lose momentum. The balance of scope, rate of change, and stakeholders involved leads to project success or failure.

When it comes to implementing improvements, the lean term is kaizen. Kaizen is not just a facilitated improvement event but any improvement made to address a problem. The previous chapter as well as this one describes how to manage improvement projects and facilitate teams. However, these concepts are just as applicable to daily improvements made at the gemba. Kaizen should happen everywhere, all the time. It is essential to ingrain the kaizen mind-set of continuous improvement. The focus is always on delivering value to our customers. Without our customers, we have no purpose to exist as a company.

Advice for RIEs
- Kaizen should not happen to people; it happens through people.
- Facilitators are there to help point the team in the right direction (where the opportunities lie). The team develops the solutions.
- Completing a few objectives is significantly better than partially starting many.
- Sometimes you have to explain the obvious because the distribution of common sense is not even.

Projects ripe for the rapid improvement approach share common characteristics:

- Problem and goal are clearly defined
- Within your scope of control
- Can be fixed quickly (i.e., solutions can be implemented within 30–60 days)
- Eliminates unnecessary work and/or reduces costs
- Strong leadership support and buy-in from key stakeholders
- Aligned with organizational values and strategic initiatives

Effective RIEs include clearly specified roles and responsibilities:

- *Sponsor:* Leadership position (e.g., vice president, director) with decision-making authority over area of focus. This individual is accountable for the success of the effort and helps remove barriers to action plan implementation. The sponsor helps drive results through oversight and support.
- *Process owner:* Person with managerial oversight (e.g., manager, supervisor) who is responsible for implementation and sustainability of the action plan.
- *Participants:* Process experts that provide content expertise and context to solve the problems and issues being addressed. These individuals also help develop and implement the action plan and build staff buy-in and engagement.
- *Facilitator:* Individual with responsibility to lead participants through the problem-solving process. He or she partners with the team to drive action plan implementation.

FACILITATION GUIDELINES

Facilitated meetings for RIEs should follow the same guidelines as earlier regarding roles, responsibilities, and ground rules. Establishing team roles helps clarify expectations and ensures that the problem-solving process can be efficiently managed (Andersen, Rovik, & Ingebrigtsen, 2014). Since RIEs are short in nature, it is important to have delegated tasks and timelines. Following are common roles within RIE teams:

- *Lead facilitator:* Guides group through problem-solving activities to achieve objectives. This person ensures everyone participates and stays focused.
- *Process checker:* This role is for a co-facilitator. The process checker maintains focus on agreed-upon processes used and helps the participants apply tools correctly. He or she also assists the lead facilitator.
- *Scribe:* The scribe is responsible for recording ideas verbatim on sticky notes, flip charts, or other provided materials. The role of scribe is assigned to a participant.
- *Timekeeper:* The timekeeper monitors time during small group activities and provides updates to keep the team on track. This is another important role during an RIE. The assigned time allocation for activities should be closely

followed to ensure the RIE meets its intended objective in the set period of time.

- *Presenter:* Again, for group-based activities, the presenter leads the presentation of the group's work. He or she is responsible for concisely summarizing the activity outcome.

Ground rules provide participants with expectations for how to behave and what to expect during an RIE. Ground rules describe how the RIE will run, how participants are expected to interact, and what behaviors are acceptable or unacceptable. They help teams self-manage and self-correct. Examples of ground rules include the following:

- Start and end on time
- Cell phones and pagers should be set on vibrate
- Vegas rules—what is said in the room stays in the room
- Open mind, leave cynicism at door
- One person speaks at a time

Facilitators provide an opportunity at the start of the RIE to review ground rules and ask participants to add others to the list. The best way to ensure compliance with ground rules is to provide participants an opportunity to define what they will be.

> *The parking lot is a tool that helps keep discussions focused. Typically a flip chart or document is posted in the room of the RIE and is used to store issues and ideas that have been captured on sticky notes. The parking lot is used when topics come up that (1) are outside the project scope, (2) contain issues that need to be addressed by a different group of stakeholders, or (3) require questions, comments, or follow-up at a later point in time. This tool helps the team stay the course and meet the RIE objectives in the allocated time.*

THE KAIZEN PROBLEM-SOLVING PROCESS

Facilitating RIEs requires a structured problem-solving approach called the kaizen problem-solving process. This five-step process leads to identification of key issues, development of effective solutions, and implementation of a well-defined action plan. The five steps are (1) brainstorm issues and barriers, (2) filter and prioritize issues and barriers, (3) brainstorm solutions, (4) filter and prioritize solutions, and (5) develop and implement the action plan (Figure 9.1). A set of tools accompanies each step to help facilitate the process. The following section reviews the five steps and associated tools. Note that only a select number of tools are presented. As stated in the introduction, there are many ways to accomplish a task, but this book presents the most effective approaches based on years of experience facilitating rapid improvements.

160 *Chapter Nine*

1. Brainstorm issues and barriers
2. Filter and prioritize
3. Brainstorm solutions
4. Filter and prioritize
5. Develop and implement action plan

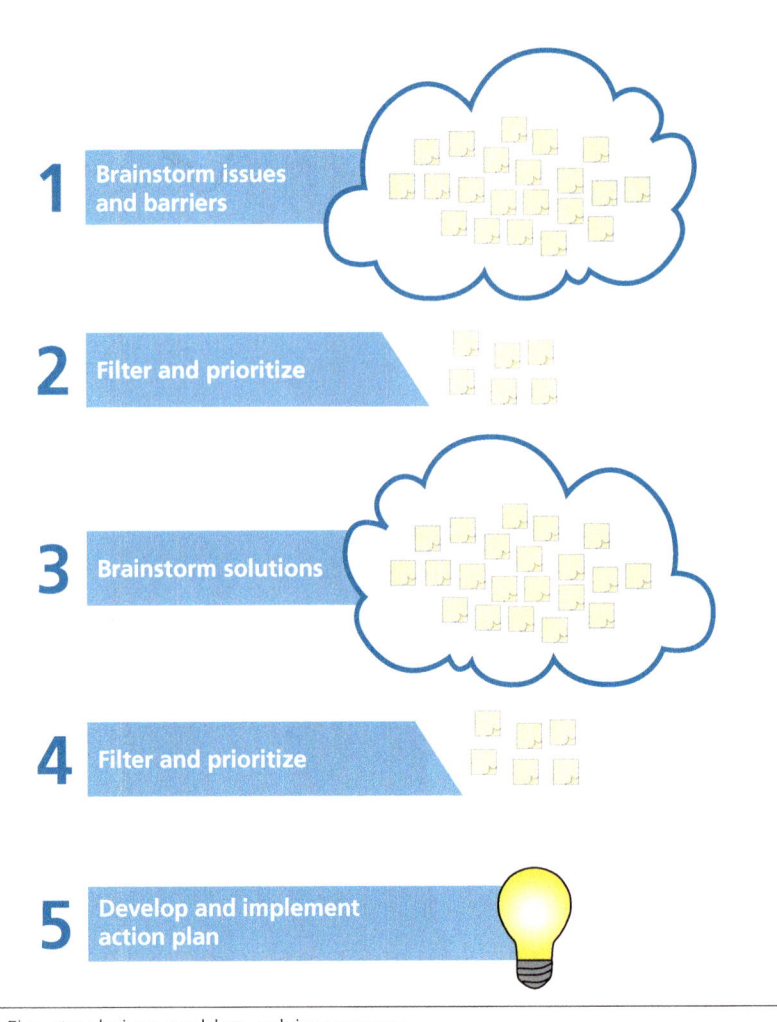

Figure 9.1 Five-step kaizen problem-solving process.

Step 1: Brainstorm Issues and Barriers

The first step of the kaizen problem-solving process is to brainstorm issues and barriers (Figure 9.2). Before discussing solutions, first identify the root causes to address. Solution development is premature if the root cause is unknown. Sometimes we search for answers without knowing the right questions. It is hard to be patient and take a step back. Think less like a firefighter and more like a fire prevention engineer. Firefighters chase down fires to put them out. The engineer designs sprinkler systems and uses specific materials to reduce the likelihood of a fire ever occurring. That is how we need to think about improvements.

Brainstorming is a divergent activity. This means any idea is accepted. During this step, you want the participants (content and process experts) to provide any potential issue or barrier that might contribute to the problem you are trying to solve. The goal is to capture as many ideas as possible regarding the topic at hand.

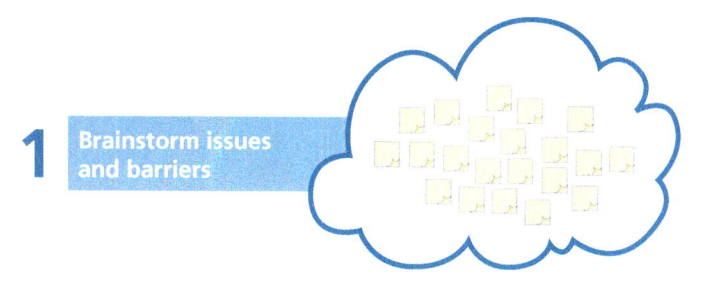

Figure 9.2 Step 1: Brainstorm issues and barriers.

Tools to Use during Step 1

Three brainstorming tools can be used during this step: (1) silent brainstorming, (2) free-for-all, and (3) the fishbone diagram.

Silent Brainstorming

- *How to do it:* Participants have 5–10 minutes of silence for this individual activity in which they write their ideas on sticky notes (one idea per note). Once everyone has written down his or her ideas, the facilitator leads the report out, a brief presentation summarizing the team's work. Each person reads one idea aloud. The facilitator takes the sticky note and places it on a blank flip chart. If other participants have the same or a similar idea, the facilitator consolidates them. The report out rotates one person, one idea at a time, until all ideas have been shared.

- *When to use it:* Silent, individual activities are a great way to diminish any dominating personalities or to provide shy, introverted personalities an opportunity to share their thoughts.

- *What it looks like:* The picture on the left in Figure 9.3 shows the team members reporting out on their ideas. The picture on the right depicts the facilitator consolidating issues and barriers by theme.

Free-for-All

- *How to do it*: The free-for-all is a dynamic brainstorming activity. The facilitator poses the question of what issues and barriers contribute to the problem and all participants openly share their ideas. It is important to assign at least one scribe during the free-for-all so that all documentation is captured. Another important consideration during this activity is the ground rules. Remember to encourage open, respectful dialogue.

- *When to use it:* This open, collaborative activity works well with groups whose members are comfortable with one another. If participants are able to leave their titles at the door and exercise an open mind, the free-for-all can be highly engaging and productive.

- *What it looks like:* Similar to silent brainstorming, the free-for-all yields a flip chart with consolidated issues and barriers.

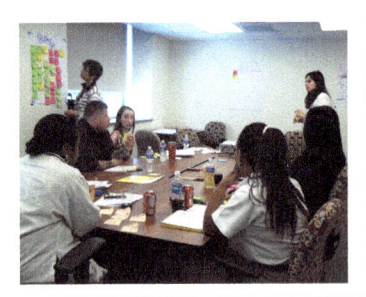

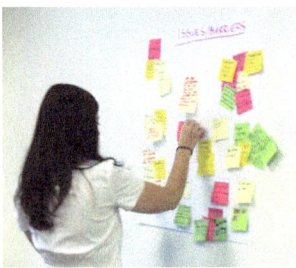

Figure 9.3 Examples of improvement teams brainstorming.

Fishbone Diagram

- *How to do it:* Chapter 7 details the fishbone diagram.
- *When to use it*: This tool provides more structure to brainstorming than either silent brainstorming or the free-for-all. The fishbone is effective if participants are slow to discuss issues and barriers or do not know where to begin. The added structure enables participants to compartmentalize the issues and barriers into predefined themes (i.e., personnel, materials/supplies, measurement, method/processes, machine/equipment).
- *What it looks like:* Figure 9.4 shows an example of a completed fishbone diagram.

Step 2: Filter and Prioritize Issues and Barriers

The second step of the kaizen problem-solving process is to filter and prioritize the issues and barriers (Figure 9.5). Step 2 is one of the most critical components of the problem-solving model. You have to differentiate between issues and barriers within your control and those outside your control before you can develop solutions.

Filtering and prioritizing are convergent activities. During this step the participants help determine which issues and barriers can be directly addressed. Subsequently, participants prioritize these issues and barriers based on the ones with the largest impact on the problem. The goal is to narrow issues and barriers to only those that we can influence.

Tools to Use during Step 2

Step 2 has two phases: (1) filter and (2) prioritize. Filtering requires one tool, the in- or out-of-control activity. Prioritization can be done through dot voting or consensus voting.

Phase 1: Filter—In or Out of Control

- *How to do it:* After the issues and barriers have been collected in step 1, the next step is to filter them. The facilitator takes one issue at a time and asks the participants whether it is "within our control" or "outside our control." The facilitator simply asks the question and moves the sticky note accordingly. The participants are responsible for categorizing the issues based on the

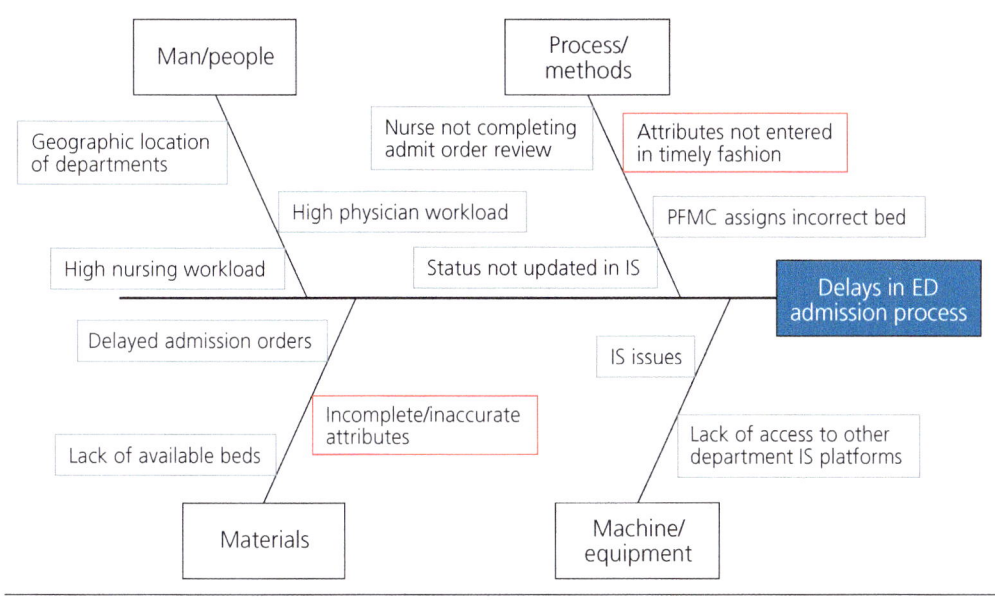

Figure 9.4 Example of a fishbone diagram.

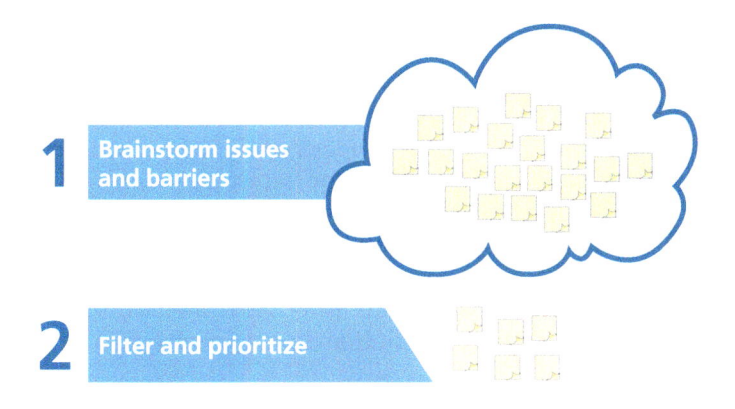

Figure 9.5 Step 2: Filter and prioritize issues and barriers.

knowledge, experience, and scope of work. If an issue or barrier seems to be partly within our control and partly outside our control, break the issue or barrier into smaller pieces. Ask participants to specifically identify those elements that are within our control and document them on a new sticky note. There should not be any sticky notes straddling the line.

- *When to use it:* Immediately after step 1.
- *What it looks like:* The flip chart should have two boxes, one inside the other (Figure 9.6). The inner box defines elements that are "in control." All issues and barriers determined to be within the group's control are placed there. Correspondingly, the issues and barriers that are outside the group's control are placed along the outside region.

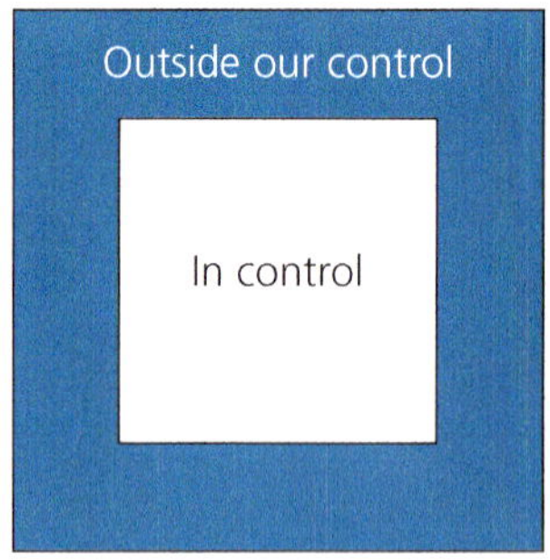

[Figure: Blue square labeled "Outside our control" with a white inner square labeled "In control"]

Figure 9.6 In-control or out-of-control template.

- *Hint for categorizing issues and barriers:* While performing the in- or out-of-control activity, facilitators continue to recategorize issues and barriers by theme (e.g., staffing, technology, process, communication). The identified issues and barriers are typically symptoms of underlying root causes. The themes provide a general summary of these symptoms and may define the potential root cause of the problem. The facilitator creates the categories and writes each one on a new sticky note and displays it above the cluster of issues and barriers. Participants review and approve the categories before phase 2. The flip chart in Figure 9.7 shows the sticky notes sorted by theme.

Phase 2: Prioritize Issues and Barriers

Once the issues and barriers have been sorted (according to whether they are within or outside our control) and categorized by theme, the next step is to prioritize them. Prioritization occurs only for issues and barriers determined to be within the group's control. During this phase, participants vote on what theme/category within their control has the most significant impact on the problem. Generally two or three prioritized themes result from the voting activity. Depending on the breadth and complexity of the prioritized themes, the facilitator might choose to focus on one or two for solution development (steps 3–5).

Dot Voting

- *How to do it:* Each participant receives four dots. The dots can be stickers, pieces of paper, or made with markers. Participants use the dots to vote on the theme/category that has the biggest impact on the problem. Participants do not vote on the individual issues or barriers identified. This is why it is important to categorize after filtering. Participants use their dots as they deem appropriate. Dots can be evenly distributed (four dots for four categories) or concentrated (four dots for one category or three dots for one and only one dot for another). The theme/category with the most dots is the priority for steps 3–5.

- *When to use it:* Dot voting is an individual activity. Participants are encouraged to go up to the flip chart and vote regardless of what their peers are considering. The dot voting strategy aims to reduce group bias.

- *What it looks like:* Figure 9.8 shows various teams using dot voting. The picture on the far right shows the dots surrounding the identified categories (orange sticky notes).

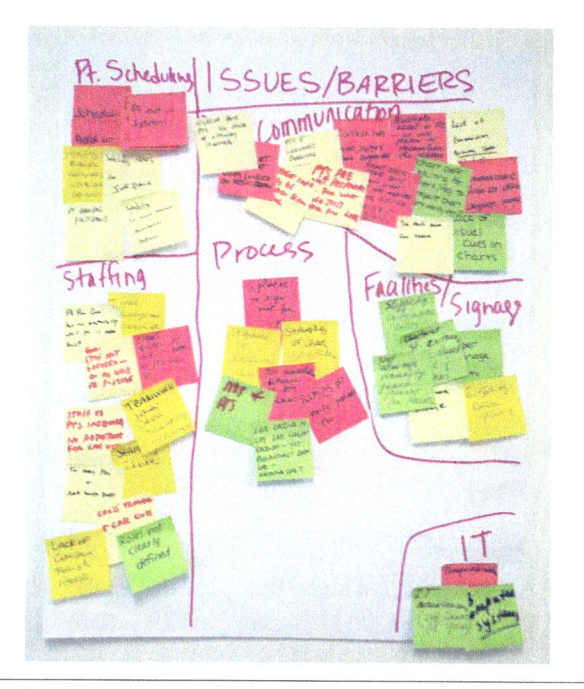

Figure 9.7 Example of categorizing issues and barriers.

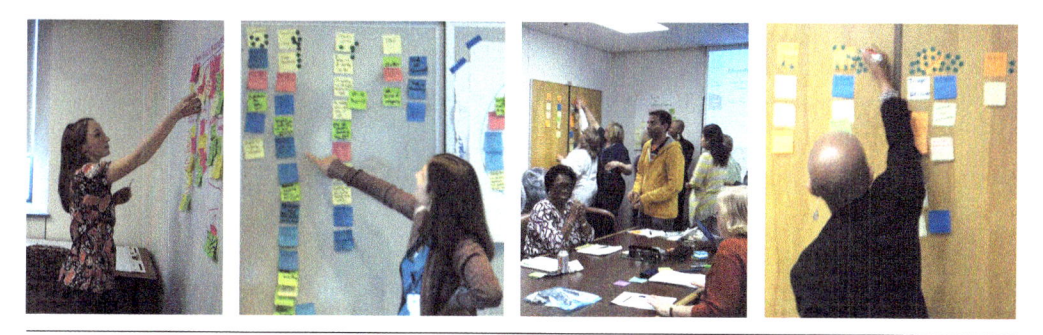

Figure 9.8 Examples of improvement teams voting.

Consensus Voting

- *How to do it:* Consensus voting is a group-based activity. The identified categories are discussed with the participants. The facilitator leads the discussion until there is agreement around the priority category of issues and barriers.

- *When to use it:* This approach is effective if there is general consensus and a clear theme throughout step 1. Similar to the free-for-all brainstorming activity, this can be a dynamic activity that requires facilitation.

- *What it looks like:* Consensus can be shown through a simple show of hands.

Step 3: Brainstorm Solutions

The third step of the kaizen problem-solving process is to brainstorm solutions (Figure 9.9). By now, the prioritized category of issues and barriers has been identified as the root cause. The team is now ready to begin solution development. As noted earlier, there might be one or two prioritized themes/categories that will be addressed during this step.

Brainstorming solutions is a divergent activity. All ideas are welcomed. As with step 1, you want the participants to share any and all ideas that could address the root cause. The objective of step 3 is to gather as many solutions as possible. Solution development entails the following (Silverstein et al., 2009):

- Substitutions—replace existing process with improved approach
- Combinations—leverage and combine steps to improve quality and efficiency
- Adoption and adaption—adopt and adapt proven best practices
- Modification—change the approach/steps to yield different results
- Elimination—remove process steps that produce errors or inefficiencies

Guidelines for Solution Development: Spear's Four Rules

Solution development requires creative insight and a logical approach for implementation. The guiding rules for this problem-solving step come from Steven Spear. Spear developed four rules based on observations at Toyota manufacturing plants. These rules serve as the foundation for solution development (Jimmerson, 2010; Spear, 2005):

1. Activities are clear and well defined. Everyone knows what he or she is supposed to do, when, and how long it should take.
2. Steps are simple and direct.
3. Flow is simple and direct. The process has as few steps and people as are needed to complete.
4. Problems are dealt with in a timely and direct manner.

> *In most areas with opportunities for improvement, the common source of issues is the violation of Spear's first rule. Staff cannot communicate and coordinate efforts effectively without clear expectations.*

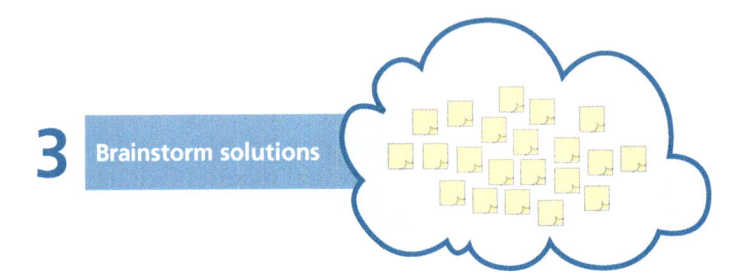

Figure 9.9 Step 3: Brainstorm solutions.

Tools to Use during Step 3

Four tools can be used during step 3: (1) silent brainstorming, (2) free-for-all, (3) direct issue-to-solution brainstorming, and (4) reverse engineering. The silent brainstorming and the free-for-all tools are conducted in the same way as described in step 1.

Direct Issue-to-Solution Brainstorming

- *How to do it:* Direct issue-to-solution brainstorming is the most effective of the solution development tools. Participants work in small groups of three or four people. Each group receives the sticky notes from the prioritized theme/category. Then, each individual note is placed in a column on flip chart paper or on a table or desk. The group brainstorms solutions to the specific issue. During this process, the group might identify a general solution that addresses several issues at once.

- *When to use it:* This tool is the suggested approach for simple, effective solution development. It provides a linear path from issue to solution, which tends to appeal to most participants.

- *What it looks like:* Figure 9.10 shows the flow of direct issue-to-solution brainstorming. First, the prioritized theme is selected. Second, the individual issues that compose the theme are placed in a column. And third, corresponding solutions are developed for each individual issue.

Reverse Engineering

- *How to do it:* The reverse engineering tool provides a different approach to problem solving. Rather than developing solutions based on the identified root causes, the reverse engineering approach takes issue identification to the next level. During this activity, the participants discuss all of the ways in which

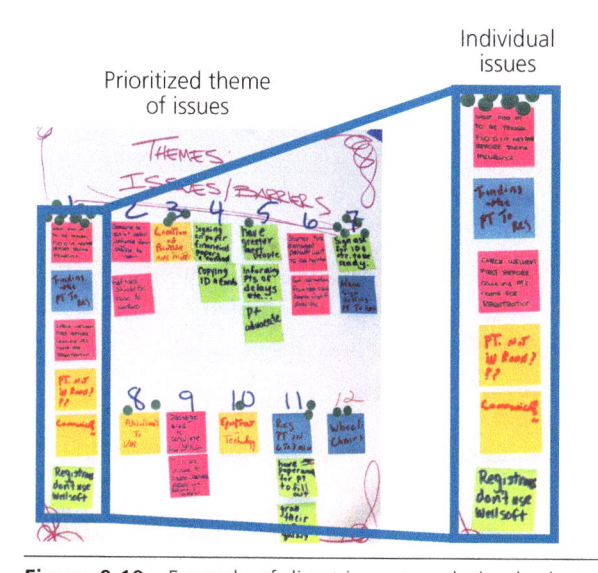

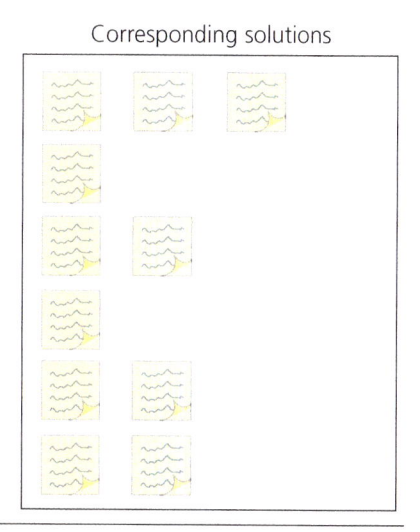

Figure 9.10 Example of direct issue-to-solution brainstorming.

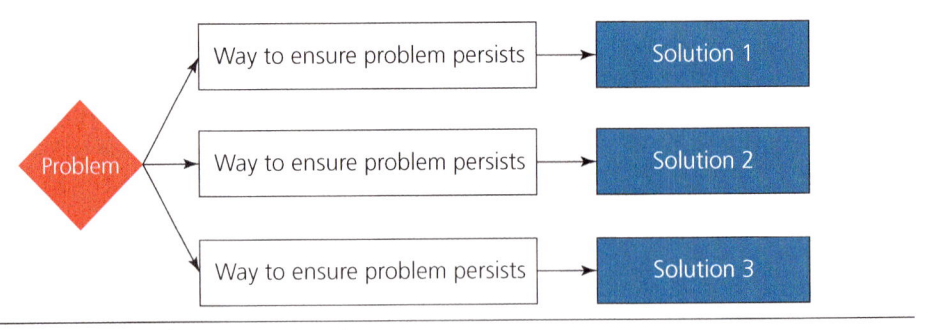

Figure 9.11 Example of reverse engineering.

they can ensure that the problem persists. Once the group brainstorms ways to achieve this, they shift focus toward solving the new problems identified.

- For example, if the problem being addressed is a loud nursing unit, one way to ensure that the condition persists is to implement a "talk loud" policy that requires staff to shout during all interactions. To counter the "talk loud" policy, the team might develop a visual management solution that obviates the need for verbal communication, thus reducing the noise level.

- *When to use it:* This tool is highly effective when groups are struggling with creative ideas.

- *What it looks like:* Figure 9.11 depicts the flow from prioritized problem to ways in which it can persist, leading to a corresponding solution.

Step 4: Filter and Prioritize Solutions

The fourth step of the kaizen problem-solving process is to filter and prioritize the solutions (Figure 9.12). Selecting what you get involved with is tricky. We live in a resource-scarce world, including our own resources (e.g., time, effort, money). There will always be more good ideas than time to implement them (McChesney et al., 2012). We have to prioritize by what will give us the biggest bang for our buck. The convergence of solutions through filtering and prioritizing leads to a high-impact action plan (step 5). The goal is to narrow solutions to those that are effective.

Tools to Use during Step 4

The main tool used during step 4 is the payoff matrix. Depending on the results of prioritization, the group might have to use dot or consensus voting to further refine the selection. Another tool that helps segment solutions is the Lamina (pronounced *la-mine-ah*) tree of low-hanging fruit.

Payoff Matrix

- *How to do it:* The payoff matrix is a simple and highly effective tool that is based on an x-axis and a y-axis. The x-axis is "Ease of implementation," which is defined as easy or difficult. The y-axis is "Impact on problem," which is defined as low or high. The facilitator asks a presenter from each group to read aloud their solutions from step 3. For each solution, the facilitator asks the

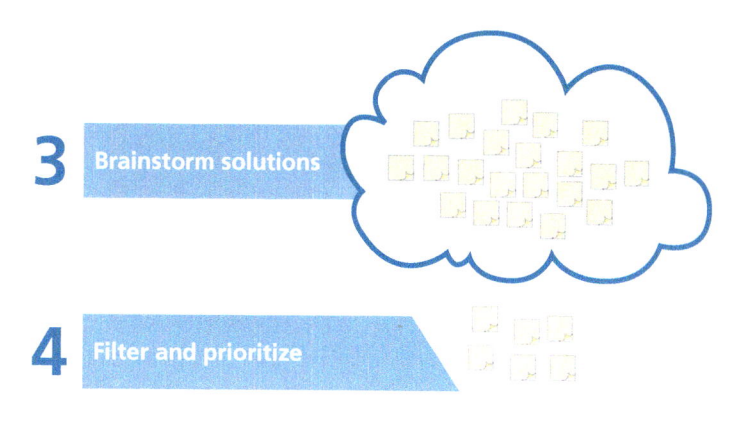

Figure 9.12 Step 4: Filter and prioritize solutions.

participants, "How easy is this to do?" and "What is the potential impact on addressing the problem?" As with the in- or out-of-control tool, the participants determine the appropriate quadrant. The goal is to differentiate and isolate solutions:

- *High impact, easy to implement:* These are the types of solutions we are looking for. Ideas that fall into this category provide the biggest impact at a relatively low cost and with little effort.

- *High impact, difficult to implement:* Solutions that fall into this category require careful consideration. It is important to understand the reason for it being categorized as difficult to implement. Are the difficulties in resource requirements (e.g., staffing, new equipment), culture, or behaviors? Depending on the factors, the team might decide to table the solution or develop a recommendation for the sponsor to provide guidance or make decisions.

- *Low impact, easy to implement:* These solutions are known as "just-do-its"—simple ideas that have a minimal positive impact and consume little or no resources.

- *Low impact, difficult to implement:* Solutions in this category should be ignored altogether. The value of the payoff matrix is in identifying the high-impact solutions. Avoid anything that is difficult with a minimal impact.

- *When to use it:* The payoff matrix is used after all solutions have been brainstormed.

- *What it looks like:* Figure 9.13 shows the four quadrants. The green quadrants indicate solutions worth pursuing for step 5, the orange quadrant (high/difficult) represents solutions that require further consideration and refinement, and the red quadrant (low/difficult) should be avoided.

Lamina Tree of Low-Hanging Fruit

- *How to do it:* The Lamina tree tool stores the low/easy solutions known as the just-do-its. Since just-do-its are simple, straightforward ideas, they do not

170 Chapter Nine

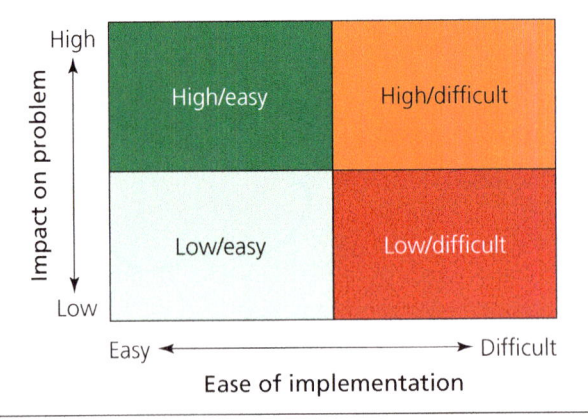

Figure 9.13 Payoff matrix.
Note: For more information on the matrix, visit http://www.mindtools.com/pages/article/newHTE_95.htm.

require thorough action plans. Therefore, the Lamina tree of low-hanging fruit serves as a temporary placeholder for these ideas.

- *When to use it:* The Lamina tree is used after the solutions have been prioritized by quadrant. The Lamina tree holds solutions from the low/easy quadrant. The solutions act as leaves on the tree—the more the better. Once action plans are developed for the high/easy and select high/difficult solutions, the solutions on the tree are assigned an action plan.

- *What it looks like:* Figure 9.14 shows a before-and-after view of the Lamina tree. (The Lamina tree of low-hanging fruit was developed by Caroline Lamina, a Jefferson lean leader [Figure 9.15].)

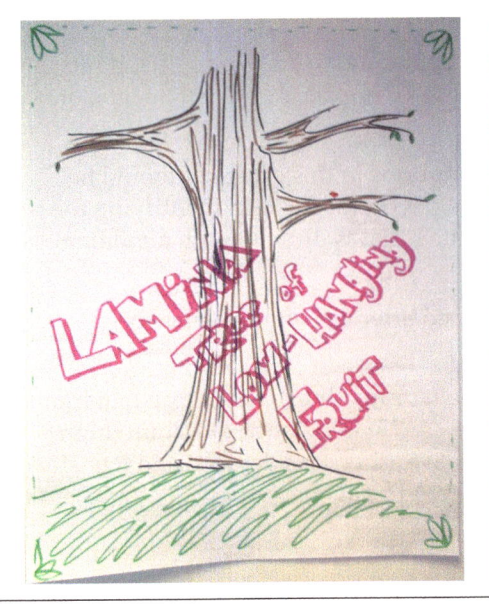

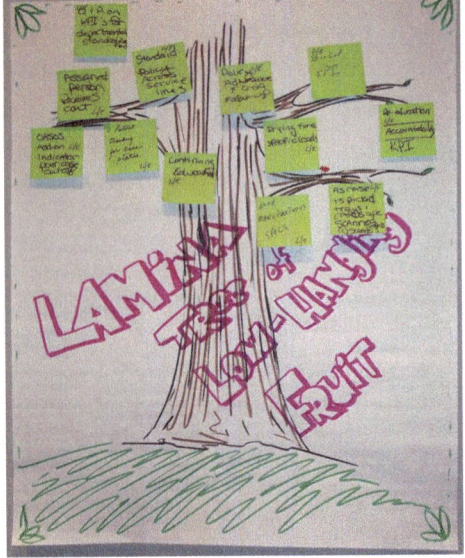

Figure 9.14 Example of Lamina tree of low-hanging fruit.

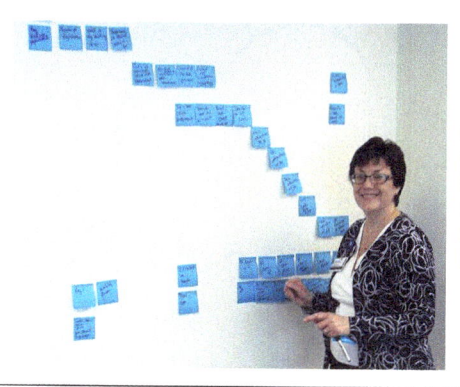

Caroline (Carrie) Lamina, anatomic pathology manager in the Clinical Lab and a Jefferson lean leader since 2010, facilitating a swimlane map. Carrie developed the tree of low-hanging fruit, hence the name.

Figure 9.15   Inventor of the Lamina tree.

Step 5: Develop and Implement the Action Plan

The final step of the kaizen problem-solving process is to develop and implement the action plan (Figure 9.16). The action plan details how tasks will be accomplished based on a set timeline.

Tools to Use during Step 5

The two tools used during step 5 are the action plan worksheet and the control phase action plan.

Action Plan Worksheet

- *How to do it:* The action plan worksheet defines how to execute the prioritized solutions. The participants take the selected solutions (high/easy and some high/difficult) and complete the worksheet.

- *When to use it:* Once the payoff matrix is complete, the prioritized solutions are removed from the flip chart. Participants can be broken into smaller groups to complete this tool.

- *What it looks like:* The action plan worksheet has two components: the action plan and recommendations. The action plan (Table 9.1) is used for tasks or solutions that do not require sponsor approval. Recommendations (Table 9.2) are used in order to provide a business case for sponsor review and decision. Each table provides specific information on the solution. "What" is the solution identified in step 4. "How and why" provides the steps to complete the task/solution along with the explanation for why it is being done as part of the project. "Resources needed" includes staff, equipment, supplies, and leadership support. "Expected outcome" outlines what will result from this solution. Ideally, the expected outcome is quantitative (i.e., performance metrics). Anytime we put a countermeasure in place for a problem, we have to measure (through observations and/or metrics) or check to see that the problem truly has been solved. The last two components, "Who" and "By when," define the responsible person and timeline for completion. The recommendation table also has "What decision needs to be made?" as an item. This helps facilitate the discussion between the RIE team and the sponsor.

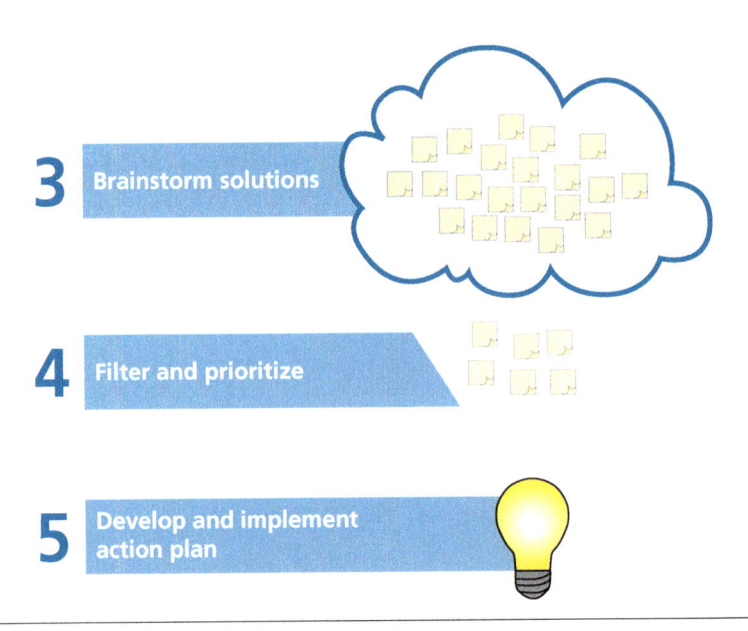

Figure 9.16 Step 5: Develop and implement an action plan.

Table 9.1 Action plan template.

What	How and why	Resources needed	Expected outcome	Who	By when

Table 9.2 Recommendation template.

What	How and why	Resources needed	Expected outcome	What decision needs to be made?	By when

Control Phase Action Plan

- *How to do it:* The Control phase action plan is a Microsoft Excel–based tool used to document post-RIE activities. The facilitator and the process owner help manage post-RIE implementation of action items. As described in the section "Control Phase" in Chapter 8, the Control phase action plan serves as the agenda for weekly status update meetings.

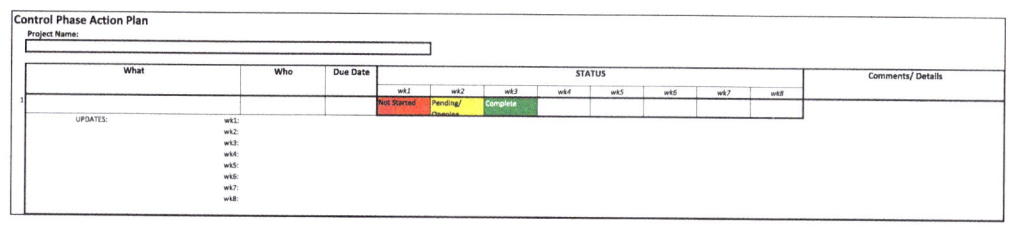

Figure 9.17 Control phase action plan screenshot.

- *When to use it:* The action plan worksheet is transferred to this tool. The control phase action plan is updated weekly and disseminated to the project team.

- *What it looks like:* The Microsoft Excel tool tracks updates using both a stoplight indicator (red = not started, yellow = in progress, green = complete) and supporting text for updates. Figure 9.17 is a blank template of the tool. Appendix C provides details for using the tool in Microsoft Excel.

The kaizen problem-solving process keeps discussions moving toward action. Each step has a specific objective that leads to a high-impact solution. Steps are completed in succession and cannot be skipped. You should not go from step 4 (developing solutions) back to step 1 (brainstorming issues and barriers). This is how things do not get resolved! After each step is complete, the facilitator gets consensus that the step is finished and the team moves forward to the next one.

Remember along the way that problem solving is a team sport. As a facilitator, you do not want to leave people behind. Ensure a level of consensus (or at least common understanding) before moving forward on discussion items. The facilitator's job is to leverage and optimize the knowledge and experience of the team. This five-step process positions them to do so.

> *Do you have to take this formal approach? No. The five-step framework is a guide to problem solving. If a problem needs immediate attention, think through the process to determine the most effective solution. Remember the four rules of solution development.*

FACILITATOR'S ROLE IN GROUP DYNAMICS

A facilitator acts like an orchestra conductor. The facilitator works with experts and forms teams to collaboratively solve problems. A good conductor harnesses the skills of many to create a unified piece of music. Similarly, a good facilitator can extract and leverage the knowledge and contributions of individuals and coordinate a focused improvement effort. The facilitator has four main roles during this process:

1. Creating and maintaining a collaborative group environment
2. Building rapport
3. Establishing and upholding expectations for behavior (ground rules)
4. Keeping progress moving forward

Improvement teams typically run through the five stages of team development: forming, storming, norming, performing, and adjourning (Table 9.3) (Tuckman, 1965). The forming stage represents the beginning of the project work (when the RIE team comes together). The facilitator helps shape expectations and defines the approach and agenda for the initiative. As conversations move into the current state issues and barriers, individuals begin challenging each other and jockeying for position. The storming stage can be emotional and frustrating. During this time, the facilitator role switches to a coaching capacity. The facilitator needs to adeptly manage conflicts, uncover root causes, and guide the team forward in the problem-solving process. Norming occurs when individuals within the team begin to build rapport and competitive cohesion. The facilitator shifts to a

Table 9.3 Stages of group dynamics.

Stage	Description	Facilitator's role	Problem-solving step
Forming	• Kickoff • Introduction of project, process, and what to expect • Might have lack of clarity about purpose or problem • Individuals may not know each other	**Direct** • Clarify roles and expectations • Provide structure • Manage discussions	**Step 1** Brainstorm issues and barriers
Storming	• Disagreements, frustration, and/or challenging people's ideas	**Coach** • Facilitate communication • Surface and address issues • Manage conflict	**Step 1** Brainstorm issues and barriers **Step 2** Filter and prioritize issues and barriers
Norming	• Leverage ground rules • Build rapport and relationships • Competitive cohesion develops ("We are the best")	**Support** • Support and consultation as needed • Passive, enabling team to establish internal roles	**Step 3** Brainstorm solutions **Step 4** Filter and prioritize solutions
Performing	• Clarity and agreement on goals • Constructive confrontation • Creative idea sharing	**Support** • Same as above	**Step 5** Develop and implement action plan
Adjourning	• Planned project close • Recognition for participation and contributions	**Delegate** • Provide handoff instructions	**Project close**

supporting role, enabling the team a degree of autonomy to establish roles and develop solutions.

As the team moves into the action plan development phase, team members collectively begin performing. The performing stage occurs when team members leverage each other's strengths and take a unified approach to accomplish the stated goal. Lastly, the adjourning stage represents the conclusion of the effort. The facilitator directs handoff conversations between the team and sponsors in order to ensure all tasks have assigned owners and associated timelines. Once all handoff items are addressed, the team can formally disband.

> *The facilitator's focus is on process: organization, communication, roles, behaviors, and decision making. Team members focus on content.*

CHAPTER CHALLENGE

Facilitate a small group discussion or project team through the five-step kaizen problem-solving process. What tools do you find to be effective? Which tools are challenging or require practice? How was the facilitation approach received by your colleagues? What was the end result?

BONUS CHALLENGE

Incorporate Spear's four rules into a meeting or project you are working on. How was it received? What value do the rules contribute?

QUESTIONS

1. What characteristics make a good RIE?
2. What roles need to be defined for an RIE?
3. Why are ground rules established? How do they contribute to the improvement team self-managing each other?
4. What is the benefit of having a structured problem-solving approach?
5. Before this chapter, did you have a clearly defined way to solve problems?
6. Why is there an emphasis on divergent thinking during step 1, brainstorm issues and barriers?
7. What is the significance of sorting issues and barriers into those that are within your control and those that are outside your control?
8. What happens if you try to address an issue or barrier that is outside your control?
9. How can Spear's four rules be applied to your work area? Are there processes or tasks that violate any of the rules? If so, what can you do to address it?

10. Why is the payoff matrix an essential tool prior to action plan development? Who determines the priorities?
11. How can you apply the problem-solving process to informal efforts?
12. What are the responsibilities of the facilitator when leading any type of RIE or even a meeting?
13. How do the stages of group dynamics affect the facilitator's role? What phase is the most vulnerable?

Chapter 10
Leading Change: Lessons from the Road

It is not necessary to change. Survival is not mandatory.

—W. Edwards Deming

Identifying how to change a process is easy; the hard part is getting people to understand the need for change and then act on it. Leading change is a difficult, uphill struggle that we all encounter in everyday life. This chapter covers the components of effective lean management and strategic change leadership, and provides insight from Jefferson's lean leaders.

Change occurs when something moves from its current state to a new future state (Figure 10.1). During the change there is a transition period. The transition state is the period of time in which the performance gap from the current state to the future state shortens. The current state defines what exists today in terms of processes, culture, and expectations. Employees are comfortable with predictable, consistent processes. The future state presents the unknown. It may be undefined and, as a result, cause hesitation, insecurity, and uncertainty. Spanning the current and future states is the transition. Transition states can be disorganized and tumultuous and can create inefficiencies. This turbulent time is the critical turning point in driving positive, sustainable change.

When a process alteration occurs, it requires thought, which takes more time and energy. Think back to when you switched from a tactile touch phone to a smartphone. At first, you had to stop and think about everything you were doing. You could no longer feel the buttons, so you had to look at what you were typing. But at some point it became automatic. It required hardwiring the new way. The transition was most likely difficult due to the change from tactile buttons to a sensitive touch screen. You became less productive and made more mistakes as you adjusted. But over time you became facile and more efficient. This example

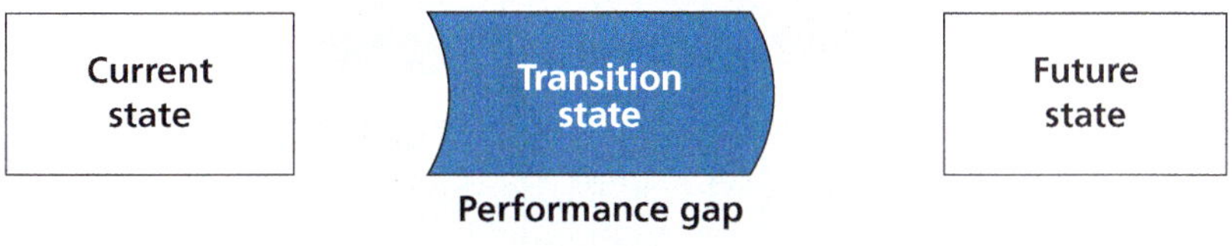

Figure 10.1 Change model.

Table 10.1 States of change at the macro and micro levels.

State	Macro level (organization, department, etc.)	Micro level (individual)
Current	How things are currently being done today	How I do my job today
Transition	How to shift from today's work to future needs	How my job will change
Future	How things will be done tomorrow	How I will fit into this new way of working

helps in describing the importance of managing the transition state. The transition requires patience, reassurance, education, communication, and support in order to make a successful leap to the future state.

Change happens at macro and micro levels (Table 10.1). In reality, there are both organizational and individual states of change. Both levels require attention and thought into the strategy to improve the likelihood of success.

LEAN MANAGEMENT

To further promote and sustain continuous improvement, the right systems need to be in place. The lean management system comprises two main components: standard work and discipline (Mann, 2010). This system provides the structure from which all lean improvement strategies can be successfully developed and deployed. An underlying philosophy in the system is discipline to adhere to standard work and accountability.

As with any system, tools and concepts accompany the lean management philosophy to create discipline and achieve results. Positive results will follow if processes are managed effectively (Chan et al., 2014). The leadership challenge is to set the tone, manage expectations, and hold staff accountable for performance (Aij et al., 2013; Kaplan, Patterson, Ching, & Blackmore, 2014).

Leaders have a pivotal role during the transition state of change. Leaders must communicate, coach, and remove barriers during this time in order to reduce resistance and static inertia. Communication is an integral component of leadership. During the transition state, employees need a degree of reassurance from decision makers and leaders. Employees want to understand the reason for change as well as the urgency behind it. Additionally, employees look for what is in it for them. At a personal level, what about the change will likely get employee buy-in? Since change happens at an individual level, employees need to personally commit to changing their role in the process and help move toward the future state. Leaders must also communicate how the change will occur, which is essentially the components of an action plan (i.e., who, what, how, why, and by when).

As a coach, a leader has to help employees manage the transition. Leaders might need to meet with staff individually and develop strategies to address personal barriers to change (e.g., lack of knowledge or skill set in the new environment). Training and education position staff to quickly adopt new processes, and reduce the time from the current state to the future state (Graban & Prachand, 2010; Langley et al., 2009). The transition state is an active period that requires frequent touch points between leadership and staff to ensure barrier removal. Resistance is a natural response to change. Active change management includes strategies to reduce or limit resistance while keeping progress moving forward.

> *A lean leader is someone who has the technical skills to drive process improvement and personal skills to support change management. Lean leaders focus on continuous improvement, gemba walks, empowering staff to solve problems, and system/process issues (asking why, not who).*

Leader Standard Work

Leader standard work is a core element of lean management. As described in Chapter 5, standard work is the basis for improvement. The responsibility of following standards does not exclude leaders. For a person in a leadership or managerial role, standard work translates to daily checklists and regular expectations. Leader standard work is the lynchpin of change management. The main components of leader standard work are gemba walks and huddles.

Gemba walks are a way to learn by seeing. The closer a leader's oversight is to the staff at the gemba, the more frequently he or she should walk (Mann, 2010). Learning to see involves looking for process variation and flow disruption, wastes, and underlying issues that limit productivity and quality. Gemba walks require going to see the actual process, learning through observation, and asking questions (Womack, 2011). When a problem arises, a good lean manager does not respond, "Come to my office and let's talk about it," but rather, "Show me." Gemba walks remove assumptions about what is happening and require verification (Liker, 2004). Gemba walks also do more than just verify issues; they help build rapport and understanding between leaders, their staff, and customers.

Gemba walks are not meant to be used solely for problems. This activity is an ongoing responsibility and leadership best practice. It helps in anticipating and preventing issues as well as verifying and solving identified problems. Leaders will sometimes implement a change without understanding the actual current state and operations of a process. As a result, the process can become more cumbersome, can become inefficient, and can increase quality-related issues—the opposite of the intention. Leaders are responsible for going to see what actually happens, engaging staff in learning about their struggles, and soliciting ideas for improvement.

Huddles are an effective way to communicate with staff. Huddles are short, standardized meetings that involve individuals from a department or team. Typically they occur before the start of a shift or during a transition/handoff of shifts. A huddle should have a standard agenda that includes the following (Mann, 2010):

- *Performance dashboard updates:* Review of key metrics progress compared with target and expectations

- *Things to be aware of:* Review of any anticipated issues or problems as well as expected customer volume and staffing issues

- *Open discussion:* Discussion of any concerns or opportunities for improvement

Staff members or the manager of the area can lead huddles. The following are questions to ask at every huddle:

1. How are we doing?
2. What opportunities do we have to improve?
3. What are we doing to improve/address them?

Discipline

The best way to improve overall performance is to establish the expectations, provide the needed education and support to achieve them, and hold employees accountable for the results. Weight management offers a great analogy for discipline. If your goal is to lose weight, what do you need to do? The answer is simple: burn more calories than you consume. The trick is not which workout or diet fad to enroll in. Rather, it is having the discipline to burn more calories than you consume, which obviously means smart eating and exercise. People who maintain a healthy weight or who can lose weight and sustain their weight loss display the discipline to do so (not counting genetic factors). It is a matter of personal will and effort. So using this analogy, in management we know what the key standard tasks are that we should be doing (e.g., gemba walks, communication). However, most leaders lack the discipline to do them.

Discipline requires a daily commitment to leader standard work (Kaplan et al., 2014). Gemba walks should be scheduled and regularly occurring, as well as spontaneous in nature. Leaders need to shift their focus from firefighting to fire prevention. Employee empowerment is central to this effort. Figure 10.2 segments roles and responsibilities for frontline staff, middle management, and senior leaders. Frontline staff have a primary focus on maintaining daily operations while participating in improvement efforts (Jimmerson et al., 2005). Middle managers should spend the majority of their time on improvement efforts. They have

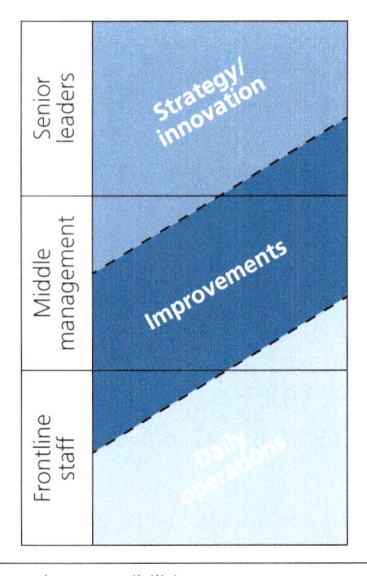

Figure 10.2 Segmenting roles and responsibilities.

additional responsibilities to monitor daily operations and participate in strategy development and innovation. Senior leaders should spend the majority of their time on strategy and innovation while contributing to improvement efforts. Lean management emphasizes the need to empower the frontline staff to problem solve at the source (Jimmerson et al., 2005). If senior leaders and middle managers are too busy fighting fires and troubleshooting at the daily operations level, there is no one setting the direction and strategy for improvement.

Empowering employees means giving them the education and tools to become problem solvers. Then, leadership needs to create a working environment that enables and promotes active problem solving (Toussaint & Gerard, 2010). There needs to be an asserted effort to develop the skill sets and competencies of staff and then empower them to improve their work. Process change is simple and straightforward. The hard part is dealing with people and the myriad reactions to change (from acceptance to passive resistance to active resistance/sabotage). Empowering staff is a scary thing for leaders because it takes control out of their hands. It is, however, liberating to delegate tasks and responsibilities to competent staff, giving the leader more freedom to concentrate on priority issues, improvement projects, and strategic initiatives.

> *Leaders need to provide staff the "what" but empower staff to determine the "how." It is the responsibility of leaders to provide direction, but the staff makes it come to life (with leadership support behind the scenes).*

LEADING CHANGE

The transition from the current state to the future state makes all the difference. Meaningful, sustainable change is not possible without a strategic approach to manage individuals through the transition (Lighter, 2013). There are strategies that position a successful change initiative. The approach models John Kotter's article "Leading Change: Why Transformation Efforts Fail" (1995). Kotter identified various reasons that initiatives and projects failed, based on common mistakes made by leadership. This section highlights the main considerations and tools to apply before, during, and after a transition (Figure 10.3).

Current state	Transition state	Future state
	Performance gap	
1. Create urgency for change	3. Define and communicate the vision	
2. Establish the guiding coalition	4. Remove barriers	6. Hardwire changes
	5. Provide feedback on progress	

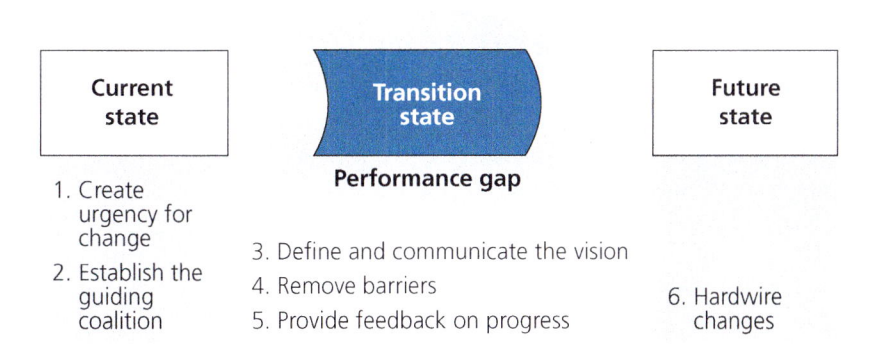

Figure 10.3 Change model with leadership responsibilities.

1. Create Urgency for Change

Without a need or sense of urgency for change, it is nearly impossible to shift static inertia to dynamic. Sometimes leaders have to make the fear of doing nothing appear more dangerous than the fear of the unknown. Using the burning platform analogy, if the platform is ablaze and disintegrating rapidly, you will jump off, even though you are afraid that sharks or other dangers might be in the water, because the option of staying on the platform is no longer viable. Getting people on board with the idea of change is challenging but essential. Overcoming inertia is the most difficult step (Womack & Jones, 1996).

Answer the following questions when evaluating the case for change (Advisory Board Company, 2011):

1. Is this a priority?
2. Do the benefits outweigh the costs?
3. Do employees have the right skill set to execute?

If you answered no to any of the questions, the initiative needs further analysis and realignment with organizational objectives.

2. Establish the Guiding Coalition

To drive change, there needs to be a core group of individuals dedicated to the objective. The guiding coalition is responsible for generating momentum and building buy-in from their peers. A guiding coalition gives you strength in numbers. These individuals can help move everyone in the same direction and build the positive, forward momentum needed to change things as well as sustain the gains. You need to have people who are passionate about the end goal in order to generate engagement and buy-in with those around them.

There are hidden leaders that have tremendous influence. Identify and leverage their network. Hidden leaders drive organizations through the power of influence. Driving improvements does not happen in isolation. Leaders need to leverage one another and build support from their colleagues and senior management (Jones & Mitchell, 2006). The guiding coalition needs to include individuals with authority (decision-making ability), expertise in various core operations, credibility both internally and externally, and leadership competencies (Kotter, 1995). These characteristics capture the central elements of change leadership.

3. Define and Communicate the Vision

The vision defines where the leader sees the organization or department going (Lighter, 2013). Without a vision, the change initiative can disband into seemingly unintegrated tasks without an end goal. Employees cannot align their individual responsibilities and tasks with the organization's strategic objectives if the direction is not defined or communicated.

The elevator speech is a highly effective tool used to concisely communicate the urgency of change, the direction for the future state, and how employees can contribute to the stated goals. The format is simple:

- Project/change description
- Why it is important

- What success looks like in the future
- What you (employee) can do to contribute

At the individual level, employees need to feel connected to the need for change (see discussion on purpose, process, and people in Chapter 1). They also need to believe that change will bring about positive outcomes. Large departments that operate 24/7 pose a unique challenge. Communication is challenging and more critical because you have to reach night shift and weekend staff, as well as part-timers. This is why communication is so important. Failure to reach these individuals can cause a change effort to halt, be less effective, or fall apart.

4. Remove Barriers

One of the main roles for leaders is removing barriers and obstacles that impede progress. Barriers include organizational structure/hierarchy, limited skills or training, inadequate staffing or information systems support, and lack of supervisory support and commitment (Kotter, 1995). These issues need to be anticipated and addressed in order to keep progress moving forward. Once inertia becomes dynamic, it is critical to ensure limited resistance to maintain the established momentum. This is where leader standard work comes into play. Through gemba walks and huddles, leaders can anticipate issues and work with staff to strategically remediate and remove barriers. Resistance also arises when there is lack of agreement on the problem or the solution (Chalice, 2007).

5. Provide Feedback on Progress

The transition state can take weeks, months, or even years. The future state can appear so distant and unattainable that employees lose sight of the goals, and energy dissipates. To counter this effect, it is essential that staff receive consistent feedback. Benefits of acknowledging success and progress include the following:

- Validation of efforts and potential sacrifices
- Recognition and appreciation of staff contributing to change
- Reinforcement and encouragement of vision and progress made to date
- Limited pushback from resistors or other individuals not supportive of the change

Again, through leader standard work and performance dashboards, key metrics should be reviewed to assess progress. Celebrate accomplishments, both large and small, along the way. These short-term wins remind staff of the progress made to date and help communicate their status along the transformation journey.

6. Hardwire Changes

Leader standard work is crucial in hardwiring gains. Hardwiring improvements comes with discipline and accountability. Leaders need to consistently perform gemba walks and ask everywhere: (1) What is the process? (2) How can you tell it is working? and (3) What are you doing to improve it? A true transformation occurs at many levels in many forms. A new paradigm might require different skills and a new mind-set that are not currently available. Hardwiring improvements is one of the most challenging responsibilities.

Changing culture with existing people poses another real challenge. If leaders train, educate, support, and hold staff accountable for their performance, staff will take care of the results (Graban & Prachand, 2010). Without a solid, unified leadership front, sustainability and progress are likely to fail. Changing the work environment is the challenge. Without hard work and discipline, nothing can be accomplished. In order to be excellent and strive for perfection, you must have the discipline, day in and day out, to do the right things, the right way, every time. Getting better is an ongoing journey and at times a struggle. But if you are persistent and disciplined, you will achieve your results. Vision and innovation are important, but structure and discipline are critical (Kenney, 2011).

LESSONS FROM JEFFERSON LEAN LEADERS

Since 2008, Jefferson has certified over 90 individuals as lean practitioners (known as lean leaders at Jefferson). Lean leaders hold full-time positions throughout the clinical and academic departments within the organization. Positions held include physicians (attendings, fellows, and residents), nurses, pharmacists, respiratory therapists, and administrators. These employees dedicate their time academically through a four-credit graduate lean certification program as well as practically through lean project assignments post-certification.

There have been nearly 100 formal lean projects at Jefferson over the last seven years, ranging from rapid improvements, to 5S events, to project-based education. Some lean leaders have been in the program since its inception, while others are newly certified. To provide readers with insight from the wealth of experience accumulated at Jefferson, the lean leaders answered three questions. Their lessons learned shed light on the importance of discipline, persistence, and dedication to improvement. The transition from "doing lean" to "becoming lean" is subtle and happens over time. Lean leaders will tell you it takes more than a year before things begin to come naturally. Project experience and content refreshers help hardwire lean thinking.

What advice do you have for individuals who want to execute lean projects?

- "It is very important to clearly identify the problem before jumping to solutions. Lean projects must be focused on eliminating waste and identifying value adding processes through the eyes of the customer. Remember, do not try and 'boil the ocean.'" Brian Glynn, RRT, clinical supervisor, pulmonary care

- "Stay committed and focused. There are still a number of people who do not believe in the benefits of lean. Do not let them discourage you." Roseann Pauline, MBA, change agent, supply chain management

- "Be prepared to face resistance. People are scared of change and fear you are assessing their individual performance. As a lean leader you need to support, reassure, and guide those participating during the entire process." Steven Gudowski, RRT, clinical supervisor, pulmonary care

- "Be sure to provide training for individuals on tools and techniques for influencing others to change. Not paying adequate attention to the people-side of change can quickly stifle any positive results that are generated from a lean project." Shane Flickinger, MHA, CLSSBB, manager, operations support

- "Ensure you have buy-in from management and leadership. You will need their support to help you build results into the culture of your organization." Nicole Jastrzembski, RN, information systems coordinator, emergency medicine

What has been a key lesson learned in your engagement with the lean program at Jefferson?

- "Put it all on the table—the good, the bad, and the ugly." Carole Harvey, educator, patient access

- "Trust the lean process to work." Caroline Lamina, anatomic pathology manager, clinical laboratory

- "Sometimes you need to put your ideas and opinions aside to allow teams to build their own solutions. But you still need to use your experience to guide them towards a good outcome." Andrew Wierzbieniec, MHSA, administrator, medical oncology

- "You must be prepared to meet resistance and develop a change management plan. Lean projects often result in a change to a process which can lead to fear and trepidation. Engaging front-line staff in the process will help overcome this resistance." Brian Glynn, RRT, clinical supervisor, pulmonary care

- "Not all staff will be supportive or engaged. Some will challenge the principles of lean. Be persistent and work towards engaging those who are interested in making changes." Jenny Bosley, RN, MS, clinical nurse specialist, performance improvement

- "Lean needs to be more than head knowledge; it needs to be part of your soul. How you live and look at life every day. To make lean a viable part of your personal or organizational culture, lean needs to be a passion . . . always striving to be the best at getting better." Robert Bartosz, MHA, executive associate and director of finance, Jefferson Graduate School of Biomedical Sciences

If an organization wanted to begin a lean journey, how do you suggest it get started?

- "Pick a few highly motivated people with great attitudes and make them lean leaders. Those few will use lean themselves and teach others in the process. This will be the start of a new lean culture at your institution." Steven Gudowski, RRT, clinical supervisor, pulmonary care

- "The best way for them to get started would be to engage their staff. Communication is key. They should also offer lean courses to the staff to give them an opportunity to see how being lean can positively affect their organization." Lisa Liciardello, BSN, RN, clinical charge nurse, nursing

- "I would suggest to not start off attempting to 'boil the ocean.' Instead, begin the journey by identifying small wins, such as creating standards, because without these no improvements can occur." Leigh Resnick, MS, RRT, manager, operations support

- "Demonstrate to employees that they will actually have the opportunity to impact their daily work by improving processes that will lead to better job satisfaction and customer satisfaction. Process improvement is a journey, not a destination." Thomas J. Louden, director of managed care reimbursement and contract compliance, managed care contracting

Everything You Need to Know

5-8-4 summarizes the book into the most salient points (Figure 10.4). If you understand the components of 5-8-4, you will be a successful problem solver and lean leader. The "5" represents (1) the five lean principles, (2) the concept that everything is 5S, and (3) the kaizen problem-solving process. First, the five lean principles provide the roadmap for creating a lean process. This framework is the model for executing lean improvements. The components within each principle describe key deliverables and considerations. Second, a core take-away of this book is that everything is 5S. The 5S approach is a systematic way to improve physical layout and system/process design. Finally, the kaizen problem-solving process is a standard approach focused on identifying the root causes within your control and developing and implementing high-impact solutions.

The "8" represents the eight wastes. In order to identify the root causes, you must have a thorough understanding of these wastes. The eight DOWNTIME wastes are the focus of lean thinking. Once you identify your customer and define value, you can begin to identify, isolate, and eliminate the NVA activity. Waste reduction and elimination is at the core of lean.

Lastly, the "4" represents Spear's four rules: (1) activities are clear and well defined, (2) steps are simple and direct, (3) flow is simple and direct, and (4) problems and issues are dealt with in a timely and direct manner. The rules provide the framework for solution development. The point is that the new solution is not more complicated than what currently exists. Integrating the 5-8-4 components provides the structure and systematic approaches necessary to drive meaningful change.

The future of healthcare is unknown. Delivery models and organizational structures will change in response to shifts in reimbursement and customer

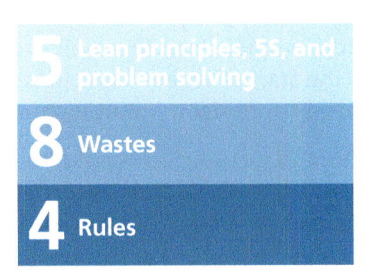

Figure 10.4 Lean thinking summarized as 5-8-4.

requirements. Lean thinking has a pivotal role in leading the way. Cost reduction and resource allocation will continue to drive decisions, making quality improvement paramount (Al, Feenstra, & Brouwer, 2005; Slobbe et al., 2011). Doing things correctly the first time helps reduce operational costs through less rework and fewer inefficiencies. Using the lean thinking philosophy for the underlying leadership system, as described in Chapter 1, aligns organizational goals with individual employees. The purpose, process, people approach promotes empowering employees to own and improve their work in order to achieve higher-level objectives. Lastly, the horizontal lean perspective (i.e., patients, products, materials, and equipment flow horizontally across functions) enhances coordination and collaboration across stakeholder groups. A systems-based viewpoint and management approach positions organizations to support and improve population health and broader health system strategies.

CHAPTER CHALLENGE

Implement leader standard work as part of your daily responsibilities (even if you do not have a formal leadership role or staff reporting to you). Conduct daily gemba walks. What are you learning from staff? What system/process issues exist that inhibit their work or threaten quality?

BONUS CHALLENGE

Implement huddles in your work area. Start regular, structured meetings to discuss current state issues and performance and anticipated concerns. How are the huddles improving communication? What improvements have been realized as a result?

QUESTIONS

1. Why is it important to manage the transition state of change?
2. What happens if the future state is not defined?
3. How does leader standard work support continuous improvement and sustainability?
4. What is the result of leaders that do not conduct gemba walks or facilitate huddles?
5. Why do senior leaders and middle management need to focus more on improvements and strategy than on daily operations? Why is empowering frontline staff difficult?
6. What elements of leading change can be difficult in your organization/department/work setting? Why?
7. How can you develop and communicate a sense of urgency? What is the significance in doing so?

8. Who can be members of your guiding coalition for positive change? What characteristics do they share? How can they leverage one another?

9. Why is performance feedback necessary during the transition state?

10. How are changes and improvements hardwired?

11. How does culture affect change efforts?

12. Which of the lessons learned shared by Jefferson lean leaders resonates with you? Why?

13. How can the 5-8-4 concept be deployed in your organization/department/work setting?

Bonus Question: What will you do differently now that you are a lean thinker?

Appendixes

The appendixes provide instructions to support the tools provided on the accompanying CD. The CD is organized by the DMAIC project phases (Figure A.1). Two documents live outside the folders: the lean DMAIC checklist and the rapid improvement event portfolio. These two documents drive rapid improvement execution. The five folders contain various tools and templates referenced in the lean DMAIC checklist. Remember, the checklist, portfolio, tools, and templates are suggested to help project execution and should be adopted and adapted to your organization, department, or work setting accordingly.

To support your use of the tools, a supplementary folder labeled "Appendix Examples" contains a case study project for improving patient flow in a physician's office. The case study employs all of the tools described in the appendix to demonstrate the appropriate use. Refer to the examples as you use each template.

> *Save as a new file any tool or template that you use. The tools and templates are "read only" so that you cannot overwrite them.*

Name
- 01_DEFINE
- 02_MEASURE
- 03_ANALYZE
- 04_IMPROVE
- 05_CONTROL
- Lean DMAIC Checklist
- Rapid Improvement Event Portfolio

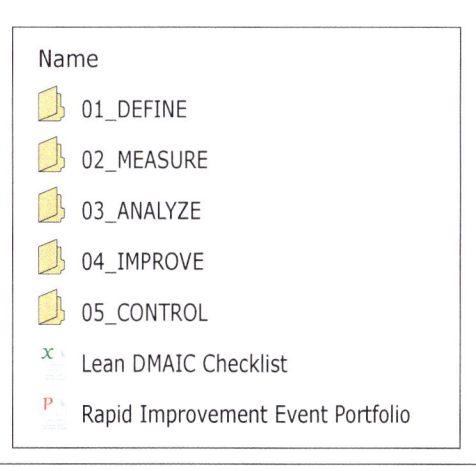

Figure A.1 Organization of CD documents.

Appendix A
Rapid Improvement Event Portfolio

The rapid improvement event portfolio is a Microsoft PowerPoint document that contains consolidated project deliverables. The portfolio aligns with the lean DMAIC checklist. Teams can document and summarize all deliverables in one location. This reduces excessive numbers of electronic files, versions, and other document control issues. Portfolio slides are segmented by DMAIC phase and described accordingly.

HIGH-LEVEL PROJECT PLAN

Before the first Define phase tool there is a high-level project plan template (Table A.1). The plan contains some of the major project deliverables along with comments and columns describing why the deliverable is important, who is responsible, and when the task needs to be completed.

DEFINE

Project Charter

Description: The project charter is a two-page document that defines the project (Figure A.2). The first page contains basic project information (title, sponsor, process owner, team members, facilitators, start date, and scope). Other components include the project description, problem, and goal as well as the potential benefits (Silverstein et al., 2009). This page gives individuals a solid understanding of what the project objective is and how success is defined. The second page of the charter reviews data sources, projects that can be leveraged or acknowledged, individuals of value (to be contacted for VOC interviews), and potential barriers to success. These elements provide a high-level environmental scan.

When to use it: At the project start with the facilitators and sponsor.

Required? Yes.

Communication Plan

Description: The communication plan aligns communication strategies with stakeholder groups (Table A.2). Each group has a specified key message tailored

Table A.1 High-level project plan.

Deliverable/action	Comments	Why are we doing this?	By when	Who will lead it
Project charter	Need to discuss with sponsor/process owners	To determine what is in and out of scope and what the project objective is	12/29	T. Brady
Communication plan	Ensure this includes department/staff upstream and downstream of the process	To ensure all stakeholders know what to expect, what they need to do, how they can help, etc.	12/29	D. Ortiz
Develop high-level process map	30,000-foot view of the process	To depict the process at a high level	1/9	M. Vaughn
Voice of customer interviews	Need to coordinate and interview appropriate stakeholders of process	To identify key themes staff indicate are contributors to the problem and tie quantitative measures to these themes	1/16	M. Vaughn
Logistics	Schedule event, identify process expert team, finalize resource requirements, prepare team packet	To ensure schedule and deliverables line up	1/16	D. Pedroia
Change leadership	Conduct change readiness assessment, conduct stakeholder analysis		1/17	T. Brady

Data analysis	Determine key metrics to monitor/data to display (no more than five); provide narrative to support graphs	To quantitatively analyze and determine root causes of the problem	1/28	M. Vaughn
Finalize fishbone diagram	Use information from VOC, observations, and data analysis	To qualitatively analyze and determine root causes of the problem	1/29	M. Vaughn
Draft improvement event agenda		To outline how to use the time with staff to achieve our project objective	1/28	T. Brady
Facilitate improvement event	Gather team of staff to identify solution to key drivers of the issues	To develop a high-impact action plan for staff to implement over the next four weeks	2/2	T. Brady
Develop control phase plan	Action plan based on facilitated session	To assign, document, update, and hold staff accountable for key action items	2/2	M. Vaughn
Draft A3 report		To document project concisely so it can be shared across all areas of the organization	2/17	T. Brady
Present A3 report to sponsor and process owner		To communicate lessons learned and project outcomes	3/6	T. Brady

Project title: Improving physician's office patient flow	
Sponsors: S. A. Moose and G. L. Lohman **Process owners:** V. Wllfork and J. Edelman **Team members:** R. Gronkowski, M. Hoomanawanui, R. Ninkovich, S. Vollmer, D. Revis **Facilitators:** T. Brady (lead), M. Vaughn, D. Pedroia (logistics), D. Ortiz (communications) **Project start date:** Dec. 29, 2014 **Project scope:** Physician's office visit from patient sign-in to checkout	**Project description/problem and goal:** **What is the problem or opportunity?** Patient throughput is inefficient. Patients wait (in waiting area or exam room) for extended periods of time. **What is the goal for the team?** Reduce patient throughput time and balance staff workloads. **Potential benefits:** **Why are you doing this?** Patient satisfaction scores are low and throughput times are too long. We are not providing excellent service to our customers and risk losing their business. **What are you expecting to come out of this?** Improved coordination and collaboration across all staff. Improved patient satisfaction. Reduced throughput time.

What are the data sources?

Office information system (OIS) and patient satisfaction surveys

How will the data be collected?

Electronically through the OIS and patient satisfaction survey tool. Reporting is automated.

Are there other completed or active projects that can be leveraged? No other projects have previously addressed patient throughput and/or satisfaction.	**Individuals of value:** B. LaFell (office manager), B. Browner (medical assistant), N. Solder (physician), D. Hightower (registrar/scheduler), P. Chung (charge nurse)

Potential barriers to success:

High volume so it is difficult for employees to take time to work on improvement projects.

No financial resources (project must be budget-neutral).

Staff has worked here for a long time. Many processes are ingrained as "the way we've always done it."

Figure A.2 Project charter.

Table A.2 Communication plan.

Group	Key message	Delivery mechanism (e-mail, phone, etc.)	Frequency	Person responsible to deliver
Patients	Changes in processes to create a better experience and meet patient needs.	Signage, newsletter	Once before improvement, once afterward	D. Ortiz (with process owners)
Administration	Changes in policy/procedure that impact workflow, coding, billing, scheduling, etc.	E-mail, weekly meeting	Weekly	D. Ortiz (with process owners)
Medical assistants	Changes in workflow, responsibilities related to discipline. What is changing, when, how, and why.	E-mail, daily huddle	At least once per week	D. Ortiz (with lead medical assistant)
Nurses	Changes in workflow, responsibilities related to discipline. What is changing, when, how, and why.	E-mail, daily huddle	At least once per week	D. Ortiz (with charge nurse)
Physicians	Changes in workflow, responsibilities related to discipline. What is changing, when, how, and why.	E-mail, daily huddle	At least once per week	D. Ortiz (with lead physician)
Registrars/schedulers	Changes in workflow, responsibilities related to discipline. What is changing, when, how, and why.	E-mail, daily huddle	At least once per week	D. Ortiz (with process owners)

to its interests, responsibilities, or needs. The delivery mechanism and frequency correspond with the nature of the group and its workflow.

When to use it: Draft with the sponsor and use throughout the duration of the project.

Required? Yes.

Waste Observations

Description: The waste observation table accompanies gemba walks and consolidates the results (Table A.3). Observations are documented and accompanied by clarifying comments.

When to use it: During or after gemba walks.

Required? Yes.

Table A.3 Waste observations.

Waste	Observations	Comments
Defects	Missing information on patient chart (demographics, insurance). Schedule is inaccurate.	
Overproduction	Chart prep (paper).	Staff prepares almost double of what is required.
Waiting	Patients wait in waiting room/exam room. Staff waits for tasks/assignments/information.	A lot of waiting by everyone. Though it seems busy, it also appears that nothing is happening because of the waiting.
Nonutilized skill/intellect	Staff waits for tasks/assignments/information. Uneven workload balance.	Medical assistants seem to be doing a lot of extra, unnecessary work.
Transportation	Patients walk a good amount.	Cannot change this due to fixed office layout.
Inventory	Patients waiting in waiting room (work-in-process—WIP).	
Motion	All staff, but mainly medical assistants, move around a lot, looking for people, information, supplies, etc.	Layout issues, no storage organization, rework from missing information.
Extra processing	Double documentation in patient charts and scheduling log.	

Waste Diagnostic Tool

Description: Figure A.3 displays the waste diagnostic tool. This tool provides a visual display of the presence and impact of waste on process flow. Each waste is evaluated along a continuum from low to high impact. The white dot is moved along the row accordingly.

When to use it: During or after gemba walks.

Required? No.

High-Level Process Map

Description: The high-level process map outlines the project scope (Figure A.4). The tool is in a modifiable table form. Process steps are added or removed as needed. However, because it is high level, the process map should not exceed eight steps.

When to use it: Before the high-level process map SIPOC (next tool). The SIPOC tool described next uses the steps defined here.

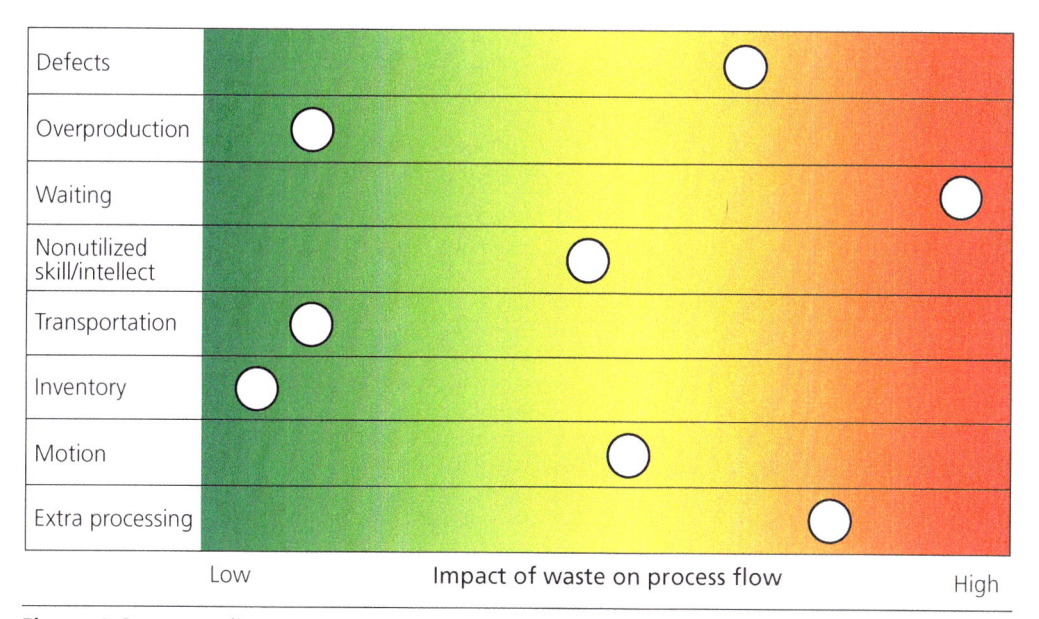

Required? Yes.

Figure A.3 Waste diagnostic.

Figure A.4 High-level process map.

High-Level Process Map SIPOC

Description: The high-level process map SIPOC details internal process requirements (Table A.4). Every step has a supplier, input, output, and customer. There are specific elements within each process step that are critical to quality (CTQ) as determined by the customer of that step. CTQ represents the factors that contribute to quality within that particular step (e.g., completed form) (Snee & Hoerl, 2003). The output of one step typically is the input to the following step (Silverstein et al., 2009). For example, a surgery patient (input) will have an IV placed (process step = placing the IV, output = patient with IV). This patient (input = patient with IV) then receives medication like a general anesthetic (process step = administer medication, output = sedated patient). To complete this tool, you have to walk the process and follow the flow of the item (i.e., patient, specimen, form). Document the details of what occurs.

When to use it: After gemba walks and process observations.

Required? Yes.

Table A.4　High-level SIPOC.

Supplier	Input	Process step	Output	Customer What is critical to quality (CTQ)?
Patient	Insurance card and license	**Sign in**	Registered patient and activated chart	Accurate/up-to-date patient information
Patient	Registered patient	**Get vitals**	Vitals taken and documented in chart	Accurate recordings of vitals (height, weight, blood pressure, temperature)
Medical assistant/ patient	Patient with vitals taken	**RN interview**	Understanding of reason for visit, history, and physical	Accurate assessment of health
Nurse	Patient history/ physical and reason for visit	**Physician exam**	Determination of illness/issue, treatment plan	Accurate assessment of health
Physician	Determination of illness/issue, treatment plan	**Receive Rx**	Prescription slip	Accurate medication, dosage, etc.
Patient	Patient with Rx	**Check out**	Scheduled follow-up appointment, patient payment	Schedule availability, accurate copay amount

Change Readiness Profile

Description: The change readiness profile provides an environmental assessment of the area within the scope (Figure A.5). Each of the six domains is evaluated along a continuum based on the current leadership abilities. The white dots move up the column from low to high depending on assessment.

When to use it: After VOC interviews and gemba walks.

Required? Optional, but strongly recommended.

System and Process Profile

Description: A profile tool that is similar to the change readiness profile evaluates systems and processes. The system and process profile depicts the potential impact of change on system or process components (Figure A.6). As with the change readiness profile, each of the six domains is evaluated along a continuum. White dots move along the column from low to high impact.

When to use it: After VOC interviews and gemba walks.

Required? Optional, but strongly recommended.

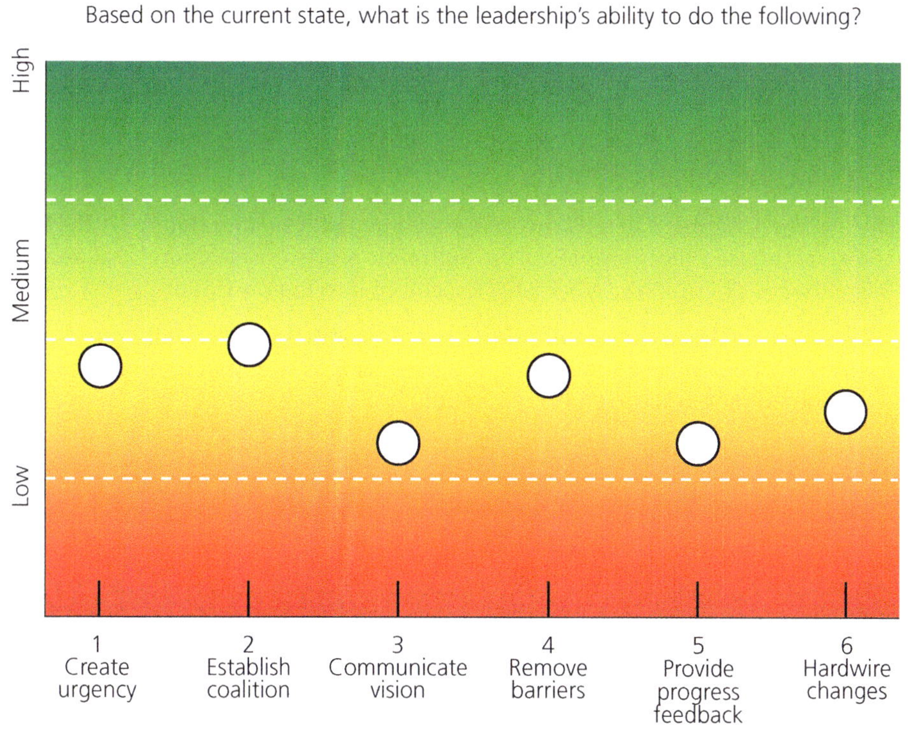

Figure A.5 Change readiness profile.

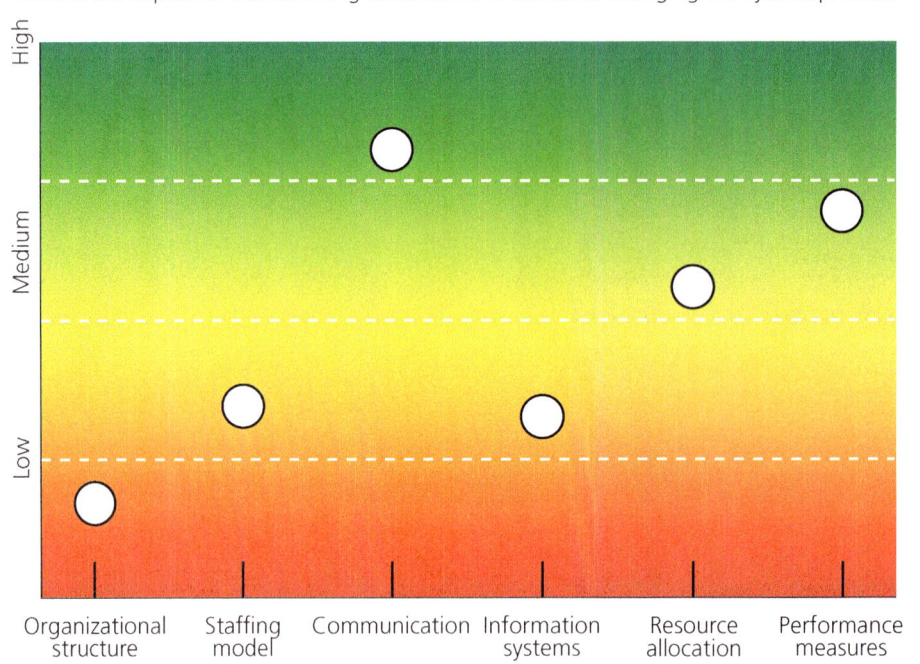

What is the impact of the following items when it comes to changing the system/process?

Figure A.6 System and process profile.

MEASURE

Process Value Analysis Results

Description: Chapter 3 details the process value analysis tool (Figure A.7). This is a gemba-based tool completed through time study observations and analysis. Paste the results from the Microsoft Excel tool into the portfolio.

When to use it: Time studies are conducted after initial gemba walks and VOC interviews. Before closely watching the process, it is essential to understand the environment and build rapport with staff.

Required? Yes (if applicable).

Workflow Value Analysis Results

Description: Chapter 3 details the workflow value analysis tool (Figure A.8). Like the process value analysis tool, this tool is gemba based. Paste the results from the Microsoft Excel tool into the portfolio.

When to use it: Time studies are conducted after initial gemba walks and VOC interviews. Workflow value analysis typically follows process value analysis. The process value analysis results will direct lean practitioners to process steps that require additional evaluation.

Required? Yes (if applicable).

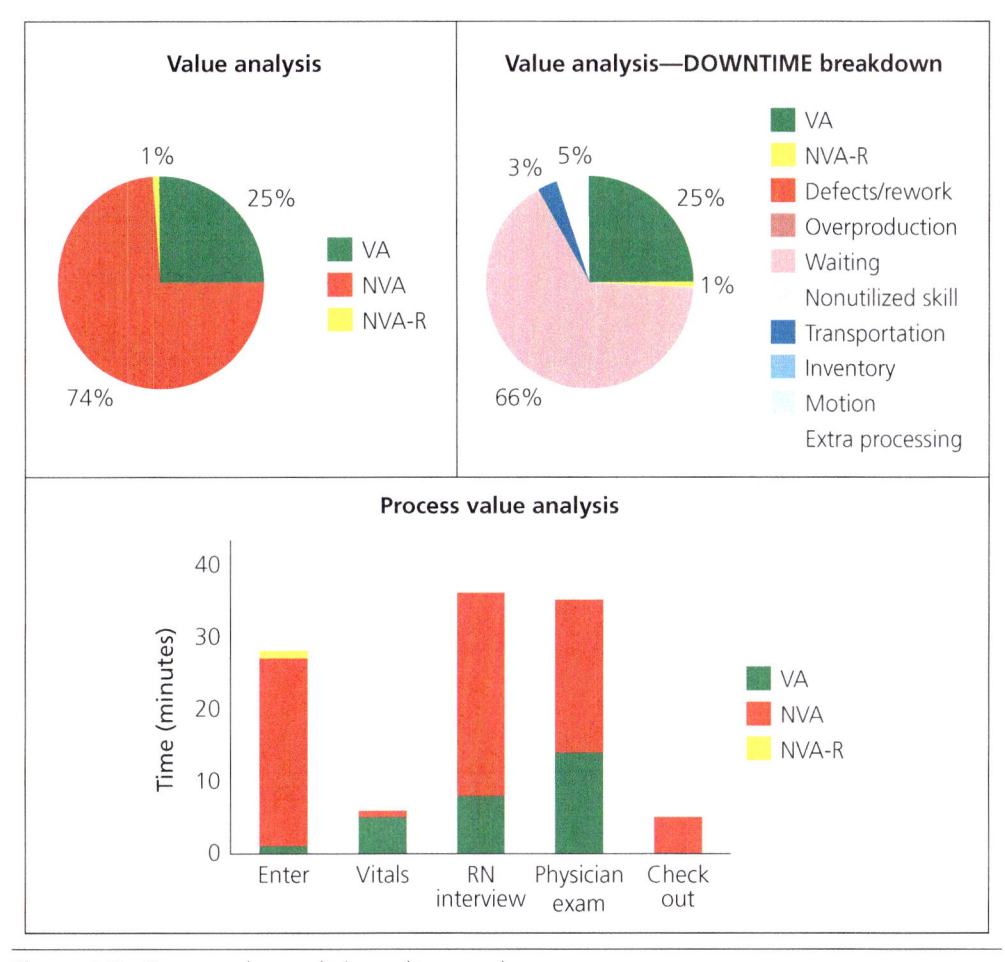

Figure A.7 Process value analysis results example.

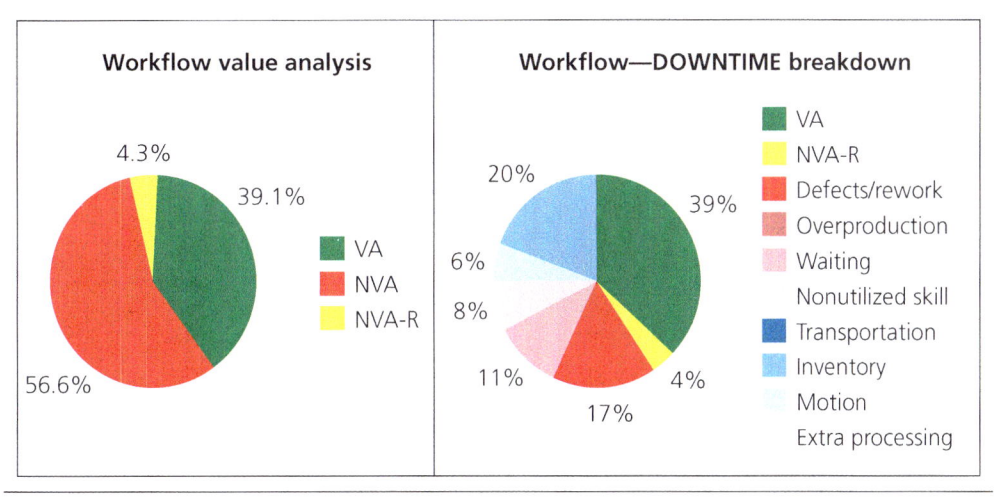

Figure A.8 Workflow value analysis results example.

Current State VSM

Description: Chapter 3 describes value stream mapping in detail. The current state VSM is a modifiable table-based process map (Figure A.9). Remember that there should be 5–8 high-level steps and fewer than 15 midlevel steps. Consolidate the map if it is too detailed. The table has a section below each midlevel process step for entering the VA/NVA cycle time and FPY. The NVA row also contains a box to enter time spent waiting, which is located between each step. Lead time, overall FPY, and value-added ratio may be entered in the bottom right-hand corner.

When to use it: After building the high-level process map (Figure A.4) and SIPOC (Table A.4).

Required? Yes.

Baseline Data for Key Metrics

Description: Improvement metrics should reflect the problem statement and objectives. Using the appropriate chart, as outlined in Chapter 7, paste the baseline data here.

When to use it: When data are available.

Required? Yes.

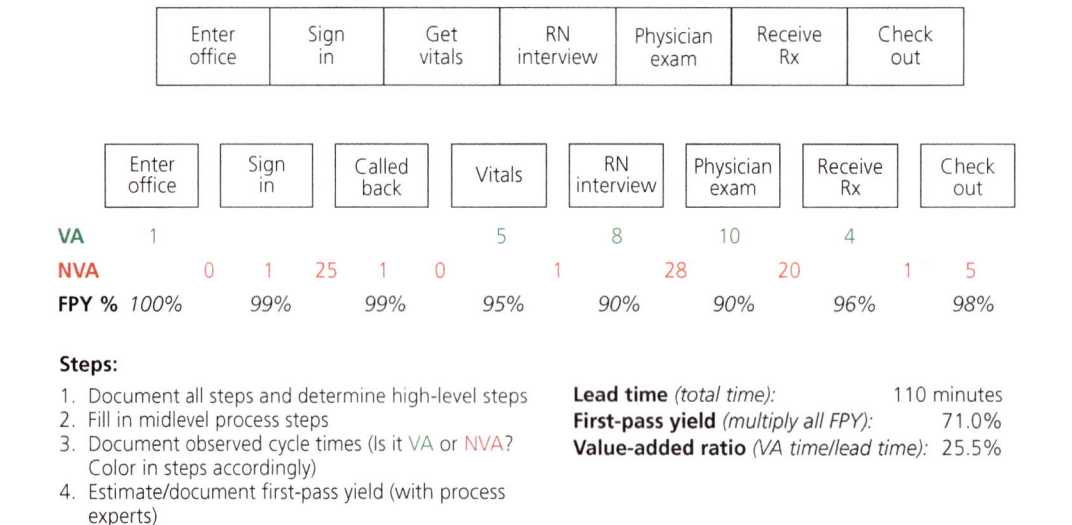

High-level steps: Enter office | Sign in | Get vitals | RN interview | Physician exam | Receive Rx | Check out

Midlevel steps: Enter office | Sign in | Called back | Vitals | RN interview | Physician exam | Receive Rx | Check out

	Enter office	Sign in	Called back	Vitals	RN interview	Physician exam	Receive Rx	Check out
VA	1			5	8	10	4	
NVA	0	1	25	1	0	1	28	20	1	5
FPY %	100%	99%		99%	95%	90%	90%	96%	98%

Steps:
1. Document all steps and determine high-level steps
2. Fill in midlevel process steps
3. Document observed cycle times (Is it VA or NVA? Color in steps accordingly)
4. Estimate/document first-pass yield (with process experts)

Lead time *(total time):* 110 minutes
First-pass yield *(multiply all FPY):* 71.0%
Value-added ratio *(VA time/lead time):* 25.5%

Figure A.9 Current state VSM template.

Voice of Customer Summary

Description: VOC interviews occur individually or in small groups. Throughout this process, key themes emerge. The table highlights these themes along with identifying the elements that are critical to quality (Table A.5).

When to use it: After completing VOC interviews, consolidate notes into more general themes and potential root causes.

Required? Yes.

Voice of Customer More of/Less of

Description: Another VOC approach, the more of/less of tool, defines stakeholder expectations (Table A.6). During VOC interviews (or even after as part of summarizing), stakeholders are asked what they want more or less of from the process. This information sheds light on areas of opportunity (less of) and potential solutions (more of).

When to use it: Either during VOC interviews as part of the questions asked or afterward during the VOC consolidation.

Required? No.

Table A.5 Voice of customer summary.

Key theme	Critical to quality (CTQ) What has a direct and significant impact on its actual or perceived quality?	Comments
Coordination	There is limited coordination across disciplines. As a result, staff doesn't know when to do what or how long tasks should take. This leads to process delays.	Occurs for all disciplines
Visual management	No visual cues signaling any information. For example, once a patient is in the exam room, you do not know how long the patient has been in there, who the patient needs to see, or what is left to do prior to discharge.	
Communication	As with coordination, communication across staff is poor. Huddles are in place, which is good.	Not having visual cues adds to the confusion
Workload balance	Uneven workloads lead to delays in processing and bottlenecks (i.e., waiting for an employee to complete several tasks).	No prioritization process, therefore nothing can be expedited

Table A.6 Voice of customer more of/less of.

More of	Less of	Comments
Visual cues		
Performance metric overviews		Charts displayed in office for monthly performance compared with goal
Communication across disciplines		
Ownership in patient experience and teamwork		
	Finger pointing	Remove "blaming" culture
	Reactive to problems rather than proactive	
	"It's not my job" response	

ANALYZE

Stakeholder Analysis

Description: The improvement team conducts stakeholder analyses internally. Stakeholders are identified (through VOC interviews, observations, and gemba walks) and listed in the table (Table A.7). Each individual or group is evaluated on its level of support for or resistance to the change initiative. Target individuals or groups that are neutral, against, or strongly against using influence strategies based on their primary issues and concerns. Alternatively, for stakeholders that are strongly supportive, develop strategies to leverage their buy-in and engagement.

When to use it: After VOC interviews and gemba walks.

Required? Optional, but strongly recommended.

Table A.7 Stakeholder analysis.

Stakeholder (name or group)	Strongly supportive	Supportive	Neutral	Against	Strongly against	Issues/concerns	Influence strategy
Patients	X					None	
Administration		X				None	
Medical assistants				X		Changes in workflow, responsibilities	Frequent communication, inclusion in problem solving, gemba walks to learn their challenges/issues
Nurses			X			Changes in responsibilities and holding staff accountable	Inclusion in problem solving
Physicians				X		No time to implement changes	Identify best time for facilitated RIE based on their availability
Registrars/schedulers	X					None	

RACI Chart

Description: The RACI chart is another stakeholder tool used to determine how to appropriately include various individuals, departments, and groups (Table A.8). The list of tasks outlines basic project deliverables or phases. The top row consists of stakeholder groups. For each task, determine whether the stakeholder group is:

- *Responsible* for doing the work
- *Accountable* for completing the task (the Responsible group typically reports to the Accountable group)
- *Consulted* as content experts
- *Informed* of the outcomes

Depending on the categorization, place the corresponding letter (R, A, C, or I) in the cell. This tool helps identify roles and responsibilities throughout the change process.

When to use it: For projects that are multidisciplinary and complex in nature with many stakeholders.

Required? Optional, but strongly recommended.

Table A.8 RACI chart.

Tasks	Stakeholder (name or group)				
	Patients	Administration	Office manager	Medical assistants, RNs, physicians	Registrars/ schedulers
Project definition		A	R		
IS technical assessment		I	R	C	C
Stakeholder analysis		I	R		
Project plan (Gantt chart)		A	R	C	C
Project implementation			A	R	R
Project results	I	A			

Data Analysis Results

Description: Determine where the opportunities are through data analysis. Chapter 1 described the difference between lagging (outcomes) and leading (process measures) metrics. Data analysis should assess the impact of leading metrics. Do the data identify the key drivers of the problem? Copy and paste analyses into this section of the portfolio.

When to use it: After establishing baseline performance and identifying leading metrics.

Required? Optional, but strongly recommended.

Fishbone Diagram

Description: Details for completing the fishbone diagram are in Chapter 7. The fishbone analysis qualitatively documents potential root causes of the problem (Figure A.10). The improvement team should populate the fishbone using VOC interviews, observations, and gemba walks.

When to use it: After VOC interviews, observations, and gemba walks, but it should be verified by content experts (employees working the process).

Required? Optional, but strongly recommended.

Fishbone Diagram

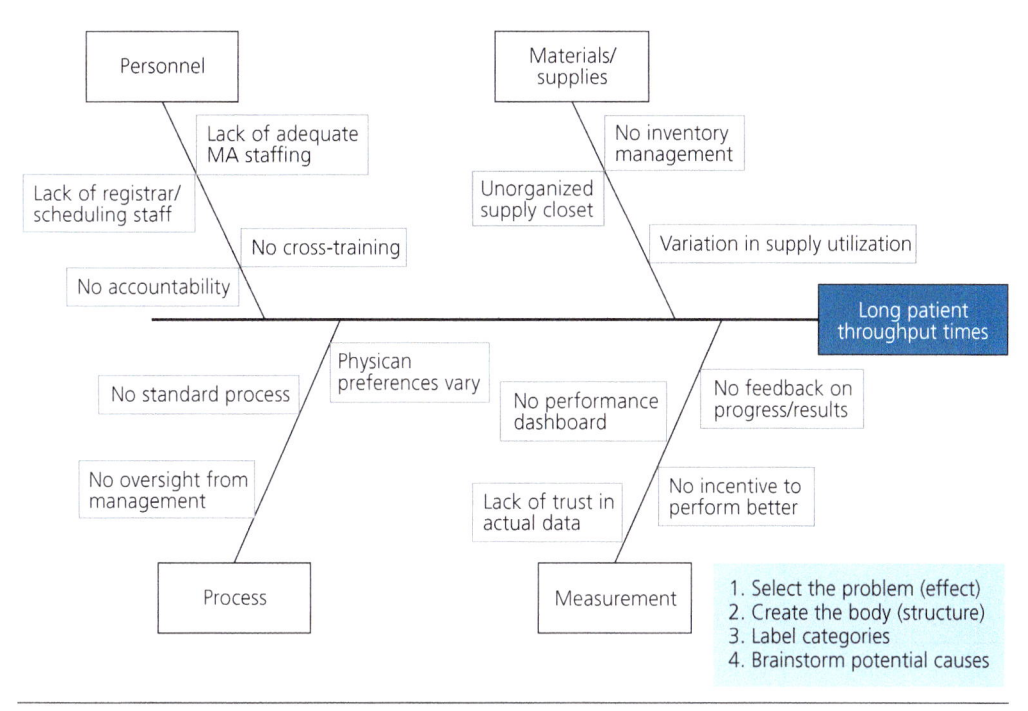

Personnel
- Lack of registrar/scheduling staff
- Lack of adequate MA staffing
- No cross-training
- No accountability

Materials/supplies
- No inventory management
- Unorganized supply closet
- Variation in supply utilization

Process
- No standard process
- Physican preferences vary
- No oversight from management

Measurement
- No performance dashboard
- No feedback on progress/results
- Lack of trust in actual data
- No incentive to perform better

Effect: Long patient throughput times

1. Select the problem (effect)
2. Create the body (structure)
3. Label categories
4. Brainstorm potential causes

Figure A.10 Fishbone diagram template.

Rapid Improvement Event Agenda

Description: Table A.9 outlines the RIE agenda. The agenda models the five-step kaizen problem-solving process and the Improve phase checklist. Facilitators need to assign sections of the agenda to one another. The "Details" column offers guidance and hints, while "Materials needed" suggests supplies. The estimated time will vary depending on the duration of the RIE.

When to use it: After the duration of the RIE has been determined.

Required? Yes.

IMPROVE

Payoff Matrix

Description: The improvement team facilitates the payoff matrix (as described in step 4 of the five-step kaizen problem-solving process in Chapter 9). The payoff matrix slide on the portfolio holds the information developed by the team afterward (Figure A.11). Not all solutions developed will become action plan items. However, there is value in documenting all ideas, so individuals outside the improvement team can see other considerations and ideas.

When to use it: The payoff matrix is used after all solutions have been brainstormed. The portfolio slide can be populated in real time or after the RIE.

Required? Yes.

Table A.9 RIE agenda template.

Title	Details	Materials needed	Estimated time
Kickoff	Goal/purpose of rapid improvement event	• Flip chart: parking lot	10 min
Intro, icebreaker	• Who the facilitators are/what we're doing • Who are you? Where do you work/what do you do?		10 min
Agenda	Review RIE agenda with participants • Current state review • Identify key issues/barriers • Develop action plan to implement future state	• PowerPoint	5 min
Current state review	Review charter, process map, data, Gemba walk observations	• PowerPoint	35 min
Step 1: Identify issues/barriers to achieving goals Step 2: Filter and prioritize	What are the biggest issues/barriers? Tools: 1) Silent brainstorming/group brainstorming/fishbone diagram–post-its 2) In/out of control 3) Dot voting	• Sticky notes • Flip chart: in/out of control	60 min
Step 3: Identify solutions Step 4: Prioritize based on impact	Based on prioritized issues/barriers, what actions/interventions can impact change? Tools: 1) Silent brainstorming/group brainstorming/direct issue-to-solution/reverse engineering 2) Payoff priority	• Sticky notes • Flip chart: payoff matrix	60 min
Step 5: Develop action plans and recommendations	Develop recommendations for next steps	• Action plan/recommendation template	45 min
Conclude session and report out	Determine next follow-up meeting (location/time/date) to review progress		20 min

High impact/easy to do	High impact/difficult to do
• Utilize visual cues (exam room flags) • Define roles and responsibilities through swimlane mapping • Survey patients on process change—solicit input on other suggestions for improvement • Do checkout upon sign-in	• Implement new information system to track financial and operational metrics • Implement financial incentives for staff based on performance to target
Low impact/easy to do (low-hanging fruit)	**Low impact/difficult to do**
• Post performance dashboard on weekly basis, review at huddles • Start employee-of-the-month award program for staff member creating/implementing positive change • Post changes as a result of patient feedback in the waiting room so patients can see that improvements are being made	• Hang signs in waiting area bathroom that define what patients need for checkout (i.e., credit card, cash)

Figure A.11 Payoff matrix template.

Action Plan and Recommendations

Description: Tables A.10 and A.11 provide the action plan and recommendation components described in step 5 of the five-step kaizen problem-solving process in Chapter 9. As with the payoff matrix, development of the action plan takes place during the RIE and is subsequently documented in the improvement portfolio. This portfolio slide is a means to document the plan and maintain a record of it along with other project deliverables.

When to use it: The action plan follows solution prioritization.

Required? Yes.

Future State VSM

Description: Chapter 3 describes future state VSMs in detail. The VSM tool for the future state is the same as that for the current state (Figure A.12). Steps for creating the future state VSM are the same.

When to use it: The future state VSM construction occurs once the solutions/interventions have been selected.

Required? No, but helpful to accompany current state VSM for comparison.

Table A.10 Action plan template.

What	How/why	Resources needed	Expected outcome	Who	When
Utilize visual cues (exam room flags)	Purchase flags to help indicate where patients are in the process	Exam room flags	Improved visual management, reduced motion, reduced LOS	R. Gronkowski	2/20
Define roles and responsibilities through swimlane mapping	Create future state swimlane map to illustrate new process flow	N/A	Clarity in staff understanding of roles/responsibilities	M. Hoomanawanui R. Ninkovich	2/18
Survey patients on process change, solicit input on other suggestions for improvement	E-mail electronic survey to solicit voice of customer	Survey	Identified opportunities for improvement	R. Ninkovich	2/23
Do checkout upon sign-in	Schedule follow-up appointment and collect copay upfront; reduces time for patient	N/A	Reduced LOS	D. Revis	3/9
Post performance dashboard on weekly basis, review at huddles	Print dashboard, post in break room, and review in huddles so staff know how they are doing	Dashboard	Staff awareness of performance	S. Vollmer D. Revis	2/23
Start "employee of the month" award program for staff members creating/implementing positive change	Staff-nominated employee, improves morale and encourages contributions to improvements	Small gift/award for selected individual	Improved staff morale	R. Gronkowski	3/2
Post changes as a result of patient feedback in the waiting room so patients can see improvements are being made	Print infographic of changes and results to communicate value-adding changes	Infographic	Improved patient satisfaction	S. Vollmer D. Revis	3/9

Table A.11 Recommendation template.

What (proposal)	How/why	Resources needed	Expected outcome	What decision needs to be made?	When
Implement new information system to track financial and operational metrics	Purchase IS software to enhance metric tracking and reporting	Finances to purchase, IT expertise to install and train	Accurate performance reporting	Approval to purchase	3/2
Implement financial incentives for staff based on performance to target	Determine targets and financial incentives for all staff, align office performance with financial incentives	Finances for incentive bonus structure	Aligned effort and improved collaboration toward common goal	Approval of finances for program	3/2

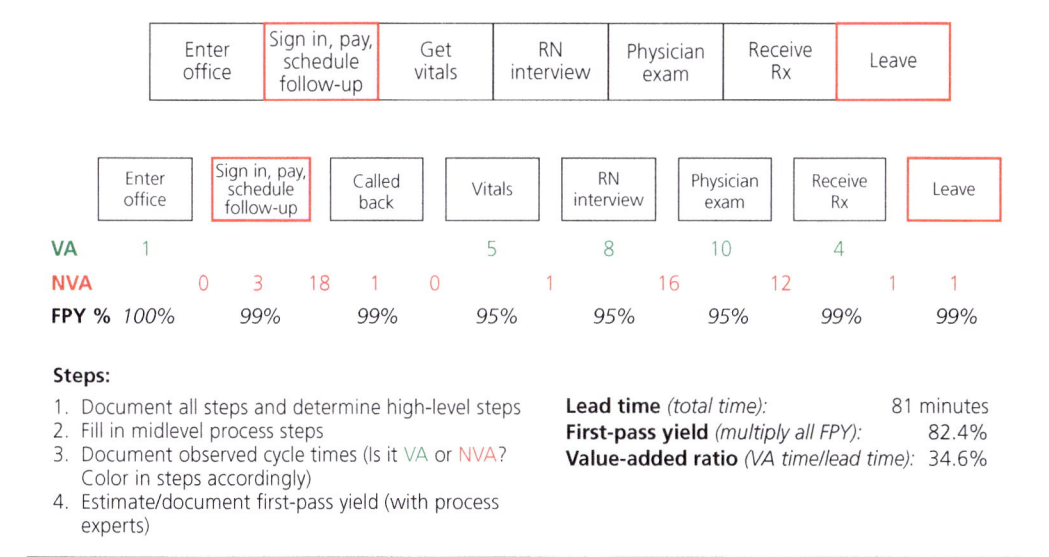

	Enter office	Sign in, pay, schedule follow-up	Get vitals	RN interview	Physician exam	Receive Rx	Leave

	Enter office	Sign in, pay, schedule follow-up	Called back	Vitals	RN interview	Physician exam	Receive Rx	Leave
VA	1			5	8	10	4	
NVA	0	3	18	1	0	1	16	12	1	1
FPY %	100%	99%	99%	95%	95%	95%	99%	99%

Steps:
1. Document all steps and determine high-level steps
2. Fill in midlevel process steps
3. Document observed cycle times (Is it VA or NVA? Color in steps accordingly)
4. Estimate/document first-pass yield (with process experts)

Lead time *(total time):* 81 minutes
First-pass yield *(multiply all FPY):* 82.4%
Value-added ratio *(VA time/lead time):* 34.6%

Figure A.12 Future state VSM template.

CONTROL

Control Phase Action Plan

Description: Appendix F provides details of the Control phase action plan.

When to use it: After the RIE as part of the Control phase team meetings.

Required? Yes.

Lessons Learned

Description: Solicit input from improvement team members (facilitators and participants) and document their thoughts. Pose the following questions: (1) What are the key lessons learned from this RIE? (2) What advice do you have for someone ready to start an RIE? and (3) What was the most gratifying part of the experience?

When to use it: After the RIE or after completing the Control phase.

Required? No, but suggested for documenting project experience.

Kaizen A3 Report

Description: The A3 report, described in the "Control Phase" section in Chapter 8, consolidates the project into a concise summary (Figure A.13). Elements from the project charter, VOC summary, process maps, data analysis, payoff matrix, and action plan inform the report. There are two versions of the kaizen A3 report in the portfolio. The first slide is a blank template for the team to complete. The second slide is a reference that contains questions and considerations to guide the team. The portfolio houses all key project deliverables. However, the kaizen A3 report should be a stand-alone document that presents the salient project components.

When to use it: At the conclusion of the project.

Required? Yes.

Improving Physician's Office Patient Flow
T. Brady, M. Vaughn, D. Pedroia, D. Ortiz

Background

The physician's office has a large volume of patients during the workweek. Patients arrive throughout the day at a variable rate. The multidisciplinary team is responsible for uneven workloads, and staffing levels are lower than desired.

Problem statement

The patient flow process is constantly interrupted by waiting. The lack of staff coordination leads to bottlenecks and compounding delays. Patient and employee satisfaction are low. As the volume of patient visits continues to rise, the need to streamline process flow/throughput is paramount.

Project/proposal objective

The goal of the project is to reduce patient length of stay (LOS) from 110 minutes to 90 minutes. This will be achieved by identifying and eliminating non-value-adding (NVA) activity and enhancing coordination across all team members.

Team members

R. Gronkowski, M. Hoomanawanui,
R. Ninkovich, S. Vollmer, D. Revis

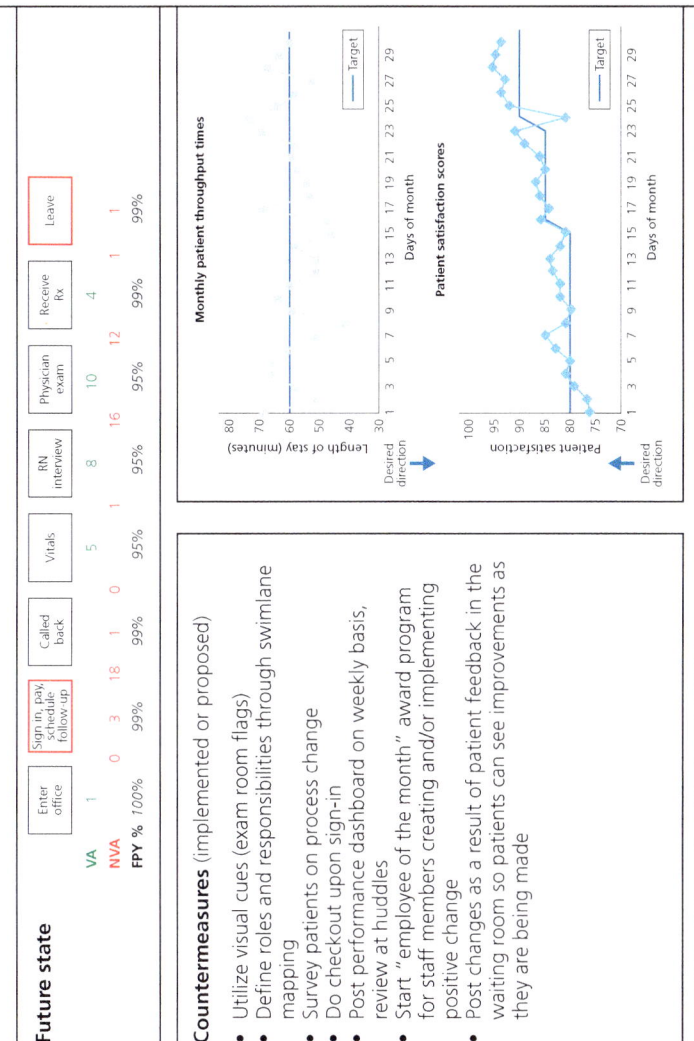

Future state

	Enter office	Sign in, pay, schedule follow up	Called back	Vitals	RN interview	Physician exam	Receive Rx	Leave
VA	1	3	1	5	8	10	4	1
NVA	0	18	0	1	16	12	1	1
FPY %	100%	99%	99%	95%	95%	95%	99%	99%

Countermeasures (implemented or proposed)

- Utilize visual cues (exam room flags)
- Define roles and responsibilities through swimlane mapping
- Survey patients on process change
- Do checkout upon sign-in
- Post performance dashboard on weekly basis, review at huddles
- Start "employee of the month" award program for staff members creating and/or implementing positive change
- Post changes as a result of patient feedback in the waiting room so patients can see improvements as they are being made

Results

Lead time: 110 minutes reduced to 81 minutes
First-pass yield: improved from 71% to 82%
Value-added ratio: improved from 26% to 35%
LOS and patient satisfaction above target

Monthly patient throughput times

Patient satisfaction scores

Next steps

Monitor results through weekly huddles.
Follow up with sponsors regarding proposed recommendations and patient feedback.

Figure A.13 Kaizen A3 report template.

Appendix B
Define Folder

DOWNTIME MATRIX

Description: The DOWNTIME matrix should accompany gemba walks and waste observations (Table A.12). It should also inform solution development.

When to use it: During observations, time studies, brainstorming issues and barriers, and solution development.

LEAN ENGAGEMENT COMMUNICATION PLAN

Description: The lean engagement communication plan (Table A.13) is a comprehensive version of the communication plan presented earlier (Table A.2). The communications lead (from the facilitator team) is responsible for overseeing execution of the plan. Table A.13 defines specific deliverables, timelines, and expectations for a lean engagement. Teams should review the plan and adapt accordingly to meet the needs of the area under review.

When to use it: Before, during, and after the RIE.

Required? Optional, but strongly recommended.

Table A.12 DOWNTIME matrix.

Waste	Definition	Examples	Potential causes	Questions to ask	Countermeasures
Defects	Rework, errors, incomplete or incorrect information	• Medication errors • Process step not performed correctly • Missing information	• Lack of understanding of what "defect-free" means • Insufficient training	• Are tasks clearly defined (who, what, when, how)? • Are errors dealt with directly and promptly or passed along?	• 5S • Visual management • Standard work • Error-proofing
Overproduction	Producing more than what is currently needed (too much or too soon)	• Medications administered early to accommodate start schedule • Printing extra copies of information just in case	• No clear understanding of what is needed, when, in what quantity • Poor communication • Inconsistent process	• Are there more supplies prepared than needed? • Is the demand known?	• Workload balancing • Standard work • Checklists • Pull systems
Waiting	Delays, waiting for anything (people, paper, equipment, information)	• Delays in bed assignments • Delays in receiving information or communication • Waiting for next process steps to begin	• Poor understanding of time required to complete a task • No visual cues to indicate next step in the process • Delays compounding one another	• Are there bottlenecks/delays in the process due to obtaining information, supplies, etc.? • Are there clear expectations for how long process steps should take?	• VSM • Swimlane map • 5S • Workload balancing • Cross-train staff
Nonutilized skill/intellect	Nonutilizing staff skills or knowledge, poor workload balance	• No cross-training • Nurses transporting patients • Physical drawing labs	• Lack of well-defined process • Unclear or undefined roles and responsibilities	• Are employees cross-trained? • Are employees encouraged to suggest/implement improvements?	• Swimlane map • Workload balancing • Standard work

Transportation	Unnecessary movement of something being processed (e.g., forms, patient, specimen, equipment)	• Placing stretcher in hall and constantly having to move it • Transporting forms from building to building or electronically to several areas	• Poor physical layout • Poor system/process design	• Are forms, patients, or materials moved to temporary locations? • Is technology being leveraged to limit physical handoffs?	• 5S • Physical layout • Visual management • Standard work
Inventory	Excessive supplies, batch processing, work in progress	• Extra/outdated manuals • Excessive supplies • Obsolete equipment	• Supply/demand not well understood • Outdated supplies/equipment not discarded • Disorganized area, unclear what is necessary/unnecessary	• Is there extra equipment/supplies lying around? • Do forms, supplies, or patients wait in groups/batches?	• 5S • Visual management • Standard work • Pull systems
Motion	Any excess movement of the employee	• Searching for anything (e.g., information, supplies, equipment, patients) • Hand-carrying paperwork to another area	• Poor physical layout • Poor system/process design	• How does the current layout impede the process flow? • Can walking be reduced by repositioning equipment, people, and/or supplies?	• 5S • Physical layout • Visual management • Standard work
Extra processing	Extra or unnecessary steps performed that do not add value to the process	• Ordering more tests than the diagnosis warrants • Entering repetitive/duplicative information	• Complex or multiple forms • Ineffective policies and procedures	• Is there more information available than what needs to be processed?	• VSM • Visual management • Workload balancing • Standard work

Table A.13 Lean engagement communication plan.

Event/item	Timing	Key messages/objectives	Delivery mechanism	Deliverables	Completed by	Recipients	Date	Comments
Kickoff	Before start of project	Review: lean approach, communication plan, kaizen event expectations (participation/engagement of *all* staff, leadership support), set target kaizen event dates	Meeting	• Process owners assigned • Communication plan approved (dates and times set for meetings) • Agreement on number of kaizen participants and their time commitment	Lean leaders	VP/department management	12/29	Establish clear expectations; identify sponsor/process owner and keep them fully engaged start to finish; review communication plan and decide how it will roll out
All-staff presentation	Before start of VOC	Purpose of project, what to expect, who the lean leaders are and what they will be doing (our DMAIC process)	Announcement at staff meeting, distribute and post team profile, hand out kaizen idea card		VP with lean leaders	All staff	1/5	Share the vision, why are we doing this?
Lean information	Start of project	What is lean, what is a kaizen event, what to expect	Handouts	• High-level overview	Lean leaders	All staff	1/5	
Weekly management update	Weekly (from start to kaizen)	Status update on project (DMAIC deliverables)	Management meetings, phone call, e-mail	• Review project status • Discuss issues, barriers, concerns • Approve charter	Lean leader/team leader	VP/department management	1/5 to 2/2	Engage department, identify and address barriers, keep progress moving forward
Staff meeting presentation	2 weeks before kaizen	What is a kaizen event; date, time, location, what to expect	Communication handout, team profile	• Collect idea cards	VP/dept. leader/lean leaders	All staff	1/20	Communicate what will happen and how they can contribute

KAIZEN

		Decision on recommendation changes	Presentation/ discussion	• Decision on recommendations • Staff education/ communication plan	Lean leaders	VP/ department management	2/2	
Kaizen action plan	End of kaizen							
Improvements/ changes communication	1 week after kaizen	Kaizen outcomes (action plan, next steps)	Short update at staff meeting, action plan handout		VP/dept. leader/ lean leaders/ kaizen team	All staff	2/9	
Action plan update	Week 2 and 4	Control phase update, issues or barriers discussion	Management meeting		Team leader for lean team	VP/ department management	2/16 to 2/27	Ensure we are on track to complete deliverables
Project results	5–8 weeks after kaizen	Project outcomes	Staff meeting		Team leader for lean team	All staff	3/9	Solicit thoughts, experiences with new changes
Report out forms	6–8 weeks after kaizen	Results: A3 report, presented by VP (kickoff), lean leaders, and representatives of kaizen team	Management update; operations meeting	• Kaizen A3 report	Lean master/ lean team	Management	3/30	Communicate success, lessons learned
Report out forms	6–8 weeks after kaizen (after MU presenta- tion)	Results: A3 report, recognition of kaizen team and lean leaders	Intranet homepage	• Intranet posting/ article	Lean master/ director of commu- nications dept.	Management	3/30	Communicate success, lessons learned

LEAN OPPORTUNITY GUIDE

Description: Table A.14 generalizes lean opportunities based on processes and performance metrics. The guide facilitates opportunity identification.

When to use it: Before project initiation to identify appropriate project selection.

Table A.14 Lean opportunity guide.

General improvement opportunities		
Staffing	Workflow Workflow balancing	Time management Productivity
Physical organization/ inventory management	Ordering processes/par levels Space allocation	Visual management Physical layout/organization
Examples of lean project metrics		
Turnaround time Cycle/processing time	Throughput time (lead time) Customer, patient, employee satisfaction	Quality output Cost savings/avoidance

Examples of department/function-specific improvement opportunities		
Business services	Timeliness and accuracy of results/reports Transactional throughput	Request turnaround time
Emergency departments	Length of stay Door to triage Door to physician	Door to disposition Door to discharge Admission order to transfer from ED
Diagnostic and ancillary departments	Patient transportation Patient registration Order to result	Request to completion Exam/procedure/testing scheduling Work assignments
Nursing and clinical units	Bed availability Bed empty to fill turnaround time	Patient flow Workload balance
Physician practice	Exam room utilization Access/scheduling	Patient flow Workload balance
Supply chain	Par levels Product standardization Space allocation/organization	Inventory locations Distribution process
Surgical services	Decontamination and sterilization processes Instrument availability Case assembly Operating room utilization	First case on-time start Scheduling process Operating room turnover Patient flow

VOC WASTE QUESTIONNAIRE

Description: VOC interviews can include questions from the "Define Phase" section in Chapter 8: (1) What is working? (2) What is not working? (3) What frustrates you at work? and (4) If you could change one or two things, what would you change and why? Or facilitators can take a targeted approach to determine specific DOWNTIME waste problems. The tool assists in facilitating discussion around waste and potential solutions (Figure A.14).

When to use it: During VOC interviews.

Required? Optional, but strongly recommended in operational areas.

Name B. LaFell		
Job title Office Manager		
Improving Physician Office Patient Flow through Lean: How can we improve throughput and eliminate waste?		
How can we improve patient throughput?	Improve coordination of staff. Enhance communication across disciplines (MAs, RNs, physicians, administrative staff).	
What frustrates you? What doesn't work well?	No visual cues to identify who is needed, where. Patients are unhappy because process is slow and inefficient. Employees don't know who is supposed to do what or how long tasks should take.	
What would you do differently?	Cross-train administrative and MA team to facilitate front-end flow. Improve visuals and communication throughout.	
Type of waste	**Please describe an example of this waste in your work environment**	**Please describe your ideas about what we can do to reduce or eliminate it**
Defects Rework, errors, incomplete or incorrect information	Patient charts missing demographic or insurance information.	Require some verification process to ensure all needed information is obtained.
Overproduction Producing more than what is currently needed (too much or too soon)	Chart prep (paper) process occurs at end of day in advance of following workday. Sometimes prepare a lot more than actual patient volume.	Prepare supplies as needed rather than in advance.
Waiting Delays, waiting for anything (people, paper, equipment, or information)	Patients wait for a long time in the waiting room and in the exam rooms.	Not sure; this is why we need help!

Figure A.14 VOC waste questionnaire.

Appendix C
Measure Folder

PROCESS VALUE ANALYSIS

Description: Chapter 3 explains use of the process value analysis tool (Figure A.15).

Required? Yes (if applicable).

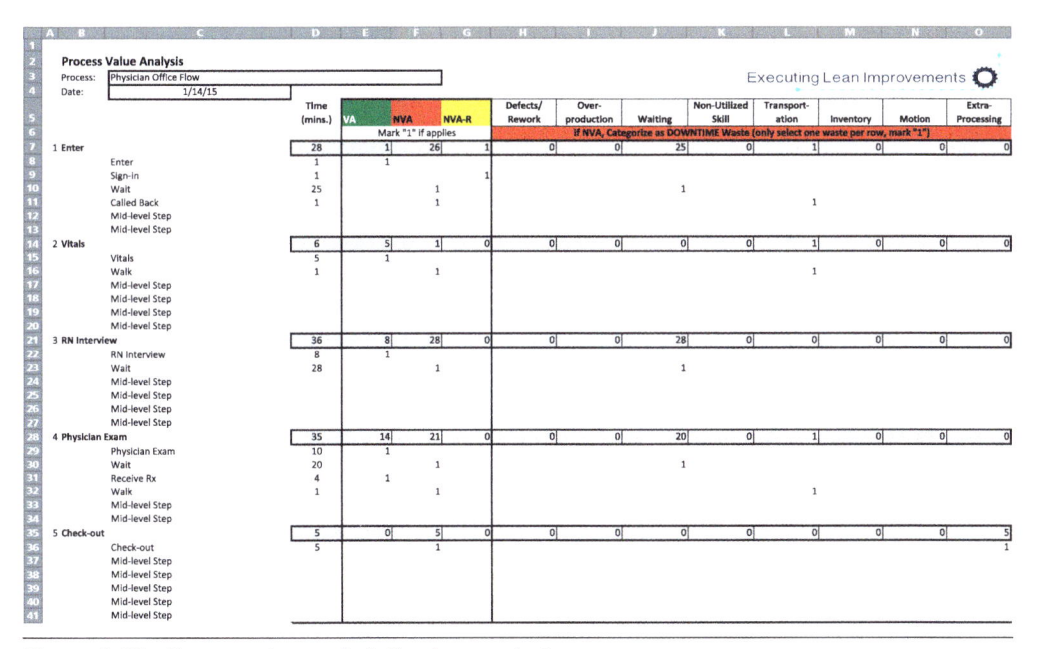

Figure A.15 Process value analysis Excel screenshot.

WORKFLOW VALUE ANALYSIS

Description: Chapter 3 describes how to use the workflow value analysis tool (Figure A.16).

Required? No.

Figure A.16 Workflow value analysis Excel screenshot.

Appendix D
Analyze Folder

5S AUDIT TOOL

Description: Chapter 4 outlines use of the 5S audit tool (Figure A.17).

Required? No.

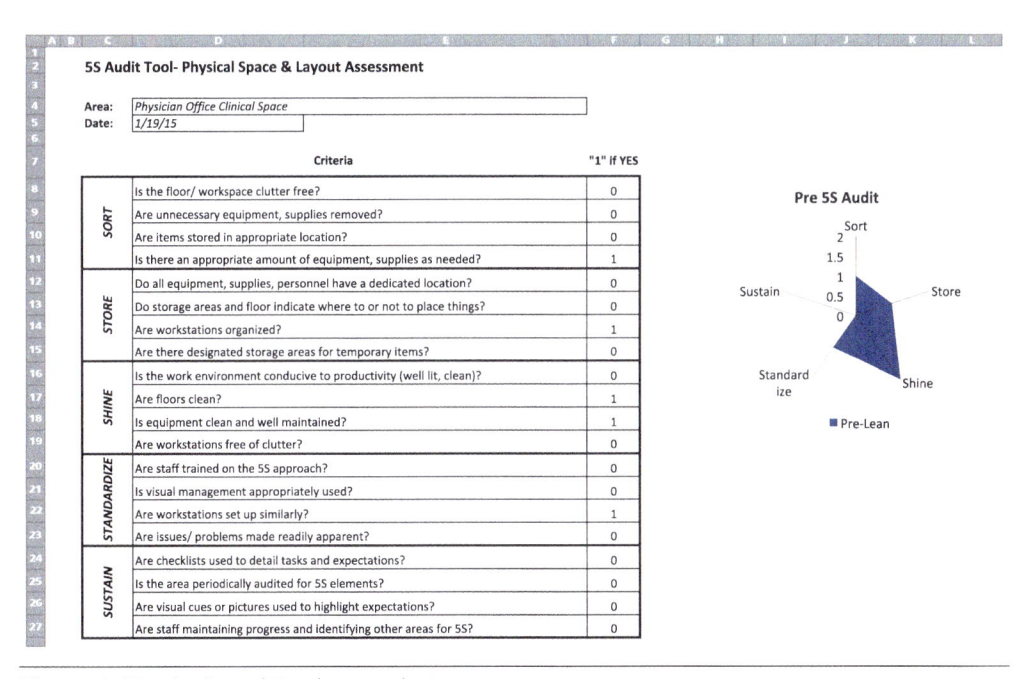

Figure A.17 Audit tool Excel screenshot.

SWIMLANE TEMPLATE

Description: Chapter 3 summarizes swimlane mapping techniques. The Microsoft Excel–based template makes it easy to document various flows by position (Figure A.18).

Required? No.

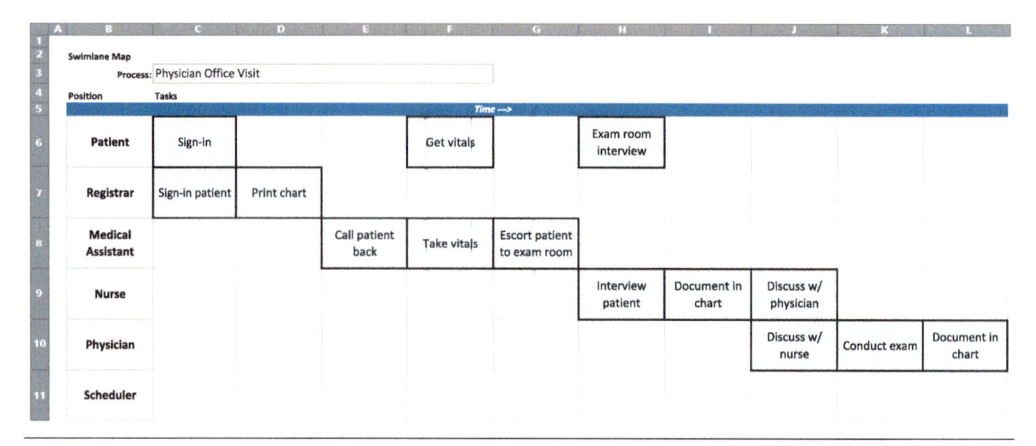

Figure A.18 Swimlane Excel screenshot.

Appendix E
Improve Folder

RIE PRESENTATION

Description: The RIE presentation drives the RIE agenda. There are placeholders throughout the slideshow for project documents (i.e., project charter, high-level process map and SIPOC, data analysis, and VOC summary). The presentation also includes the five-step kaizen problem-solving process. Each step has slides for the associated tools. Facilitators can modify the presentation to include only the tools they select to use.

When to use it: During the RIE, the presentation contains content for the current state review as well as instructions for using the various problem-solving tools.

Required? Yes.

RIE FACILITATOR EVALUATION FORM

Description: Distribute evaluations to RIE participants at the conclusion of the event (Figure A.19). Participants complete the form, hand it in, and then adjourn. Facilitators review the evaluations as part of a debrief. Ideally, the team conducts a self-evaluation using the same form before reviewing participant feedback.

When to use it: At the conclusion of the RIE.

Required? No, but strongly encouraged.

Rapid Improvement Event
Facilitator Evaluation

Event title: _____ **Date:** _____

In order to assess and improve the effectiveness of the facilitators, please provide open and honest feedback on the event you attended.

Thank you for your participation!

Facilitator's ability to:	Poor 1	Satisfactory 2	Good 3	Excellent 4
Lead the event				
Clearly explain objectives, teach content, and describe next step				
Listen and communicate with the team				
Manage time				
Motivate and engage participants				

The event:	Strongly disagree 1	Disagree 2	Agree 3	Strongly agree 4
Included the right people				
Achieved the objectives				
Was worth my time and efforts				

What two aspects of the event were most valuable for you?

-
-

What two suggestions could you offer to improve future events?

-
-

Figure A.19 RIE facilitator evaluation form.

Appendix F
Control Folder

KAIZEN A3 REPORT

Description: The "Control" section in Appendix A explains kaizen A3 reports. Figures A.20 and A.21 demonstrate how to document improvement projects.

Required? Yes.

CONTROL PHASE ACTION PLAN

Description: The Control phase action plan is a Microsoft Excel–based tool (Figure A.22). The contents derive from the action plan worksheet and approved recommendations. Each action item has its own row (indicated by a number in column B). "What" refers to the action item. Columns F–M detail the update meetings during the Control phase team meetings. Specific dates can replace generic ones. "Comments/details" in column N stores the "How/why," "Resources," and "Expected outcome" from the action plan worksheet.

The Control phase action plan serves as the agenda for the team meetings. The team reviews every action item. The person responsible (column D, "Who") provides an update. Update summaries are documented in the row with the corresponding meeting date. "Status" is indicated by "Not started," "In progress," or "Complete." Stoplight colors provide visual management for action item progress.

Figure A.23 shows an example of the Control phase action plan in use. The first item, "Utilize visual cues (exam room flags)," was completed after week 3. Progress was made during weeks 1 and 2. Rows 9–12 include verbatim updates from the individual responsible for completing the assigned task. These updates are critical pieces of information that enable the project lead to track progress over time, and reduce the likelihood of participants being unprepared since everything is appropriately documented.

The second action item in Figure A.23 demonstrates another effective way to use the tool. From a quick glance, it is clear that nothing has been initially accomplished, as indicated by two consecutive updates in red. The verbatim updates in rows 19 and 20 tell a story of inaction (i.e., "No update"). Action items that are slowly developing or have not started require energy to shift inertia. At a high level, this tool enables effective identification of vulnerable or underperforming areas. As the action plan list grows to 8–15 or more items, the stoplight indicators supply a quick visual cue for areas of focus and concern.

230 *Appendix F*

Standardizing Phlebotomy Work Baskets
Carrie L.; Glenn D.; Roseann P.; Beth-Ann S.; Scott G.

Background
The 5S lean team conducted organizational audits of work areas throghout the Center City campus. Opportunities were identified, evaluated, and prioritized based on resource requirements, scope, timeline, and need. Phlebotomy work baskets were selected for the first 5S area of focus given their clinical importance and inventory management struggles.

Problem statement
Variation in phlebotomy cart and baskets leads to oversupplying and risks expiration. Current inventory management issues and internal audits for expired supplies indicate an opportunity for standardization and improvement.

Project objective
Through the 5S approach (sort, store, shine, standardize, sustain), we will remove all unused, outdated, or unnecessary equipment and standardize the cart/basket layout.

Kaizen team
Dominique S., Damien F., Stephen M., Damond B., Hans A., Carrie L., Glenn D. Roseann P., Beth-Ann S., Scott G., Dennis D.

Sort
The group was divided into two teams to sort the baskets and determine what supplies were necessary and in what quantity.

Store
The two teams decided on locations for the supplies within the baskets.

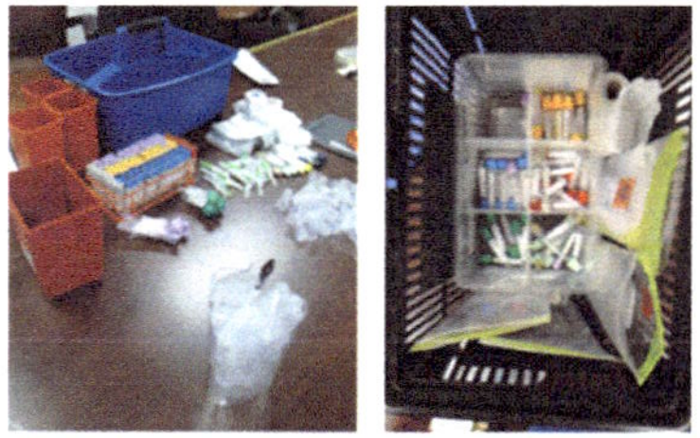

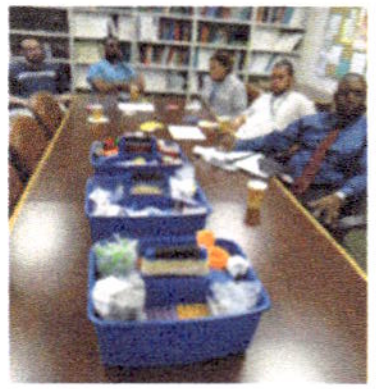

Shine
The two teams shined and cleaned the baskets. Excess inventory was removed from each basket.

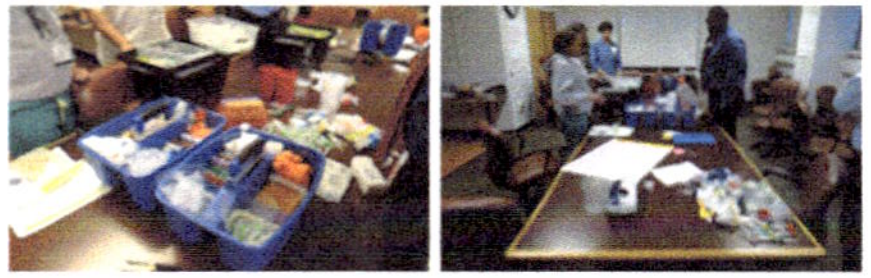

Standardize

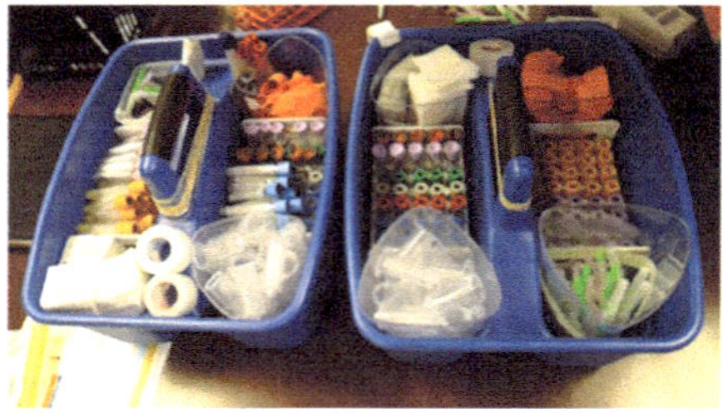

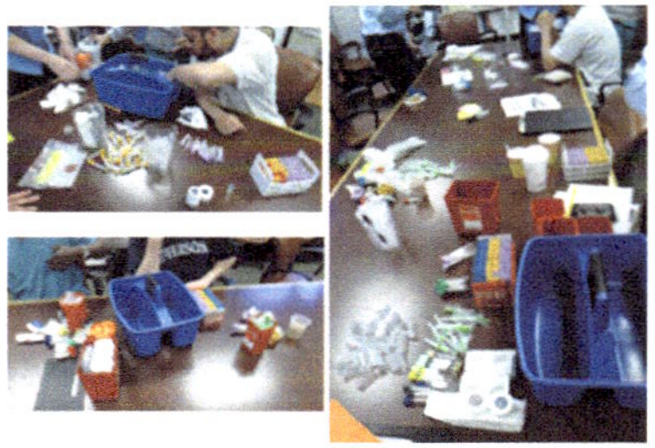

Sustain
Build awareness on why the change was needed. Benefits include baskets that are interchangeable, visually organized, and quicker to stock at the end of the shift; less waste of expired tubes and supplies; and better control of inventory.

Next steps: Solicit additional input from phlebotomists, standardize all carts/baskets.

Figure A.20 Kaizen A3 report example: Phlebotomy 5S event.

Improving Decision Making During Rapid Responses
Brian G., Michael L., Kathleen P., Linda S.

Background
The purpose of the rapid response team (RRT) system is to improve patient care by providing prompt recognition, early advanced assessment, enhanced communication with physicians, and appropriate intervention to patients with perceived changes in or deterioration of their condition. The RRT comprises staff nurse, RRT physician, surgeon, anesthesiologist, ICU nurse, respiratory therapist, and primary team physician.

Problem statement
There is a lack of standardization and lack of consistency of workflow during the rapid response process. There is a lot of potential for duplication of work along with excessive staff at patient bedside during the process. Without a standardized workflow there is also the potential to miss key processes and/or equipment.

Project/proposal objective
The project objective is to standardize workflow during a rapid response and facilitate efficient and accurate decision making. Implementation of a standardized process will improve the time rapid response was initiated to patient disposition along with notification of RRT to attending physician. This process will be implemented at the Center City campus initially and then will eventually be implemented across campuses.

High-level process map (SIPOC)
The group was divided into two teams to sort the baskets and determine what supplies were necessary and in what quantity.

Suppliers	Inputs	Process	Outputs	Customer (CTQ)
Patient or process of RRT	Patient requires immediate attention	**Clinical decline detected**	Unit RN activates pager for RRT	Clinical decline detection; timely and accurate
Unit nurse	Unit RN activates pager for RRT	**RRT called**	RRT paged	Appropriate team identified for RRT
Pager operator	RRT paged	**RRT arrives**	Management of patient initiated by RRT	Identify specific criterion for evaluation
RRT	Management of patient initiated by RRT	**Patient assessed**	RRT evaluates patient/identifies focus	Consistent measures
RRT, lab, radiology	RRT evaluates/ identifies issue(s)	**Etiology or organ system identified**	Treatment plan developed and outlined	Standardize role
RRT, pulmonary, pharmacy	Treatment plan developed and outlined	**Treatment initiated**	Team assesses response to treatment	Rx evaluation timely and accurate
RRT, ICU staff, bed manager	Team assesses response to treatment	**Disposition identified**	Patient arrives at appropriate clinical setting	Documentation from RRT

The high-level process map SIPOC illustrates the current rapid response process with multiple suppliers and duplication of processes.

Analyze qualitative data

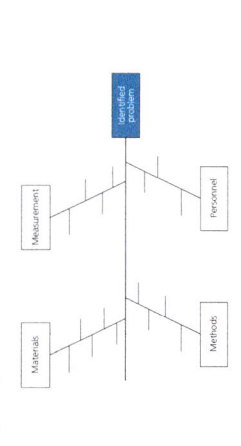

The fishbone diagram depicts the four major areas that are affected due to lack of standardization.

Countermeasures
- Implement RRT checklist to guide the rapid response process including time-specific checkpoints
- Implement availability of medical record at bedside via workplace on wheels, physical chart
- Assess crowd control at bedside
- Conduct brainstorming session with key players
- Revise current debriefing process to include questionnaire

Results
Metrics to be monitored:
- Time rapid response was initiated to patient disposition
- Notification of RRT to attending physician
- % RRT with completed RRT checklist
- Qualitative data from debriefing questionnaire

Next Steps
- Finalize RRT checklist along with debriefing questionnaire—December 30, 2013
- Educate RRT on process—January 2–15, 2014
- Promote awareness of new process on multidisciplinary level—January 2–15, 2014
- Initiate RRT checklist, at City Center campus—January 15, 2014
- Monitor progress and communicate findings—January 15–February 15, 2014
- Refine process based on findings—February 15–18, 2014
- Implement across campuses—March 1, 2014

Figure A.21 Kaizen A3 report example: Rapid responses.

232 *Appendix F*

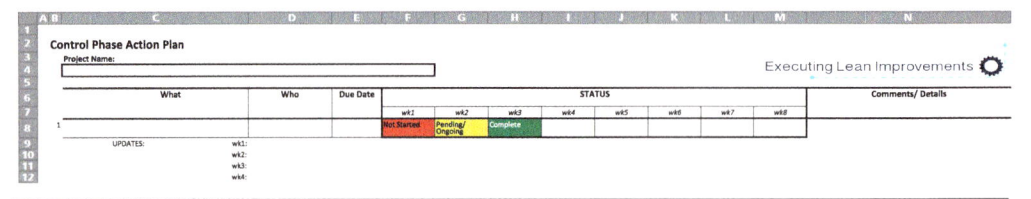

Figure A.22 Control phase action plan screenshot.

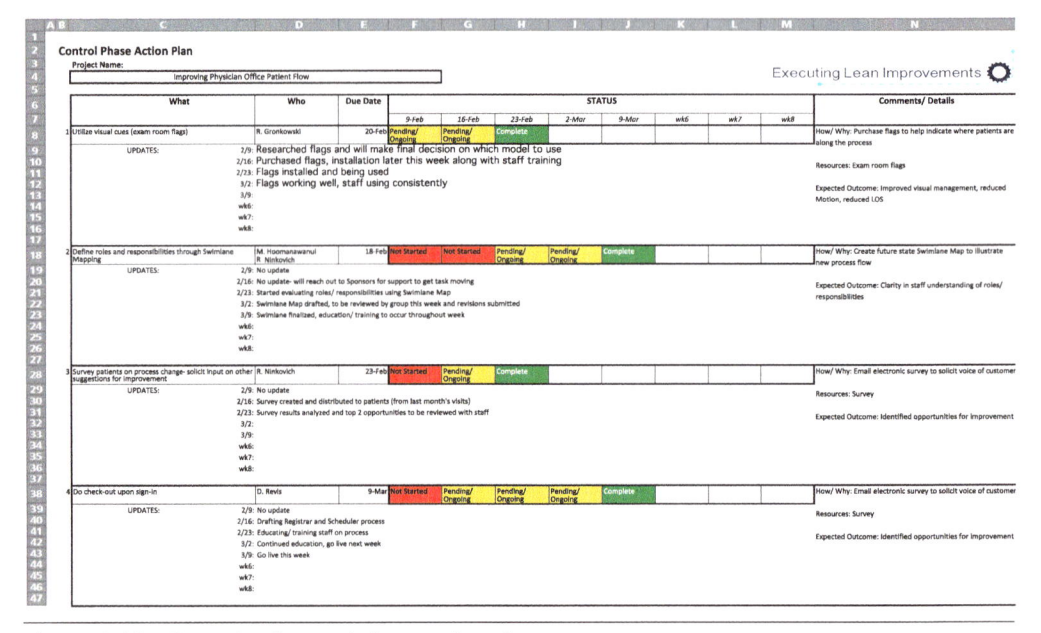

Figure A.23 Example of control phase action plan.

When to use it: The action plan worksheet transfers to this tool. The Control phase action plan is updated weekly and disseminated to the project team.

Required? Yes.

CONTROL PHASE ACTION PLAN—GANTT TEMPLATE

Description: The Gantt chart is a project management tool used to outline project deliverables (Jacobs & Chase, 2008). The tool is a horizontal bar graph depicting the sequence and duration of project tasks (Figure A.24). Column B lists tasks, and columns C–F, respectively, list the responsible party, status, and start and end dates. Columns H–N contain the appropriate time intervals for the project (i.e., days, weeks, months). To create the graph, calculate the duration to complete individual tasks as start date minus end date. The blue bar represents the task duration, beginning on the start date and concluding at the defined end date. Simply enter "1" in the cells that make up the task duration (they will automatically turn dark blue). Gantt charts provide a high-level project timeline and communication visual. The bars defining task duration enable quick

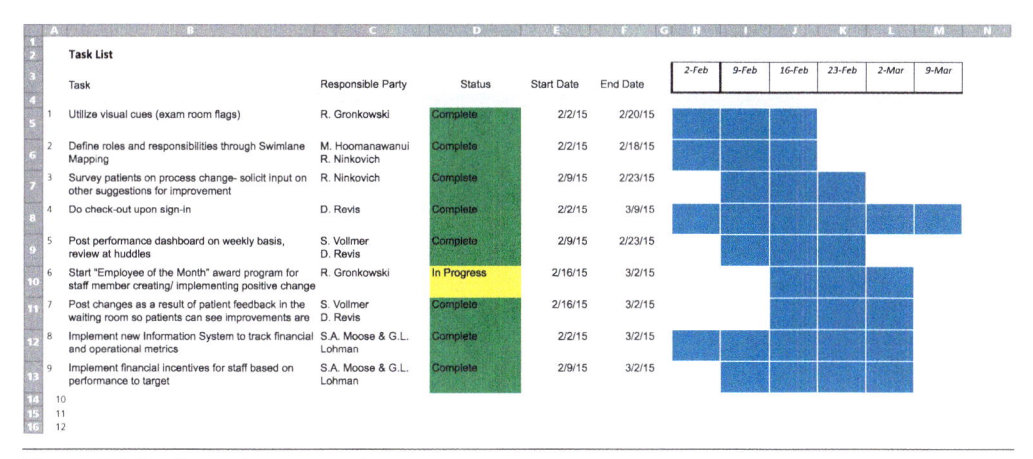

Figure A.24 Gantt chart screenshot.

identification of proper sequences (i.e., run in parallel versus progressively) as well as the rate-limiting steps that need to be closely monitored. In other words, if a particular task is delayed, will the entire project be negatively affected?

When to use it: Accompanying the Control phase action plan, the Gantt chart is an effective communication tool for senior leaders regarding the project status and timeline.

Required? Optional, but strongly recommended.

References

Advisory Board Company. (2011). *Leading change: Implementing improvements in the health care organization.* Washington, DC: Author.

Aij, K. H., Simons, F. E., Widdershoven, G. A., & Visse, M. (2013). Experiences of leaders in the implementation of lean in a teaching hospital—barriers and facilitators in clinical practices: A qualitative study. *BMJ Open, 3*(10), e003605-2013-003605. doi:10.1136/bmjopen-2013-003605

Al, M., Feenstra, T., & Brouwer, W. (2005). Corrigendum to "Decision makers' views on health care objectives and budget constraints: Results from a pilot study." *Health Policy, 74,* 109–111.

Andersen, H., Rovik, K. A., & Ingebrigtsen, T. (2014). Lean thinking in hospitals: Is there a cure for the absence of evidence? A systematic review of reviews. *BMJ Open, 4*(1), e003873-2013-003873. doi:10.1136/bmjopen-2013-003873

Armstrong, S., Fox, E., & Chapman, W. (2013). To meet health care's triple aim, lean management must be applied across the value stream: Comment on "Management practices and the quality of care in cardiac units." *JAMA Internal Medicine, 1–2,* 692–694. doi:10.1001/jamainternmed.2013.4080

Aronson, S., & Gelatt, K. (2006). *"Lean" models at health care institutions* (Original inquiry brief). Washington, DC: The Advisory Board Company.

Ballé, M., & Régnier, A. (2007). Lean as a learning system in a hospital ward. *Leadership Health Services, 20,* 33–41.

Bass, I. (2007). *Six Sigma statistics with Excel and Minitab.* New York, NY: McGraw-Hill.

Berwick, D. M., Nolan, T. W., & Whittington, J. (2008). The triple aim: Care, health, and cost. *Health Affairs (Project Hope), 27*(3), 759–769. doi:10.1377/hlthaff.27.3.759; 10.1377/hlthaff.27.3.759

Bicheno, J., & Holweg, M. (2004). *The lean toolbox* (4th ed.). Buckingham, UK: PICSIE Books.

Bradley, E. H., Curry, L. A., Spatz, E. S., Herrin, J., Cherlin, E. J., Curtis, J. P., . . . Krumholz, H. M. (2012). Hospital strategies for reducing risk-standardized mortality rates in acute myocardial infarction. *Annals of Internal*

Medicine, 156(9), 618–626. doi:10.1059/0003-4819-156-9-201205010-00003; 10.1059/0003-4819-156-9-201205010-00003

Bradley, E. H., Herrin, J., Wang, Y., Barton, B. A., Webster, T. R., Mattera, J. A., . . . Krumholz, H. M. (2006). Strategies for reducing the door-to-balloon time in acute myocardial infarction. *The New England Journal of Medicine, 355*(22), 2308–2320. doi:10.1056/NEJMsa063117

Breakthrough Management Group International. (n.d.). *Lean master training materials*. Retrieved from https://www.bmgi.com/

Brennan, T. A., Gawande, A., Thomas, E., & Studdert, D. (2005). Accidental deaths, saved lives, and improved quality. *The New England Journal of Medicine, 353*(13), 1405–1409. doi:10.1056/NEJMsb051157

Chalice, R. (2007). *Improving healthcare using Toyota lean production methods* (2nd ed.). Milwaukee, WI: ASQ Quality Press.

Chan, H., Lo, S., Lee, L., Lo, W., Yu, W., Wu, Y., . . . Chan, J. (2014). Lean techniques for the improvement of patients' flow in emergency department. *World Journal of Emergency Medicine, 5*(1), 24–28. doi:10.5847/wjem.j.1920-8642.2014.01.004

Classen, D. C., Resar, R., Griffin, F., Federico, F., Frankel, T., Kimmel, N., . . . James, B. C. (2011). "Global trigger tool" shows that adverse events in hospitals may be ten times greater than previously measured. *Health Affairs (Project Hope), 30*(4), 581–589. doi:10.1377/hlthaff.2011.0190; 10.1377/hlthaff.2011.0190

Curry, L. A., Spatz, E., Cherlin, E., Thompson, J. W., Berg, D., Ting, H. H., . . . Bradley, E. H. (2011). What distinguishes top-performing hospitals in acute myocardial infarction mortality rates? A qualitative study. *Annals of Internal Medicine, 154*(6), 384–390. doi:10.1059/0003-4819-154-6-201103150-00003; 10.1059/0003-4819-154-6-201103150-00003

de Souza, L. (2009). Trends and approaches in lean healthcare. *Leadership in Health Services, 22*(2), 121–139.

de Souza, L., & Pidd, M. (2011). Exploring the barriers to lean health care implementation. *Public Money Management, 31*, 59–66.

Delisle, D. R. (2013, October). *Systematically improving operating room patient flow through value stream mapping and kaizen events*. American Society for Quality: Making the Case for Quality.

Delisle, D. R., & Freiberg, V. (2014). Everything is 5-S: A simple yet powerful lean improvement approach applied in a pre-admission testing center. *Quality Management Journal, 21*(4), 10–22.

Delisle, D. R., & Jaffe, K. (2015). Let it flow: Improving perioperative patient flow using lean improvement strategies. *Six Sigma Forum Magazine*.

Dentzer, S. (2011). Still crossing the quality chasm—or suspended over it? *Health Affairs (Project Hope), 30*(4), 554–555. doi:10.1377/hlthaff.2011.0287; 10.1377/hlthaff.2011.0287

Farrokhi, F. R., Gunther, M., Williams, B., & Blackmore, C. C. (2013). Application of lean methodology for improved quality and efficiency in operating room instrument availability. *Journal for Healthcare Quality*. doi:10.1111/jhq.12053

Gawande, A. (2009). *The checklist manifesto: How to get things right*. New York, NY: Picador.

Graban, M. (2012). *Lean hospitals* (2nd ed.). Boca Raton, FL: CRC Press.

Graban, M., & Prachand, A. (2010). Hospitalists: Lean leaders for hospitals. *Journal of Hospital Medicine, 5*(6), 317–319. doi:10.1002/jhm.813

Graban, M., & Swartz, J. (2012). *Healthcare kaizen: Engaging front-line staff in sustainable continuous improvements*. Boca Raton, FL: CRC Press.

Grout, J. (2007). *Mistake-proofing the design of health care processes*. Rome, GA: Agency for Healthcare Research and Quality.

Hina-Syeda, H., Kimbrough, C., Murdoch, W., & Markova, T. (2013). Improving immunization rates using Lean Six Sigma processes: Alliance of Independent Academic Medical Centers National Initiative III Project. *The Ochsner Journal, 13*(3), 310–318.

Hrebiniak, L. (2013). *Making strategy work: Leading effective execution and change* (2nd ed.). Upper Saddle River, NJ: FT Press.

Imai, M. (1997). *Gemba kaizen*. New York, NY: McGraw-Hill.

Institute for Healthcare Improvement. (2005). *Going lean in health care*. Cambridge, MA: Author.

Jacobs, F., & Chase, R. (2008). *Operations and supply management: The core*. New York, NY: McGraw-Hill.

Jimmerson, C. (2010). *Value stream mapping for healthcare made easy*. New York, NY: Taylor & Francis Group.

Jimmerson, C., Weber, D., & Sobek, D. K., II. (2005). Reducing waste and errors: Piloting lean principles at Intermountain Healthcare. *Joint Commission Journal on Quality and Patient Safety/Joint Commission Resources, 31*(5), 249–257.

Joint Commission on the Accreditation of Healthcare Organizations. (2006). *Doing more with less: Lean thinking and patient safety in health care*. Oakbrook, IL: Author.

Jones, D., & Mitchell, A. (2006). *Lean thinking for the NHS*. London: NHS Confederation.

Kaplan, G. S., Patterson, S. H., Ching, J. M., & Blackmore, C. C. (2014). Why lean doesn't work for everyone. *BMJ Quality & Safety, 23*(12), 970–973. doi:10.1136/bmjqs-2014-003248

Kenney, C. (2011). *Transforming health care: Virginia Mason Medical Center's pursuit of the perfect patient experience*. New York, NY: Productivity Press.

Kohn, L., Donaldson, M., & Committee on Quality of Health Care in America, Institute of Medicine. (2000). *To err is human: Building a safer health system*. Washington, DC: The National Academies Press.

Kotter, J. (1995). Leading change: Why transformation efforts fail. *Harvard Business Review, 73*(2), 59–67.

Langley, G., Moen, R., Nolan, K., Nolan, T., Norman, C., & Provost, I. (2009). *The improvement guide: A practical approach to enhancing organizational performance* (2nd ed.). San Francisco, CA: Jossey-Bass.

Lawal, A. K., Rotter, T., Kinsman, L., Sari, N., Harrison, L., Jeffery, C., . . . Flynn, R. (2014). Lean management in health care: Definition, concepts, methodology and effects reported (systematic review protocol). *Systematic Reviews, 3*, 103-4053-3-103. doi:10.1186/2046-4053-3-103

Lean and Six Sigma International Board. (2011). *Overview of Lean Six Sigma.* Retrieved from http://image.slidesharecdn.com/01-overviewofleansixsigma-121114045047-phpapp01/95/01-overview-of-lean-six-sigma-25-638.jpg?cb=1352890536

Lean Enterprise Institute. (n.d.). *Principles of lean.* Retrieved from http://www.lean.org/WhatsLean/Principles.cfm

Leape, L. L., & Berwick, D. M. (2005). Five years after *To err is human*: What have we learned? *JAMA, 293*(19), 2384–2390. doi:10.1001/jama.293.19.2384

Lighter, D. (2013). *Basics of health care performance improvement: A Lean Six Sigma approach.* Burlington, MA: Jones & Bartlett Learning.

Liker, J. (2004). *The Toyota way: 14 management principles from the world's greatest manufacturer.* New York, NY: McGraw-Hill.

Liker, J., & Meier, D. (2006). *The Toyota way fieldbook: A practical guide for implementing Toyota's 4 Ps.* New York, NY: McGraw-Hill.

Maister, D. (1985). *The psychology of waiting lines.* Retrieved from David Maister website: http://www.columbia.edu/~ww2040/4615S13/Psychology_of_Waiting_Lines.pdf

Mann, D. (2010). *Creating a lean culture* (2nd ed.). New York, NY: Taylor and Francis Group.

Martens, L., Goode, G., Wold, J. F., Beck, L., Martin, G., Perings, C., . . . Baggerman, L. (2014). Structured syncope care pathways based on Lean Six Sigma methodology optimises resource use with shorter time to diagnosis and increased diagnostic yield. *PloS One, 9*(6), e100208. doi:10.1371/journal.pone.0100208

Martin, L., Neumann, C., Mountford, J., Bisognano, M., & Nolan, T. (2009). *Increasing efficiency and enhancing value in health care: Ways to achieve savings in operating costs per year* (IHI Innovation Series white paper). Cambridge, MA: Institute for Healthcare Improvement.

Mazur, L., McCreery, J., & Rothenberg, L. (2010). Facilitating lean learning and behaviors in hospitals during the early stages of lean implementation. *Engineering Management Journal, 24*, 11–22.

McChesney, C., Covey, S., & Huling, J. (2012). *The 4 disciplines of execution.* New York, NY: Free Press.

McConnell, K., Lindrooth, R. C., Wholey, D. R., Maddox, T. M., Bloom, N. (2013). Management practices and the quality of care in cardiac units. *JAMA Internal Medicine, 173*(8), 684–692. doi:10.1001/jamainternmed.2013.3577

Meyer, H. (2010). Life in the "lean" lane: Performance improvement at Denver Health. *Health Affairs, 29*(11), 2054–2060. doi:10.1377/hlthaff.2010.0810

Nakajima, S. (1988). *Introduction to TPM*. Cambridge, MA. Productivity Press.

Neufeld, N. J., Hoyer, E. H., Cabahug, P., Gonzalez-Fernandez, M., Mehta, M., Walker, N. C., . . . Mayer, R. S. (2013). A Lean Six Sigma quality improvement project to increase discharge paperwork completeness for admission to a comprehensive integrated inpatient rehabilitation program. *American Journal of Medical Quality, 28*(4), 301–307. doi:10.1177/1062860612470486

Niemeijer, G. C., Trip, A., de Jong, L. J., Wendt, K. W., & Does, R. J. (2012). Impact of 5 years of Lean Six Sigma in a university medical center. *Quality Management in Health Care, 21*(4), 262–268. doi:10.1097/QMH.0b013e31826e74b7

Øvretveit, J. (2005). Leading improvement. *Journal of Health Organization Management, 19*, 413–430.

Palmer, B. (2004). *Making change work: Practical tools for overcoming human resistance to change*. Milwaukee, WI: ASQ Quality Press.

Pande, P., & Holpp, L. (2002). *What is Six Sigma?* New York, NY: McGraw-Hill.

Project Management Institute. (2008). *A guide to the project management body of knowledge* (4th ed.). Newtown Square, PA: Author.

Rother, M. (2010). *Toyota kata: Managing people for improvement, adaptiveness, and superior results*. New York, NY: McGraw-Hill.

Rycroft-Malone, J., Kitson, A., Harvey, G., McCormack, B., Seers, K., Titchen, A., & Estabrooks, C. (2002). Ingredients for change: Revisiting a conceptual framework. *Quality Safety Health Care, 11*, 174–180.

Shojania, K. G., & Grimshaw, J. M. (2005). Evidence-based quality improvement: The state of the science. *Health Affairs (Project Hope), 24*(1), 138–150. doi:10.1377/hlthaff.24.1.138

Shortell, S. (1998). *Assessing the implementation and impact of clinical quality improvement efforts: Abstract, executive summary and final report*. Rockville, MD: Agency for Health Care Policy and Research.

Shortell, S. M., Rundall, T. G., & Hsu, J. (2007). Improving patient care by linking evidence-based medicine and evidence-based management. *JAMA, 298*(6), 673–676. doi:10.1001/jama.298.6.673

Shortell, S. M., & Singer, S. J. (2008). Improving patient safety by taking systems seriously. *JAMA, 299*(4), 445–447. doi:10.1001/jama.299.4.445; 10.1001/jama.299.4.445

Silverstein, D., Samuel, P., & DeCarlo, N. (2009). *The innovator's toolkit: 50+ techniques for predictable and sustainable organic growth*. Hoboken, NJ: John Wiley & Sons.

Slobbe, L., Smit, J., Groen, J., Poos, M., & Kommer, G. (2011). *Cost of illness in the Netherlands 2007: Trends in healthcare expenditure 1999–2010*. Retrieved from the National Institute for Public Health and the Environment website: http://www.rivm.nl/dsresource?objectid=rivmp:61294&type=org&disposition=inline&ns_nc=1

Smith, B. (2003, April). Lean and Six Sigma: A one-two punch. ASQ *Quality Progress*, 37–41.

Snee, R., & Hoerl, R. (2003). *Leading Six Sigma: A step-by-step guide based on experience with GE and other Six Sigma companies.* Upper Saddle River, NJ: FT Press.

Sobek, D., & Smalley, A. (2008). *Understanding A3 thinking: A critical component of Toyota's PDCA management system.* Boca Raton, FL: Productivity Press.

Spear, S. J. (2005). Fixing health care from the inside, today. *Harvard Business Review, 83*(9), 78–91, 158.

Swensen, S. J., Dilling, J. A., Harper, C. M., Jr., & Noseworthy, J. H. (2012). The Mayo Clinic Value Creation System. *American Journal of Medical Quality, 27*(1), 58–65. doi:10.1177/1062860611410966

Takahashi, Y., & Osada, T. (1990). *TPM total productive maintenance.* Tokyo, Japan: Asian Productivity Organization.

Tapping, D., Kozlowski, S., Archbold, L., & Sperl, T. (2009). *Value stream management for lean healthcare.* Chelsea, MI: MCS Media.

Teich, S. T., & Faddoul, F. F. (2013). Lean management—The journey from Toyota to healthcare. *Rambam Maimonides Medical Journal, 4*(2), e0007. doi:10.5041/RMMJ.10107

Toussaint, J., & Gerard, R. (2010). *On the mend.* Cambridge, MA: Lean Enterprise Institute.

Tuckman, B. (1965). Development sequence in small groups. *Psychological Bulletin, 63*(6), 384–399.

Vermeulen, M. J., Stukel, T. A., Guttmann, A., Rowe, B. H., Zwarenstein, M., Golden, B., . . . Schull, M. (2014). Evaluation of an emergency department lean process improvement program to reduce length of stay. *Annals of Emergency Medicine, 64*(5), 427–438. doi:10.1016/j.annemergmed.2014.06.007

Wachter, R. M. (2004). The end of the beginning: Patient safety five years after *To err is human. Health Affairs (Project Hope)*, Suppl Web Exclusives, W4-534–545. doi:10.1377/hlthaff.w4.534

Womack, J. (2011). *Gemba walks.* Cambridge, MA: Lean Enterprise Institute.

Womack, J., & Jones, D. (1996). *Lean thinking.* New York, NY: Free Press.

Womack, J. P., & Jones, D. T. (2005). Lean consumption. *Harvard Business Review, 83*(3), 58–68, 148.

Wysocki, B. (2004, April 9). To fix health care, hospitals take tips from factory floor. *Wall Street Journal.*

Zidel, T. (2012). *Lean done right.* Chicago, IL: Health Administration Press.

Index

Note: Page numbers followed by *f* or *t* refer to figures or tables, respectively.

A

action plan worksheets, 171, 172*t*
Analyze folder (Appendix D)
    5S audit tool, 225, 225*f*
    swimlane template, 226, 226*f*

B

bar chart examples, 130*f*
barriers
    brainstorming, 160–162, 163*f*
    filtering/prioritizing, 162–165, 164–165*f*
    leader removal of, 183
batching in pull systems, 108–109, 108–109*f*
brainstorming, 160–162, 163*f*, 166–168, 167–168*f*
business process design, 2*t*

C

case studies
    Clinical Lab Flow, 25–28
    Evaluating Gastroenterology Physician's Office Visit, 88–91
    Inpatient Admission from the Emergency Department, 122–123
    Operating Room Performance Dashboards, 131–132
    OR/SPCC Value Stream Mapping Event, 57–59
    Patient Flow in the Patient Testing Center, 54, 73–80
    Patient Flow through the Short-Procedure Unit (SPU), 152–155
    Patient Transportation, 107
    Pharmacy Batching, 110
    Pharmacy Inventory, 112–114
    Presurgery Patient Flow, 16–17
    Rapid Changeover in the OR, 94–95
change leadership, 177–189
    change model, 177*f*, 181*f*
    creating urgency for change, 182
    defining/communicating vision, 182–183
    discipline, 180–181
    establishing guiding coalition, 182
    5-8-4 summary, 186–187, 186*f*
    hard-wire changes, 183–184
    leader standard work, 179–180
    leading change, 181–184
    lessons from Jefferson lean leaders, 184–186
    macro/micro levels of change, 178*t*
    role in lean management, 178–181
    roles and responsibilities, 180*f*
change management, 3
change model, 177*f*, 181*f*
change readiness profile tool (DMAIC), 141, 141*f*, 150, 199, 199*f*
checklists, 99, 136–137, 138*f*
communication plans, 139–140, 147, 149, 191, 195*t*, 196
consensus voting, 165
Control folder (Appendix F), 229–233
    Control phase action plan, 229, 232*f*
    Gantt charts, 232–233, 233*f*
    kaizen A3 reports, 229, 230–231*f*
Control phase action plans, 172–173, 173*f*, 212, 229, 232*f*
current state
    defined, 32, 38
    mapping of, 32–37, 32–37*f*, 143
    VSMs, 202, 202*f*
customer demand, 86–87, 87*f*
customer value, 13*f*, 14–15*t*, 15*f*, 22
cycle time, 38, 44

D

dashboards. *See* performance dashboards
defects, in DOWNTIME matrix, 18*t*, 20
Define folder (Appendix B), 215–221
    DOWNTIME matrix, 215, 216–217*t*
    lean engagement communication plan, 215, 218–219*t*
    lean opportunity guide, 220, 220*t*
    VOC waste questionnaire, 221, 221*t*
direct issue-to-solution brainstorming, 167, 167*f*
DMAIC (Define, Measure, Analyze, Improve, Control), 133–156
    Analyze phase, 144–145, 144*f*
    case study: Patient Flow through the Short-Procedure Unit (SPU), 152–155
    change readiness profile tool, 141, 141*f*, 150
    Control phase, 148–149*f*, 148–150
    Define phase, 138–142, 139*f*, 141–142*f*
    Improve phase, 145–148, 146*f*
    kaizen, 133–136, 134–136*f*
    kaizen A3 reports, 150, 151*f*
    kata model, 134–135, 135*f*
    lean DMAIC checklist, 136–137, 138*f*
    Measure phase, 142–144, 143*f*
    Plan-Do-Check-Act (PDCA) cycle, 133–136, 134*f*
    run chart examples, 149*f*
    systems and process profile tool, 141, 142*f*, 150
dot voting, 164
DOWNTIME (Defects, Overproduction, Waiting, Nonutilized skill or intellect, Transportation, Inventory, Motion, Extra processing), 17, 18–19*t*, 20–22, 23–24*f*, 186
DOWNTIME matrix, 215, 216–217*t*

E

elevator speeches, 145
error-proof processes, 123–126, 126*f*
experts/stakeholders, 144, 145, 204, 205*t*
extra processing, 19*t*, 21

F

facilitators, 173–175, 174*t*, 227, 228*f*
financial impact calculations, 149–150
first-pass yield (FPY), 37, 37*f*, 38, 44
fishbone diagrams, 120, 121–122*f*, 122, 162, 163*f*, 206, 207*f*
5-8-4 summary, 186–187, 186*f*
five principles of lean, xxiv*f*. *See also specific lean principles*

5S
    audit tool, 64–65, 65–66*f*, 225, 225*f*
    e-mail and electronic information applicability, 66–67
    examples of, 64*f*
    explanation of, 62–63, 62*t*, 186
    organizing physical space, 63*t*, 65*f*
    organizing systems/processes, 63*t*
    phases of, 62
5 Whys method, 119–120, 120*f*
flow. *See* lean principle #3: establish flow
free-for-all brainstorming, 161
future state, 38
future state VSMs, 209, 211*f*

G

Gantt charts, 232–233, 233*f*
gemba activity, 50, 183
ground rules, 159
group dynamics, 173–175, 174*t*

H

high-level process maps, 33*f*, 197, 197*f*
high-level project plans, 191, 192–193*t*
hoshin kanri, 6, 6*f*
human error, 126

I

idle time, 92
Improve folder (Appendix E)
    RIE facilitator evaluation form, 227, 228*f*
    RIE presentation, 227
inventory, in DOWNTIME matrix, 19*t*, 21
inventory management
    kanban card template, 111, 112*f*
    par levels, 111–112
    in pull systems, 110–112, 112*f*

J

just-in-time production. *See* lean principle #4: implement pull

K

kaizen, 44, 133–136, 157. *See also* DMAIC (Define, Measure, Analyze, Improve, Control); rapid improvement events (RIEs)
kaizen A3 reports, 150, 151*f*, 212, 213*f*, 229, 230–231*f*

kaizen problem-solving process, 159–170
    explanation of, 147, 160f, 186
    five steps of, 159, 160f
    Step 1: brainstorm issues and barriers, 160–162, 163f
    Step 2: filter/prioritize issues and barriers, 162–165, 164–165f
    Step 3: brainstorm solutions, 166–168, 167–168f
    Step 4: filter/prioritize solutions, 168, 170–171f
    Step 5: develop/implement action plan, 171–173, 172t, 173f
kanban card template, 111, 112f
kata model, 134–135, 135f
key performance indicators (KPIs), 6

L

lagging metric, 6
Lamina tree of low-hanging fruit, 168, 169–170, 170f, 171f
layout and work area design, 67–69
    explanation of, 62t, 67–69
    using spaghetti diagrams, 67, 68–71f, 69
lead time, 38, 44
leader standard work, 179–180
leadership systems, 4, 5f. *See also* change leadership
leading metric, 6
lean engagement communication plans, 215, 218–219t
lean fundamentals, 61–81. *See also specific fundamentals*
    case study: Patient Flow in the Patient Testing Center, 73–80
    5S, 62–67, 62t, 63t, 64f
    layout and work area design, 62t, 67–69, 67–71f
    roadmap for lean process, 61f
    visual management, 62t, 70–72, 72f, 80
lean opportunity guides, 7–8t, 220, 220t
lean principle #1: define value, 9–29
    case study: Clinical Lab Flow, 25–28
    case study: Presurgery Patient Flow, 16–17
    determining scope, 9–12, 10f, 12f
    identifying waste, 17–28, 17f, 18–19t, 22–24f
    providing customer value, 12–17, 13f, 14–15t, 15f, 22
    in roadmap for lean process, 10f
lean principle #2: map the value stream, 31–60
    case study: OR/SPCC Value Stream Mapping Event, 57–59

case study: Patient Flow in the Patient Testing Center, 54
constructing swimlane map, 44, 47–49f
data collection and analysis, 50–56, 52–56f
explanation of value stream map, 38–39, 40f
map the current state, 32–37, 32–37f
process value analysis, 51–53, 52–53f
in roadmap for lean process, 31f
steps for building value stream map, 39, 41–43f, 45–46f
workflow value analysis, 54–56, 55–56f
lean principle #3: establish flow, 83–100
    case study: Evaluating Gastroenterology Physician's Office Visit, 88–91
    case study: Rapid Changeover in the OR, 94–95
    checklists, 99
    determining customer demand, 86–87, 87f
    process balancing, 87, 88f, 92–93, 92f
    rapid changeover, 93
    roadmap for lean process, 83f
    standardize the work, 96–99, 98t, 99f
lean principle #4: implement pull, 101–115
    case study: Patient Transportation, 107
    case study: Pharmacy Batching, 110
    case study: Pharmacy Inventory, 112–114
    creating pull systems, 102, 104–106f
    inventory management, 110–112, 112f
    push systems, 103–104, 103–104f
    reducing batching, 108–109, 108–109f
    single-piece flow, 108, 108–109f
lean principle #5: strive for perfection, 117–132
    case study: Inpatient Admission from the Emergency Department, 122–123
    case study: Operating Room Performance Dashboards, 131–132
    error-proof processes, 123–126, 126f
    identifying root causes, 117–122, 119–122f
    performance dashboards, 128–131, 129t, 130–131f
    roadmap for lean process, 118f
    sustainability of improvements, 127–131
    threats to sustainability, 128t
lean thinking, 1–8
    horizontal process flow, 5f
    leadership system, 4, 5f
    performance improvement methodologies, 1–3, 2t
    philosophy of, 3–6
    roadmap for lean process, 7, 7–8t
    strategy deployment, 6f
Lean-Six Sigma, xx

M

macro/micro levels of change, 178t
McQuaid, David P., xix–xxi
Measure folder (Appendix C)
    process value analysis, 223, 223f
    workflow value analysis, 224, 224f
methodologies. *See* performance improvement methodologies; *specific methodologies*
Microsoft Excel
    Control phase action plan, 172–173, 173f, 229, 232f
    5S audit tool, 64, 225f
    performance dashboards, 128
    process value analysis, 22, 51, 143, 200, 223f
    swimlane template, 226f
    workflow value analysis, 55, 143, 200, 224f
Microsoft PowerPoint, 191
midlevel process maps, 33f
motion, in DOWNTIME matrix, 19t. *See also* spaghetti diagrams

N

Nash, David B., xv–xvii
nonutilized skill/intellect, in DOWNTIME matrix, 18t, 20
non-value-adding (NVA) activity, 14–15t, 14–16
non-value-adding regulatory (NVA-R) requirement, 14–16, 14t, 15f

O

operational metrics, 128
overproduction, in DOWNTIME matrix, 18t, 20

P

par levels, in inventory management, 111–112
payoff matrix, 168–169, 170f, 207, 209f
people, as a component of lean, 4, 5, 5f
perfection. *See* lean principle #5: strive for perfection
performance dashboards, 128–132
    bar chart examples, 130f
    examples of, 131t
    performance update table, 129t
    pie graph examples, 131f
    run chart examples, 130f
performance excellence framework, 5–6, 5f
performance improvement methodologies, 1–3, 2t
performance update table, 129t

pie graph examples, 131f
Plan-Do-Check-Act (PDCA) cycle, 133–136, 134f
problem-solving. *See* kaizen problem-solving process
process, as a component of lean, 4–5, 5f
process balancing, 87, 88f, 92–93, 92f
process value analysis, 51–53, 52–53f, 143, 150, 200, 201f, 223, 223f
project charters, 191, 194f
project management, 3
The Psychology of Waiting Lines (Harvard Business School report), 84–86
pull systems. *See* lean principle #4: implement pull
purpose, as a component of lean, 4, 5f
push systems, 103–104, 103–104f

Q

quality assurance, 2t

R

RACI charts, 205, 206t
rapid changeover, 93
rapid improvement event (RIE), 157–176
    agenda for, 207, 208t
    defined, 133, 145
    facilitation guidelines, 158–159
    facilitator evaluation forms, 227, 228f
    facilitator's role in group dynamics, 173–175, 174t
    ground rules, 159
    kaizen problem-solving process, 159–170, 163–165f, 167–168f, 170–171f, 172t, 173f
    presentations, 227
    roles and responsibilities, 158
rapid improvement event portfolio (Appendix A), 191–213
    action plan and recommendations, 209, 210–211t
    baseline data for key metrics, 202
    change readiness profile tool, 199, 199f
    communication plans, 191, 195t, 196
    Control phase action plan, 212
    current state VSMs, 202, 202f
    data analysis results, 206
    fishbone diagrams, 206, 207f
    future state VSMs, 209, 211f
    high-level process maps, 197, 197f
    high-level project plans, 191, 192–193t
    kaizen A3 reports, 212, 213f
    lessons learned, 212

payoff matrix, 207, 209*f*
process value analysis results, 200, 201*f*
project charters, 191, 194*f*
RACI charts, 205, 206*t*
RIE agenda, 207, 208*t*
SIPOC, 198, 198*t*
stakeholder analysis, 204, 205*t*
systems and process profile tool, 199, 200*f*
voice of customer (VOC) summary, 203, 203–204*t*
waste diagnostic tool, 197, 197*f*
waste observations, 196, 196*t*
workflow value analysis results, 200, 201*f*
reallocation of work, 92–93
regulatory requirements, 14–16
reverse engineering, 167–168, 168*f*
roadmap (five principles of lean), xxiv*f*, 7. *See also specific lean principles*
root cause analysis, 117–122
    fishbone diagrams, 120, 121–122*f*, 122
    5 Whys method, 119–120, 120*f*
run charts, 130*f*, 149*f*

S

Shewhart, Walter A., 133
shine, in 5S, 62–63, 63*t*, 64–65*f*
Shingo, Shigeo, 126
silent brainstorming, 161
single-piece flow, 108, 108–109*f*
SIPOC (Supplier, Input, Process, Output, Customer), 11, 12*f*, 143, 198, 198*t*
Six Sigma, 2*t*
sort, in 5S, 62–63, 63*t*, 64–65*f*
spaghetti diagrams, 67, 68–71*f*, 69
Spear's four rules, 166, 186
stakeholders. *See* experts/stakeholders
standard work template, 98*t*
standardize, in 5S, 62–63, 63*t*, 64–65*f*
standardize the work, 96–99, 98*t*, 99*f*
store, in 5S, 62–63, 63*t*, 64–65*f*
sustain, in 5S, 62–63, 63*t*, 64–65*f*
sustainability of improvements, 127–131, 128*t*
swimlane maps, 44, 47–49*f*, 171*f*, 226, 226*f*
systems and process profile tool (DMAIC), 141, 142*f*, 199, 200*f*

T

Takt time, 86–87, 87*f*, 92, 92*f*
Thomas Jefferson University School of Population Health. *See also* case studies
    certification of lean leaders, 184
    lessons from Jefferson lean leaders, 184–186
    scope of, xv–xx, 184
threats to sustainability, 128*t*
total quality management, 2*t*
Toyota Kata (Rother), 134
Toyota Motor Corporation, 3, 124, 126, 150, 166
transportation, in DOWNTIME matrix, 19*t*, 20–21. *See also* spaghetti diagrams

U

U-shaped orientations, 69, 69*f*

V

value. *See* lean principle #1: define value; lean principle #2: map the value stream
value-adding (VA) activity, 14–16, 14–15*t*, 15*f*
value-adding ratio, 38, 44
vision statements, 145, 182–183
visual cue "noise," 72
visual management, 62*t*, 70–72, 72*f*, 80. *See also* performance dashboards
voice of customer (VOC)
    interviews, 140, 143, 145
    summary, 203, 203–204*t*
    waste questionnaire, 221, 221*t*
VSM. *See* lean principle #2: map the value stream

W

wait time
    defined, 20
    in DOWNTIME matrix, 18*t*
    reducing via flow, 84–86
    in VSM calculations, 44
waste, 17–28
    diagnostic tool, 197, 197*f*
    in DOWNTIME matrix, 17, 17*f*, 18–19*t*, 20–22, 23–24*f*
    observations, 196, 196*t*
    preliminary waste diagnostic tool, 21, 22*f*
    VOC waste questionnaire, 221, 221*t*
waste walks, 140
work area design. *See* layout and work area design
workflow value analysis, 54–56, 55–56*f*, 143, 200, 201*f*, 224, 224*f*
work-in-process (WIP), 92
workload balance charts, 92–93, 92*f*

About the Author

Dr. Dennis R. Delisle is the director for operations support for Thomas Jefferson University Hospitals and an adjunct faculty member at Thomas Jefferson University's School of Population Health. Dennis holds certifications as a Lean Master, Six Sigma Black Belt, and Project Management Professional. Dennis is a trained examiner for the Keystone Alliance for Performance Excellence and co-leads Jefferson's Performance Excellence program, utilizing the Malcolm Baldrige National Quality Award Criteria. He is responsible for the strategic deployment and education of performance excellence tools and methodologies throughout the enterprise, which includes over 180 active Lean-Six Sigma facilitators. Dennis developed and teaches undergraduate and graduate courses in operational excellence.

Dennis is a fellow of the American College of Healthcare Executives. He received his undergraduate degree in biology from Syracuse University, his master of health services administration from The George Washington University, and his doctor of science degree in health systems management from Tulane University. Dennis grew up in Branchburg, New Jersey, and currently resides in Philadelphia, Pennsylvania.